MANUAL TREATMENT FOR TRAUMATIC INJURIES

XU MENGZHONG

FOREIGN LANGUAGES PRESS

First Edition   1997
Second Printing   2000

Translated by   Cui Shuyi
                   Cui Shuzhi

Home Page:
http://www.flp.com.cn
E-mail Addresses:
Info@flp.com.cn
Sales@flp.com.cn

ISBN 7-119-01795-0

©Foreign Languages Press, Beijing, 1997
Published by Foreign Languages Press
24 Baiwanzhuang Road, Beijing 100037, China
Printed by Foreign Languages Printing House
19 Chegongzhuang Xilu, Beijing 100044, China
Distributed by China International Book Trading Corporation
35 Chegongzhuang Xilu, Beijing 100044, China
P.O. Box 399, Beijing, China
Printed in the People's Republic of China

CONTENTS

Chapter 1
GENERAL INTRODUCTION TO MANUAL TREATMENT

1. Classification and Mechanism of Manual Treatment Effect

Hand manipulations have an important place in the diagnosis and treatment of sports injuries. In the long history of traditional Chinese medicine, massotherapy was widely applied in treating a great variety of diseases, especially injury to bone articulations and soft tissues, and rich clinical experience has been garnered.

Being different in approach but equally satisfactory in curative effect, massotherapy and acupuncture share the same theory in diagnosis and treatment and are very much alike in choosing the corresponding points along the various meridians and collaterals. There are detailed accounts of manual treatment in traditional Chinese medicine records. The general introduction to manual treatment in *Yi Zong Jin Jian* (*Golden Mirror of Medicine*) states, "The principle of manual treatment for disorders is to apply manipulations to the injured bones or tendons to ensure full recovery and rehabilitation of the disorder. However, the manipulations for different disorders, whether serious or slight, should vary. The curative effects, whether cure and recovery, are satisfactory, quick or slow, leaving any after-effects or not, all depend on whether the manipulations are properly applied."

In the past several decades, thanks to the great efforts made by Chinese medical workers in studying and updating the legacy of traditional Chinese medicine, manual treatment, which has been widely applied in sports medicine, has been developed into a branch of medicine with unique characteristics.

1) Classification of Manual Treatment

(1) Manipulations for Reduction

This refers to applying reduction to fracture dislocations with manipulations. Some sports injuries involve fracture, such as fracture of forearm, fracture of tibia and fibula and fracture of metacarpal bone. All these fractures need timely correction to effect anatomical reduction and functional restoration of the fracture ends. Only effective reduction can ensure union of the fracture and recovery of function. The principles of treatment for fractures include fine reduction, proper local strapping and correct functional exercises. The three are closely related. Applying these principles may speed the reduction of the fracture, promote recovery of functions of the affected limb and ensure the athlete's early participation in training and competition. Manipulations for fracture reduction in common use include eight types, namely, traction, pulling, pressing, pushing, hold-carrying, palpation, lifting and rejoining.

(2) Manipulations for Articular Reduction

Articular dislocation includes complete dislocation, subluxation and disturbance of small joints. Articular dislocations, especially subluxation and disturbance of small joints, are often seen in athletes. Complete dislocation includes subluxation of capitulum radii and subluxation of sacro-iliac joint. And disturbance of small joints includes that of small lumbar joints and of foot and ankle joints. All types of joint dislocation require manual reduction, and the earlier the better. For most cases, the reduction can be achieved with just one treatment and the pain be relieved promptly after one successful reduction. Unlike fracture and injury of soft tissues, subluxation and disturbance of small joints may be successfully reduced though they are apt to relapse afterwards and have to be treated again. Self-protection is therefore necessary.

(3) Massage Manipulations

Massage has proved to be a most important manual treatment method, very effective in treating acute and chronic soft tissue injuries, some types of bone and cartilage injuries, and in overcoming fatigue. Many Chinese medical workers are thus devoting great attention to clinical and theoretical studies of massage. Given a wide variety of commonly used manipulations, each school has its own unique features, so that to date not unified classification has been made. At present, however, it is generally recognized that manipulations in common use include: pushing, grasping, pressing, palm-rubbing, rolling and rotating, scrubbing, shaking, pulling, traction, vibrating, striking, restoration, stamping, and plucking.

2) Curative Effects and Principles of Massage for Sports Injuries

(1) Relieving Muscle Cramp and Activating Collaterals

Meridians and collaterals circulate throughout the human body, from exterior to interior and from top to toe. They serve as specific conduits for circulation and linkage of qi (vital energy) and blood. Physiologically, meridians and collaterals have the functions of promoting the circulation of qi and blood and coordinating yin and yang. Pathologically, they have the functions of resisting disease and reflecting symptoms. In the prevention and cure of disease, they have the functions of conducting, inducing and coordinating deficiency and excess. The pain suffered from sports injury is caused by the meridians and collaterals being blocked. "When the conduits are patent, there is no pain, while they are blocked, there is pain." In accordance with this principle, acupoints are along the related meridians and collaterals are pressed and massaged to relieve the pain and cure the disease.

Injury of tissues is signalled by pain at the muscle, ligament, fascia, synovia, cartilage and bone; it causes tension and spasm in the muscle. This is a natural protective reaction of the human body telling it to reduce activity of the injured region and so prevent aggravation of the injury. If the injury is not treated promptly local exudative edema occurs in time inducing fibrosis, adhesion and stiffness of the muscle. These pathological changes may stimulate or constrict the peripheral nerves and blood vessels, causing constant pain and local obstruction in the circulation of blood, which in turn leads to further strained muscles with reduced function, resulting in a vicious cycle. Massage as a curative therapy relaxes muscles, relieves pain and overcomes fatigue brought on by physical training. The principles of relaxing soft tissues with massage are as follows:

a) Promotion of local circulation of blood and lymph, raising local temperature to relax the musculature and repair injured musculature directly.

b) Sedation and pain relief focuses on manipulating certain acupoints of the injured parts to stop pain according to the principle of "stopping pain by causing pain." For example, strong stimulation on acupoint Huantiao (GB 30) for sciatica, pluck the exterior epicondyle of humerus for tennis elbow, and pluck the piriformis for injury of this muscle. Beneath some acupoints lie nerve trunks, e.g., the clavicular section of the brachial plexus under the acupoint Quepen (ST 12), the sciatic nerve under Huantiao (GB 30), the posterior tibial nerve under Weizhong (BL 40), and the median nerve under Quze (PC 3). Constricting the nerve may temporarily block the conducive function of the nerve, while digit-pressing on certain points may kill pain and produce the anaesthetic effect.

c) Massage provides positive stimulation to strained muscle and relaxes the muscle. For example, muscular tension of the triceps muscle and the deltoid muscle of the upper arm may be relaxed by pressing and grasping. Myospasm and pain may be eased by passive traction and extension of the muscles. Myospasm in the gastrocnemius may be relieved by passive dorsiflexion of the ankle joint, pulling the leg muscles and then pushing, pressing and kneading the muscle bellies.

(2) Restoring and Treating Injured Muscles and Tendons and Reducing Dislocated Joints

Malposition of muscles and fasciae is often seen in sports injuries and causes pain and dysfunction, which we call "Jin Tiao Cao" in traditional Chinese medicine. Cords and tubercles may be palpated in case of arrangement disturbance of muscle fibre. The symptoms may be relaxed by pressing and plucking manipulations to regulate and restore the muscle fibre. Slipping of tendon may cause serious dysfunction of the joint, and there may be tenderness at the slipped tendon when felt with hand. The slipped tendon may be reduced and symptoms relaxed by manual treatment. At the acute state in injuries of the superior clunial nerves, cords may be palpated at the border of the wing of ilium. With the reduction of the superior clunial nerves by manual treatment, symptoms will be eased accordingly. Articular synovial incarceration manifests as pain and motor impairment caused by incarceration of synovium in the articular space. By performing traction, pulling and rotation, the synovium will slip out of the joint, ensuring a reduction, and the symptoms will disappear.

(3) Promoting Blood Circulation by Removing Blood Stasis

3

Any tissue injury leads to bleeding, edema and exudate from the tissue. If not treated promptly and the swelling persists, haematoma formation will reduce the elasticity of the tissue and cause cicatricial adhesion in it, thus directly affecting its function.

a) Start massage treatment the day after the injury. Apply kneading, rubbing and pushing to raise skin temperature and promote the circulation of blood and lymph so as to increase the number of white cells, enhance the phagocytosis of white cells and clear away local necrotic tissues and extravasated blood. The direct mechanical effect of the manual treatment may help the dispersion of fluid in the affected area, afford better absorption and the subsidence of swelling. Squeeze-press the joint to ensure the hydrarthrosis and haemarthrosis to flow into tissues outside the joint and thus avoid articular adhesion.

b) Promote circulation of qi and blood. Angiectasis and accelerated blood flow in the tissues resulting from massage may enhance the nutrition supply to local tissues and help repair those injured.

c) Passive movements of the limbs may pull straight the spasmodic tissues and prevent tissue adhesion. For example, periarthritis of shoulder, also called frozen shoulder, involves blockage of qi and stasis of blood caused by exposure to cold, wind and dampness. This may be treated with soft and gentle manipulations at the early stage, while at the late stage such manipulations as pulling, traction, shaking and plucking are used to enlarge the range of shoulder movement, restore elasticity of muscles, remove adhesion and finally dispel the blockage and stasis.

(4) Reducing and Restoring Malposition of Bone Joints

This applies to subluxation and malposition of joints, excluding dislocation of large joints. For instance, no special change is shown by X-ray examination for subluxation of the sacro-iliac joint, so reduction of this joint and elimination of the symptoms may be achieved by manual treatment. Disorders of small ankle joints are another example. As there are many small joints in the ankle region, disorder in the relationship among them is liable to occur during physical training, causing pain and weakness of the foot. Traction and squeeze-pressing manipulations may help the ankle joints to restore to their normal conditions and relieve the pain.

2. Application of Massage Manipulations

1) Selection

(1) Selection of Manipulations Depends on the Disorder and Its Various Stages

According to the principle of determining treatment based on the differentiation of symptoms and signs in applying traditional Chinese medical massage, given the removal of the pathogenic causes of disease, permanent cure can be achieved. As for general rules in the treatment, the manipulations performed should vary individually and be governed by time and place. In acute articular contusion, for example, the principle of treatment at the early stage is to prevent swelling, stop bleeding and spasmolysis and eliminate pain. The main manipulations are pressing, palm-rubbing, kneading and scrubbing, while avoiding strong manipulations. At the late stage when articulation is impeded with pain not apparent, the principle of lubricating the joint and relaxing muscles and tendons to promote blood circulation should be adopted. For this, such manipulations as pressing, rotating and pulling are applied to relax articular adhesion and improve articular function.

As for cervical spondylopathy of the nerve root type, the principles of treatment are spasmolysis and relieving pain, while correcting improper position of the cervical vertebrae. The manipulations should be pressing at the tender area or corresponding acupoints, and traction and rotate-pulling the neck region; while the principles of treatment for cervical spondylopathy of the vertebral artery type are to restore consciousness and improve vision, calm the mind and allay excitement, as well as to relax muscles and tendons to promote blood circulation, For this the main manipulations are pushing, kneading, pressing and traction, while rotate-pulling is not recommended.

The goal of treatment can only be achieved by selecting the appropriate manipulating methods according to specific injuries and acupoints. For instance, kneading, pressing and plucking manipulations should be performed for sprain of the posterior muscle group of thigh with force being applied at the tender spots, supplemented by the pressing at the acupoints Huantiao (GB 30) and Weizhong (BL 40). Selecting the right manipulating methods and correctly locating the affected region are important in curing an injury. However, the curative effects will not be satisfactory if good manipulating methods are not combined with precisely locating the tender spots and acupoints. Likewise, though the affected region is precisely located, the curative effect will be little if the force does not penetrate to a deeply located ischial tuberosity and the belly of muscle.

(3) Selecting Manipulating Methods According to Local Anatomic Characteristics

Manual treatment should focus on the affected area and those surrounding it. In selecting the right manipulating methods, priority should be given to the anatomic characteristics and pathological changes of the manipulated area. For massage of the head, since the craniofacial region is basically a bony structure with less and thin muscle, such manipulating methods as palm-rubbing, pushing, kneading and finger-percussing rather than striking and vibrating are recommended. Since the lumber and back regions are muscular, with the bones and articulations deeply embedded, heavy manipulations are the main choices. Massage is forbidden for injured areas with signs of inflammation so as to avoid spreading the inflammation.

Huangdi Neijing: *Su Wen* (*The Yellow Emperor's Canon of Internal Medicine: Plain Questions*) states: To treat heat syndromes with methods of cold or cool nature, cold syndromes with hot-natured methods, stagnation and accumulation of pathogen by diffusion, stasis by dissipation, fatigue by warmth, disease of deficiency type by reinforcing method, and exogenous pathogen by dispelling.

These principles are still of considerable guiding significance.

2) Proper Application of Manipulating Strength

(1) Manipulating Strength

Proper application of manipulating strength requires accurate location of site and appropriate degree of manipulating strength, neither over-using or under-using such strength. The suitable degree of strength depends on the actual condition of the injury. It is wrong to exert strong force blindly as it would cause pain to the patient during treatment and produce adverse reaction in the affected tissues. If injury to be ankle joint, for example, the principles of treatment are to relax the muscles and tendons and activate the flow of qi and blood in the meridians and collaterals, and promote blood circulation by removing blood stasis. Heavy manipulation in such cases would only aggravate the ankle ligament injury and worsen local swelling and blood stasis. While the strength exerted on muscular regions may be stronger for deep penetration, the method of rhythmic stepping up may be used. The force applied on well-developed muscles and deep foci should normally be fairly strong, while it should be lighter otherwise. The curative effects depend very much on the proficiency of the massagist in manipulation. An experienced massagist can deliver a fairly light force deep and penetrating, an inexperienced operator is unable to do this however strong the force. Severe pain or skin abrasion may result. Skill in manipulation requires repeated practice. "Practice makes perfect" is not accomplished overnight.

(2) Manipulating Sites

First locate the tender spots, areas that are painful on pressure, and corresponding acupoints. Tender spots in sports injury are often found at the initial and end points of muscles. The tender area at the belly of muscles, the initial or end point of ligaments, and the attaching point of fasciae are limited and apparent. Laceration of muscular fascia, injury of ligament and abrasion of tendon sheath may all be a focus, with tenderness there. Stimulation by such foci leads to muscular tension or myospasm, and protracted muscular tension results in insufficient blood supply to the muscle itself. In turn, tissue anoxia and metabolic disturbance enlarge the tenderness area which, in some cases, spreads to positions far from the original focus. In the case of incarceration of lumbar synovium, in addition to the tenderness at the incarcerated areas, there is pain in the entire lumbar region, which may radiate to the lower limbs where there may be corresponding tenderness. The original tender spot is often at the focus site, so accurately locating the tender spot, which is also the key manipulating site, may aid in diagnosis and treatment. Locating acupoints for massage includes that for two types, i.e., points along the meridians and the A Shi points. In treating sciatica, e.g., digitally press acupoints Huantiao (GB 30), Weizhong (BL 40) and Chengshan (BL 57), as well as the A Shi point.

The degree of manipulating strength varies with different locations. For deep tender areas, the manipulation should be strong and the area small. If the manipulated area is too large, the deep tender area is not reached however strong the manipulation is. For example, satisfactory effect in deep tenderness in the lumbar region is possible by slow finger-tip or elbow-tip pressing, but impossible by palm-pressing, which does not deliver the strength to the tender area. When the tender area assumes a cord-shape, such as in the case of injury of the superior clunial nerves, the tenderness is not at any certain point but in a cord-shaped area. In this case, the strength should not be exerted at a single point but along the whole cord by plucking manipulation to restore the muscles with superficial and gentle strength. To sum up, the manipulation sites and their depth vary with the disease condition and habits of the massagist.

Acupoints are of great importance in the treatment of sports injuries. Stimulation of different points may achieve such curative effects as activation of qi and blood flow in the meridians and collaterals. Pressing acupoint Quepen (ST 12) may temporarily block the blood flow through the subclavian artery, while sudden release of the pressure will increase the impact of the blood flow to the upper limbs, bringing warmth to the area and dredging the small blood vessels to improve blood supply to the upper limbs. Pressing acupoint Weizhong (BL 40) may block the conductive function of the posterior tibial nerve to relieve pain in the lower limbs and relax muscular spasm. However, the mechanism of point stimulation effect must not be interpreted merely in terms of blood and lymph circulation and the nervous system. The therapeutic mechanism of the meridians and collaterals, which constitute a unique and comprehensive system of their own, awaits further research and exploration.

(3) Manipulating Time

In order to achieve good therapeutic effect, the importance of manipulating time must be appreciated. This includes selecting different manipulations according to the stage of the injury, the number of days for one course of treatment, and the length of time each treatment is given. Dislocation of shoulder joint requires immediate manual reduction. Over massage on soft tissues should be avoided in tissue injury cases, as it would only worsen the condition. Massage of the shoulder, back and arm muscles may be started three days after the reduction to promote the flow of qi and blood, prevent amyotrophy and enhance restoration of shoulder tissues. Two weeks later initial abduction of shoulder joint should be performed to prevent articular adhesion for early restoration of the joint function. The length of time for each treatment varies, as for example the manipulating time for tennis elbow should not be too long, while to relax the lumbar muscles it may take 20-30 minutes.

3) Hand Sensation of Manual Treatment

For correct diagnosis and successful treatment, it is important to palpate and inspect the diseased region and its adjacent tissues carefully so as to thoroughly understand the situation.

(1) Hand Sensation of Fracture

Swelling and tenderness in the soft tissues often accompany a fracture. Where there is fracture displacement, fracture ends and various malformations of displacement as well as the degrees and trend of the displacement may be palpated, and these provide the main basis for manual reduction. When the affected limbs is moved, there is a friction sensation and bone crepitation sound, with abnormal movement of the limb. When the fracture is complicated by injury of nerves and blood vessels, the pulse feels weak, the affected limb moves slowly and the skin temperature is lowered. In incomplete fracture or bone rupture cases, only local swelling and tenderness occur.

(2) Palpation of Joint Dislocation

Dislocation malformation and displacement may be discovered by palpation. With dislocation of shoulder joint, e.g., the shoulder region feels empty, the shoulder square and tender. In dislocation of large joints, changes in distal nerves and blood vessels of the affected limb require examination. With subluxation and malposition of a joint, local swelling and tenderness in the joint will disappear on palpation after manual reduction. A typical case is the subluxation of the capitulum radii.

(3) Palpation of Soft Tissue Injury

a) Tension of muscle: Overtraining may cause large-area muscle tension. Sprain of muscles may cause local tension in the sprained muscle group, accompanied by tenderness. When only one side is injured, the extent of tension may be checked by contrasting it with the normal site.

b) Flaccidity of muscle: As a manifestation of amyotrophy, the muscles feel flaccid and soft, the volume of muscle is less and muscular contraction weakens. Amyotrophy of the quadriceps muscle of thigh caused by pathological changes in the knee joint is an example.

c) Scleroma in muscle: With acute muscle injury and disturbance of arrangement of muscle fibre, scleroma and tenderness may be palpated and can be treated with satisfactory result. Scars left from myofibrosis caused by old injuries may also form scleromas, which are rather difficult to cure.

d) Transverse groove of muscle: Transverse groove is palpable with rupture of muscle. Marked symptoms are found with a complete rupture of the muscle, while for partial rupture no marked transverse groove but only tenderness is palpable.

e) Swelling and thickening of soft tissues: Swelling in soft tissues to varying degrees accompanies various acute injuries, while tissue thickening is often palpable in chronic strain, such as in synovitis of knee joint. With swelling and thickening in deep tissue layers, repeated palpation is needed. For instance, thickened bursa at transverse process is palpable in the syndrome of the third lumbar vertebral transverse process.

f) Scleroma in tissues: Traditional Chinese medicine attributes the scleroma palpated at the surface of the body to stagnation of qi and blood and blockage in the meridians and collaterals. It is fairly difficult and needs careful searching to palpate well the scleroma which may or may not be located at acupoints. The treatment should be mainly directed at dispelling the scleroma.

g) Cord in tissues: This is also caused by stagnation of qi and blood. The soft tissues are felt to be cord-like with tenderness, such as when caused by displacement of the musculatures of nerves, ligaments and fasciae. The sensation of cord, most distinguished in a case of slipped tendon, may also be palpated with local muscular tension. Hand sensation for tendons includes mass of tendon or localized nodular hyperplasia of soft tissues with eminence, displacement of muscle and tendon, hypertrophy of muscle and tendon as well as indurative tendon, which respectively indicate such changes as scleroma, slipped tendon, thickening and induration.

3. Effect of Manual Treatment for Sports Injuries

1) Emergency Treatment for Injuries Sustained in Physical Training

Such injuries as systremma, light sprain of ankle joint and disturbance of small wrist joints sustained in physical training should be given emergency treatment on the spot, allowing the physical training to continue. The manipulations must be brief and well defined. Certain serious traumas need also to be given timely manual treatment to relieve pain promptly and minimize sequelae. Articular dislocation needs timely manual reduction, fracture needs timely reduction and strapping, and contusion of soft tissue requires timely pressure-bandaging.

2) Preventing Sports Injury

After physical training or competition, muscles often feel tight and need timely relaxation massage. If not given promptly, the muscle may be pulled during ensuing physical training. For instance, long-term tension of the triceps calf muscle may lead to peritendonitis or even rupture of the Achilles tendon. Peritendonitis may be prevented after removal of muscular tone.

3) Overcoming Fatigue

Massage for athletes to relax muscles may overcome not only physical but also mental fatigue. Among all the current physiological methods of relaxation, massotherapy is the most widely accepted of all.

4) Curing Different Sports Injuries

Manual treatment is not a panacea for all sports injuries. However, as a factor in comprehensive treatment, manual manipulation has excellent curative effect in acute sports injuries. It may stop pain promptly while treating dislocation and subluxation of joints, disorder of small joints, acute lumbar sprain and incarceration of meniscus of the knee joint. In chronic sprain, manual treatment must be performed repeatedly in combination with physiotherapy, acupuncture and moxibustion as well as medication.

4. Massage Manipulation Methods

1) Pressing

Pressing is done with thumb, palm or elbow. The force applied is exerted not only on the skin but may penetrate deep into the muscles, bones and viscera to dispel blood stasis and stop pain. Being an important manipulation in on-the-point massage, pressing is commonly used in the treatment of sports injuries.

a) Digit Pressing

This is pressing the tender area or acupoints with the thumb, the force generating from the thumb belly. Avoid exerting force with the thumb tip, as the nail would cause pain to the skin, while the force would not reach deep tissue layers. In case the force of one thumb is not enough, overlap with the other thumb to perform the pressing or flex the phalangeal joint at a right angle and overlap with the palm of the other hand on the phalangeal joint to add more force. The pressing may also be applied by flexing the index finger and pressing on the local area with the dorsal aspect of the first phalangeal joint. With the area stimulated being accurate and strength adjustable, digit-pressing manipulation has the effect of relaxing muscles and tendons and activating the flow of qi and blood in the meridians and collaterals and treating pain by causing pain. (See Figs. 1, 2, 3 and 4)

b) Palm Pressing

This manipulation is applied to muscular regions, such as the lumbodorsal, the thigh and the lower leg. A pre-treatment preparatory manipulation and one of the key manipulation methods for relaxing muscles, palm-pressing may be performed with the whole palm, palm base, or the major and minor thenars. The movement should be slow and even so that the force penetrates. If the force is not sufficient, the massagist may straighten both elbows and overlap both palms to press downward with the help of body weight to increase the force. (See Figs. 5, 6 and 7)

c) Elbow-tip Pressing

This method is applied when the digit-pressing force does not reach deep sites. With great pressure and strong stimulation, it is often adopted to stimulate the ischial tuberosity and deep layer lumbar muscles. If the pressing force is still not strong enough, the massagist may increase the force by holding the opposite edge with one hand and pressing downward with the help of the upper part of the body. (See Fig. 8)

2) Palm Rubbing

This is performed by rubbing the skin surface of the affected part in a straight line or by spiral motions back and forth with the palmar side of hand or with the

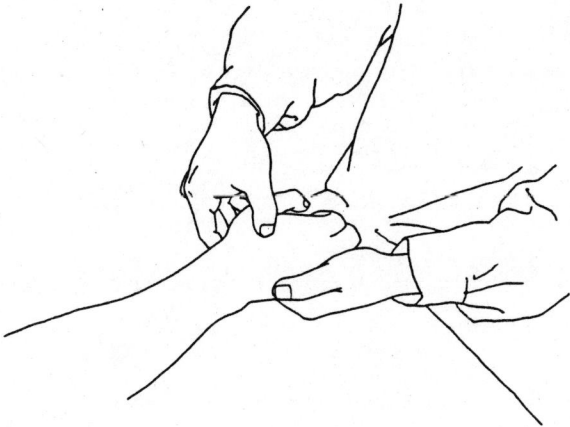

Fig. 1

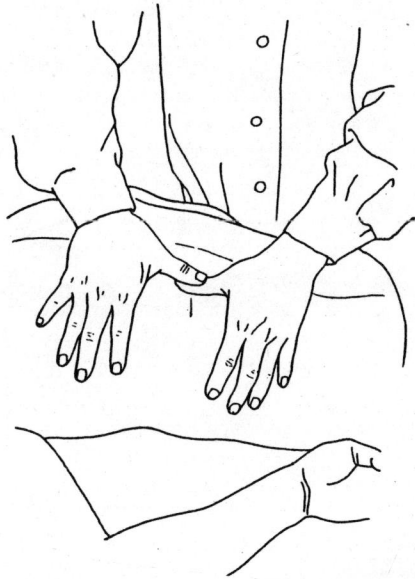

Fig. 2

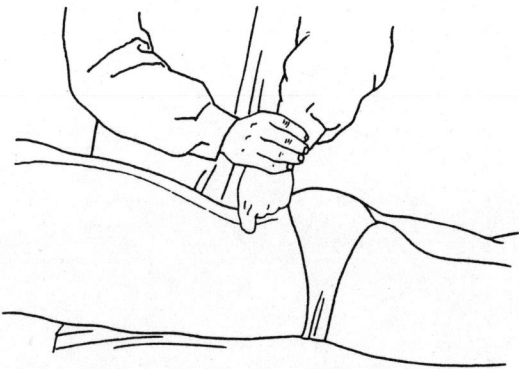

Fig. 3

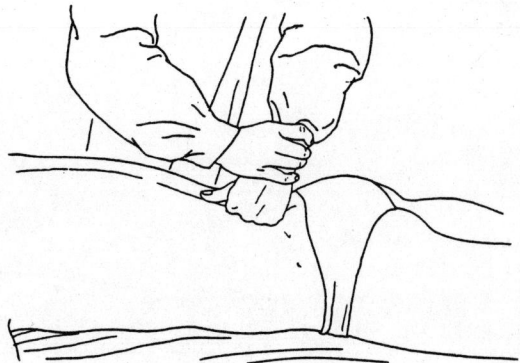

Fig. 4

Fig. 5　Palm Pressing

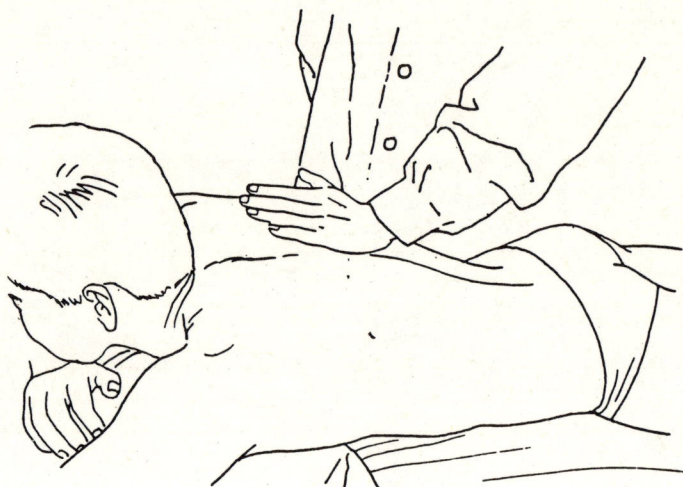

Fig. 6　Palm Pressing

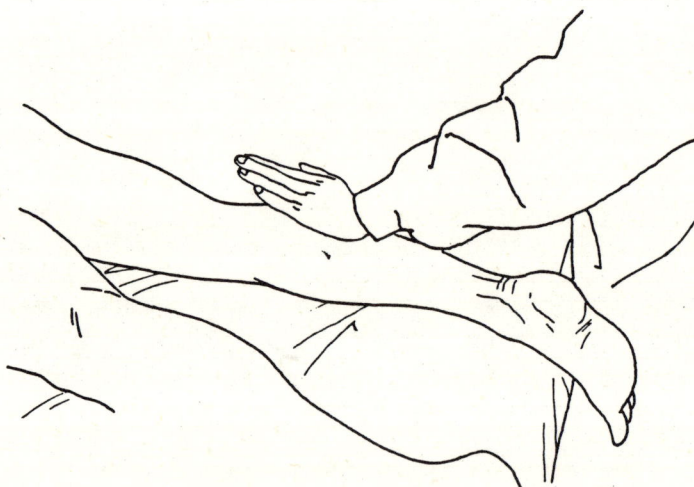

Fig. 7　Palm Pressing

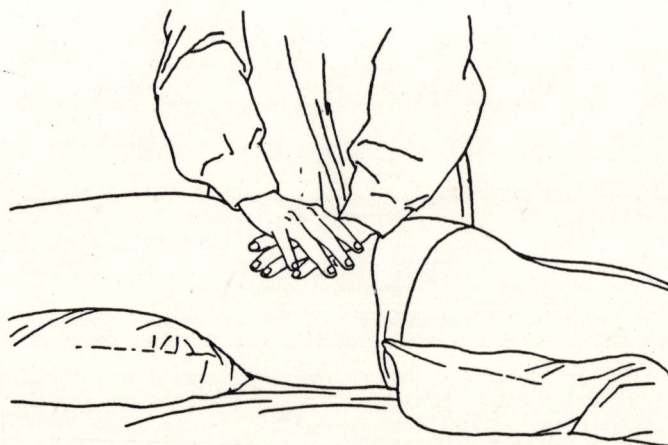

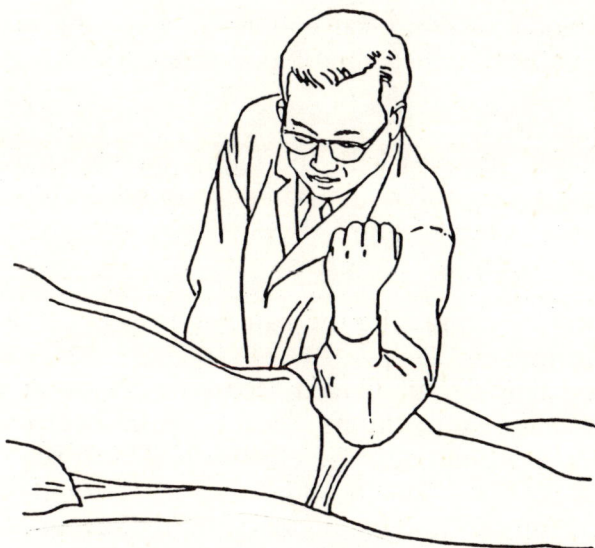

Fig. 8   Elbow-tip Pressing

belly of fingers, the force being merely skin-deep or reaching subcutaneous tissues. Some massagists apply certain external medicines to the skin before performing large-area palm-rubbing directly on the lumbodorsal region.

a) Stroking Manipulation

This is a skin-deep palm-rubbing manipulation with slow and gentle movement. It has the effects of tranquillizing the mind, spasmolysis, detumescence, pain-killing and controlling excitation. Clinically, stroking is often performed in combination with other manipulations or as a preparatory movement for manual treatment.

b) Kneading Manipulation

A commonly used method for treating sports injuries, this is applied by placing the palm or finger belly on the skin to perform even and rotating motion with the force penetrating to deep locations. Palm-kneading is subdivided into palm-base, whole-palm, and major-thenar and minor-thenar kneading. In this operation, exert force with the palm, relax the wrist, and perform small-margin rotation with the wrist and forearm. Since the area manipulated is large and stimulation mild and comfortable, it is normally used to relax muscles. Finger-kneading means performing soft and small-margin rotating kneading on acupoints or tender areas with the thumb and index finger to promote the flow of qi and blood.

c) Knead-pinching Manipulation

With the hand pincer-like and the thumb and four fingers applied closely on the skin, exert coordinated force with the palm and fingers, kneading first and then pinching with smooth movements. This method is normally applied on the four limbs. For example, in relaxing the triceps muscle of calf, hold the muscle belly in the hand and knead-pinch it from top downward to improve the functions of

13

tissues, nerves and blood vessels, clear and activate the meridians and collaterals, promote blood circulation by dispelling blood stasis, relieving muscular tone and overcoming fatigue.

d) Foulage Manipulation

Squeeze the skin and muscles with the palms facing each other and perform swift foulage with the acting force just skin-deep to generate heat by friction until the skin turns red and its temperature rises.

3) Pushing

Pushing is performed by pressing the palm or fingers on the skin and forward pushing in a straight line.

This manipulation may be subdivided according to the area and depth of the site of pathological change into thumb pushing, palm-base pushing, fist pushing and, if necessary, flat pushing with the elbow tip. The force should be deep and slow, pressing while pushing. For the lumbodorsal and abdominal regions, push from top downward; for the thoracic region from the center outward; and for the limbs from the distal to the proximal end. Light force reaches only subcutaneous tissues, while heavy force may penetrate to deep layers of muscle and tissue. Large-area manipulation provides positive stimulation to relax muscles. For muscle cramp, the massagist may cross both arms, push the lumbodorsal region with both palms in opposite directions to prolong the relaxation of muscles and subcutaneous tissues and so remove stagnation of qi and relieve muscle cramp and activate the meridians and collaterals. (See Fig. 9)

4) Grasping

Pinch the affected part or acupoints with the thumb, index finger and middle

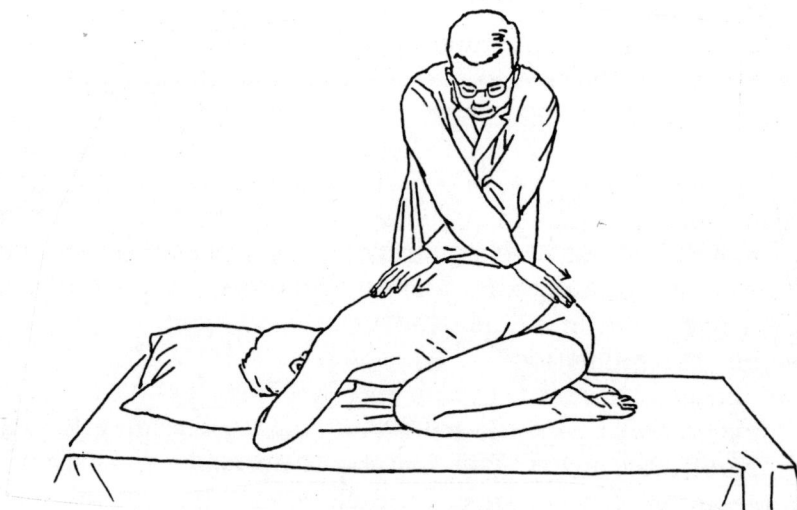

Fig. 9   Pushing

14

finger, adduct the fingers hard gradually and maintain consistent kneading while pulling the skin, subcutaneous tissues and muscles upward. Being a heavy-stimulating manipulation, this grasping method is often applied to the neck, shoulder, limbs, lumbar and back muscles as well as the sacro-iliac muscle in the treatment of headache, stiff neck, lumbar and backache and muscular tension of the limbs. This method has the following actions: clearing and activating the meridians and collaterals, inducing resuscitation and restoring consciousness, calming excitation and relieving pain.

5) Scrubbing

Place the palm, the major thenar or the minor thenar tightly on the skin and perform direct scrubbing in all directions until the skin feels hot. Similarly with foulage, the force is fairly superficial and weak and the stimulation light. The movements should be consistent with a frequency of 50 to 100 times per minute and the pressure uniform and moderate. Avoid harsh movement so as not to cause scorching pain or even abrasion of the skin. The scrubbing method is used to promote blood circulation by removing blood stasis, expelling pathogenic wind and clearing away cold. Persistent scrubbing of the lumbosacral region may cure rheumatic lumbago and deficiency of the spleen and kidney, so to strengthen the body.

6) Shaking

Hold the distal end of the limb, the joint of which is to be shaken in one hand, and the proximal end with the other hand, and shake the limb to produce passive motion of the joint. This method may also be performed by holding the patient's hand in both hands and shaking the upper limb to produce passive motion of the shoulder. The force is increased and the extent enlarged gradually, keeping the manipulation gentle. As an effective method for restoring articular functions, it may relieve rigidity, separate adhesions and prevent amyotrophy around the joint. This manipulation is often used in the treatment of scapulohumeral periarthritis.

7) Pulling

Somewhat similar to shaking, the pulling method is performed with both hands by pulling the joint hard in the same direction or the opposite direction to enable rotation, flexion or extension of the joint. It is often applied in treating disorders of small joints and in cervical spondylosis. Because the neck region is the site of many important tissues (nerves, blood vessels and spinal cord), indications must be well chosen for applying pulling in this region, and careful manipulation and accurate movements are essential. Forceful pulling should be avoided. Manipulation in the neck region should be performed only by experienced massagists. To treat disorders of small back joints and synovial incarceration, lateral pulling may be used, while for subluxation of lumbosacral joint, apply posterior-stretching pulling. This method can cure the disordered small joints and improve joint function.

8) Traction

Apply traction to the distal end of the limb from the affected area with one or both hands. Fracture and dislocation have first to be pulled for reduction of dislocation. Traction has the function of enabling passive prolongation of the tightened muscles to achieve reduction. Traction should be applied consistently, not on and off or momentarily.

9) Striking

This is striking a certain area of the body with fingers, palm or fist. It may take the forms of beating, patting or tapping. Easy to perform, striking should be done with moderate strength, too light fails to provide sufficient stimulation while too heavy aggravates the pain. The massagist must have the wrist relaxed, with movement flexible, strength uniform and frequency moderate. Such striking excites nerves, promotes flow of qi and blood and relieves fatigue.

10) Restoring

Hold the limb with the hand to regulate and restore the tissues along the line of tissue fibre or that of the meridians and collaterals, with alternate movements of gripping and loosening. This method is often used to restore contused tendons and muscles in combination with flicking-plucking manipulation. For example, in treating superior clunial nerve injury, apply flick-plucking first, then regulate and restore the superior clunial nerve along its length.

11) Stamping

For this, the massagist stamps on certain regions of the patient with the bare feet. As a therapeutic measure for treating sport injury, this is used mainly to relax muscles. The stamping should be uniform and light, avoiding sudden exertion to prevent further injury. (Scc Fig. 10)

5. Acupoints in Common Use

Acupoint is the common name for *shuxue* (points). The *shuxue* situated along the course of the twelve regular meridians, which when added with the Ren and Du are known as the fourteen regular meridians, and acupoints along them are known as acupoints on regular meridians. *Shuxue* that are not included in the fourteen regular meridians are called extraordinary points as they have specific therapeutic effects. Those points which have no fixed location or proper names but are selected by eliciting tenderness or pain are called A Shi (Oh, yes) points. These are commonly used in treating sports injuries.

The meridians are for the circulation of qi and blood, while *shuxue* serve as small pools of qi and blood circulation and may reflect symptoms. Located on the surface of the body, *shuxue* have close links with the viscera, organs and tissues of

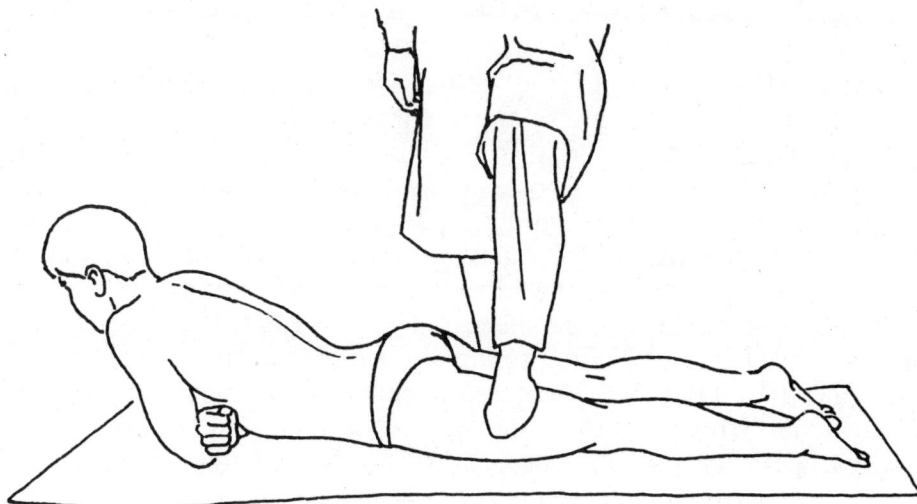

Fig. 10   Stamping

the body, and onset of a disease may be indicated by abnormal reactions at certain points. Diagnosis is thus possible by palpating with various manipulations to feel such local changes as tenderness, allergy, swelling, scleroma, temperature, as well as tension or flaccidity and protrusion or depression of muscles. *Shuxue* may help in preventing and treating disease, as they are not only reservoirs of qi and blood and pernicious energy, but also sites for prevention and treatment of disease with massotherapy as well as acupuncture and moxibustion. Clinically, corresponding acupoints along the meridians are selected in treating a disease. Massage at those points may serve as an analgesic in relieving pain.

Acupoints are the key locations for performing such manipulations as digit-pressing, digit-nipping, digit-kneading, digit-hitting and push-pressing. Stimulation on these acupoints may serve as treatment and in health care. Examples are pressing Weizhong (BL 40) for myospasm (cramp) of the lower leg and Neiguan (PC 6) for motion and altitude sickness may relieve symptoms and uneasiness.

1) Commonly Used Points on the Head and Neck

(1) Baihui (DU 20): On the midline of the head, at the cross point of the line connecting the apexes of the ears. Under Baihui are the galea aponeurotica, the anastomotic rete of the superficial temporal artery and vein and the occipital artery and vein, and also the greater occipital nerve and frontal nerve branches.

Indications: Headache and neck pain.

Manipulations: Pushing, pressing and digital hitting.

(2) Yintang (EX-HN 3): At the midpoint between the medial ends of the eyebrows. Under Yintang are branches of the supratrochlear nerve and the facial nerve.

Indications: Dizziness, headache, insomnia and cold due to pathogenic wind.

17

Manipulations: Digital hitting, pressing, pinching, kneading and flat-pushing with fingers.

(3) Taiyang (EX-HN 5): In the depression one finger breadth behind the midpoint between the lateral end of the eyebrow and the outer canthus.

Indications: Headache; also used for excitation of athletes.

Manipulations: Digital hitting, pressing, pinching and kneading.

(4) Renzhong (DU 26): At the junction of the upper 1/3 and middle 1/3 of the philtrum, under which are the orbicular muscle of mouth, blood vessels of upper lip, the facial nerve branch and the infra-optical nerve branch.

Indications: First-aid for coma, shock and heat stroke.

Manipulations: Digital hitting, pressing and nipping.

(5) Xiaguan (ST 7): In the depression between the zygomatic arch and the mandibular notch. Under Xiaguan are the parotid gland, the masseter muscle, the transverse facial artery and vein; deep down are the mandibular artery, vein and branches of the mandibular nerve and the facial nerve.

Indications: Toothache and mandibular arthritis.

Manipulations: Pressing and kneading.

(6) Jiache (ST 6): One finger breadth anterosuperior to the angle of mandible, in the depression where the masseter muscle is prominent. Under these are the masseter muscle, blood vessels, branches of the trigeminal nerve and the great auricular nerve.

Indications: Toothache, difficulty in opening the mouth, and pain and soreness of the neck muscles.

Manipulations: Digital hitting, pressing and kneading.

(7) Fengchi (GB 20): At the level of point Fengfu (DU 16), to the back of the mastoid process of the neck, in the depression between the upper end of the sternocleidomastoid and trapezius. In the depth are the splenius muscle of head and the lesser occipital nerve branch.

Indications: Headache, stiff neck, sprain of neck muscles, fever due to exogenous pathogen, pain and soreness in the shoulder and back.

Manipulations: Digital hitting, grasping, palm-rubbing and pushing.

(8) Fengfu (DU 16): About 3 cm. above the midpoint of the posterior hairline, directly below the external occipital protuberance. Under Fengfu are the nuchal ligament, the nuchal muscle, branch of the occipital artery, the interspinal venous plexus, branches of the third cervical and the greater occipital nerves.

Indications: Headache, dizziness, stiff neck and cervical spondylopathy.

Manipulations: Digital hitting, pressing and kneading.

(9) Tianding (LI 17): Above the upper fossa of the clavicle, at he posterior border of the sternocleidomastoid. Under Tianding is the platysma, in whose depth are the trapezius muscle, the great auricular nerve, the lesser occipital nerve and the accessory nerve, while still deeper is the phrenic nerve.

Indications: Pain in the neck, shoulder and arm.

Manipulations: Pressing and kneading.

(10) Quepen (ST 12): In the center of the upper fossa of the clavicle; under Quepen are the platysma and the subclavian artery.

Indications: Pain in neck, shoulder and arm. It is also used to relieve pain and for analgesia in the upper arm.

Manipulations: Pressing and kneading. Digital pressing may block the blood flow in the subclavian artery, then releasing the blood flow may produce and impact on the upper limb, thus promoting blood circulation by removing blood stasis. (See Figs. 11 and 12)

2) Commonly Used Points on the Upper Limbs

(1) Jianyu (LI 15): On the shoulder, between the acromion and the greater tuberosity of humerus, in the depression anterior and inferior to the acromion when the arm is in full abduction. Under Jianyu spread the deltoid muscle, posterior humeral circumflex artery and vein, cutaneous and muscular branches of the axillary nerve, and the supraclavicular nerves.

Indications: Periarthritis of shoulder, rotator cuff injury and subdeltoid bursitis.

Manipulations: Digital hitting, kneading and pressing.

(2) Jianliao (SJ 14): Posteroinferior to the acromion, about 3 cm. to the back of Jianyu, under which are the deltoid muscle, the posterior humeral circumflex artery and the muscular branch of the axillary nerve.

Indications: The same as for Jianyu (LI 15).

Manipulations: Digital pressing and kneading.

(3) Binao (LI 14): Slightly to the front of the terminal point of the deltoid muscle. Under Binao spread the lateral head of the triceps brachii, the deltoid muscle, the deep brachial artery, the posterior humeral circumflex artery, dorsal

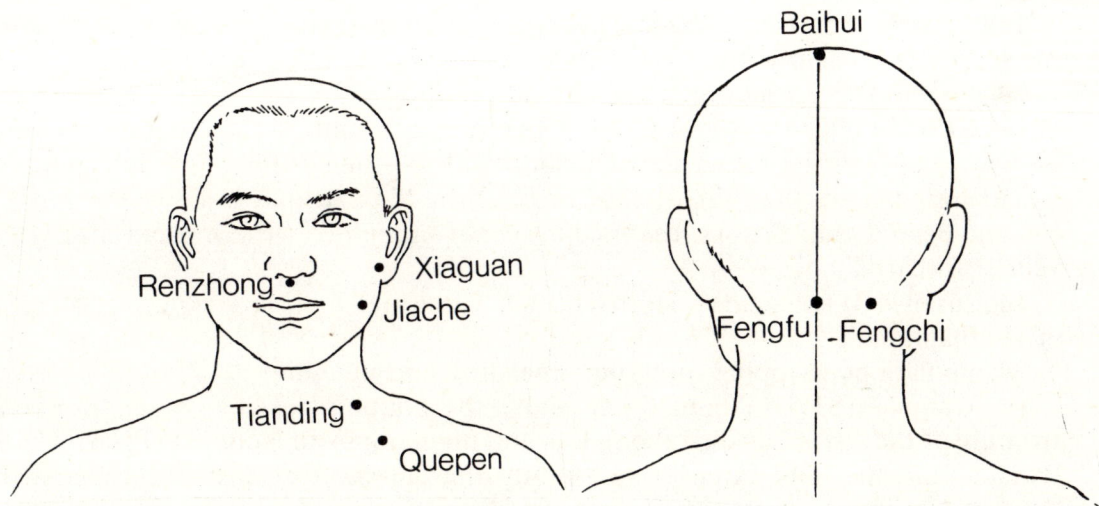

Figs. 11-12 Commonly Used Points on the Head and Neck

cutaneous nerve of arm, while deep down is the radial nerve.

Indications: Pain of shoulder and arm, and weakness of the upper limbs.

Manipulations: Digital pressing, kneading, pinching and grasping.

(4) Tianjing (SJ 10): In the depression about 3 cm. above the olecranon, to the back of the elbow. Beneath Tianjing spread the tendon of the brachial triceps, muscular branches of the radial nerve and the dossal cutaneous nerve of arm, and the cubital arterial and venous network.

Indications: Impaired flexion and extension of elbow joint, and painful neck and lumber sprain.

Manipulations: Digital pressing, kneading and nipping.

(5) Chize (LU 5): Midway between the cubital crease and the radial side of the tendon of brachial biceps. Under it are the humeroradial articulation, the biceps muscle of arm, the brachioradial muscle, the cephalic vein, the lateral cutaneous nerve of forearm and the median nerve.

Indications: Pain of shoulder and arm.

Manipulations: Pressing and kneading.

(6) Quchi (LI 11): On the radial side of the transverse striature of the elbow. Under it are the external epicondyle of humerus, the humeroradial articulation, the brachioradial muscle, the radial extensor muscle of wrist, the dorsal cutaneous nerve of forearm, and deep down the radial nerve trunk.

Indications: Pain in shoulder, elbow and lateral side of forearm, tennis elbow.

Manipulations: Nipping and kneading.

(7) Hegu (LI 4): On the dorsum of hand between the first and second metacarpal bones, approximately midway of the second metacarpal bone on the radial side. Under Hegu are the first interosseous muscle, the radial artery, the radial and median nerve branches.

Indications: Toothache, headache, mandibular arthritis and pain in the first metacarpophalangeal joint. Strong stimulation has the effect of excitation.

Manipulations: Kneading, pressing and nipping.

(8) Neiguan (PC 6): About 6 cm. above the midpoint of the cubital transverse striature, between the radial flexor tendon and the long palmar muscular tendon. Under Neiguan are the radial flexor muscle, the long palmar muscle, the superficial and deep digital flexors, the median nerve branch and the median artery and vein of forearm.

Indications: Wrist sprain, stomachache, vomiting, motion sickness and spasm of the diaphragm.

Manipulations: Nipping, pressing, kneading and pushing.

(9) Waiguan (SJ 5): About 6 cm. above the midpoint of the dorsal transverse striature of the wrist, between the radius and ulna, opposite Neiguan (PC 6). Under Waiguan are the long extensor of thumb, the common extensor of fingers, the interosseous artery and vein of forearm, the interosseous nerve and dorsal cutaneous nerve of forearm.

Indications: Wrist sprain, tenosynovitis of extensor carpi muscle and hypochondriac pain.

Manipulations: Nipping, pressing, kneading and pushing.

(10) Yangxi (LI 5): On the radial side of the wrist when the thumb is pointed upward, in the depression between the tendons of short and long extensor muscles of the thumb. Under Yangxi are the radial artery branch, the radial nerve's superficial branch and the lateral cutaneous nerve of forearm.

Indications: Headache, sprain of metacarpophalangeal point and injury of wrist soft tissues.

Manipulations: Nipping and kneading.

(11) Yangchi (SJ 4): On the transverse striature of the carpal dorsum. Under it are the common extensor tendon of fingers and the proper extensor tendon of the small finger, dorsal carpal venous network, the dorsal carpal artery, the dorsal cutaneous nerve of forearm and the ulnar nerve branch.

Indications: Common cold, rheumatism, pain in shoulder and arm with immobility, spasm of various muscles of forearm and injury of wrist joint.

Manipulations: Nipping and kneading.

(12) Houxi (SI 3): On the ulnar side proximal to the fifth metacarpophalangeal joint, at the end of the transverse striature. Under Houxi are the abductor of the small finger, dorsal artery and vein of the fingers and ulnar nerve branch.

Indications: Stiff neck, spasm of elbow and arm, pain in the fingers and lumbar sprain.

Manipulations: Nipping. (See Figs. 13 and 14)

3) Commonly Used Points on the Chest and Abdomen

(1) Danzhong (RN 17): At the junction of the anterior mid-chest and the connecting line between nipples. At the sternum are the arterial and venous branches in the thoracic cage and the fourth intercostal nerve branch.

Indications: Asthma, hiccup and contusion of muscles of the chest and hypochondrium.

Manipulations: Pressing, pushing and nipping.

(2) Zhongwan (RN 12): On the anterior midline of the abdomen, about 12 cm. above the umbilicus. The superior epigastric artery and vein and branch of the seventh and eighth intercostal nerves are in the linea alba.

Indications: Stomachache, abdominal distention and injury of abdominal muscles.

Manipulations: Pressing and kneading.

(3) Guanyuan (RN 4): On the anterior midline of abdomen, about 9 cm. below the umbilicus. In the linea alba are the superficial epigastric artery and vein, branches of the inferior epigastric artery and vein, and branch of the 10th intercostal nerve.

Indications: Among the many indications for this point are sprain of abdominal muscles, abdominal pain, diarrhoea, dysmenorrhoea, irregular menstruation, sem-

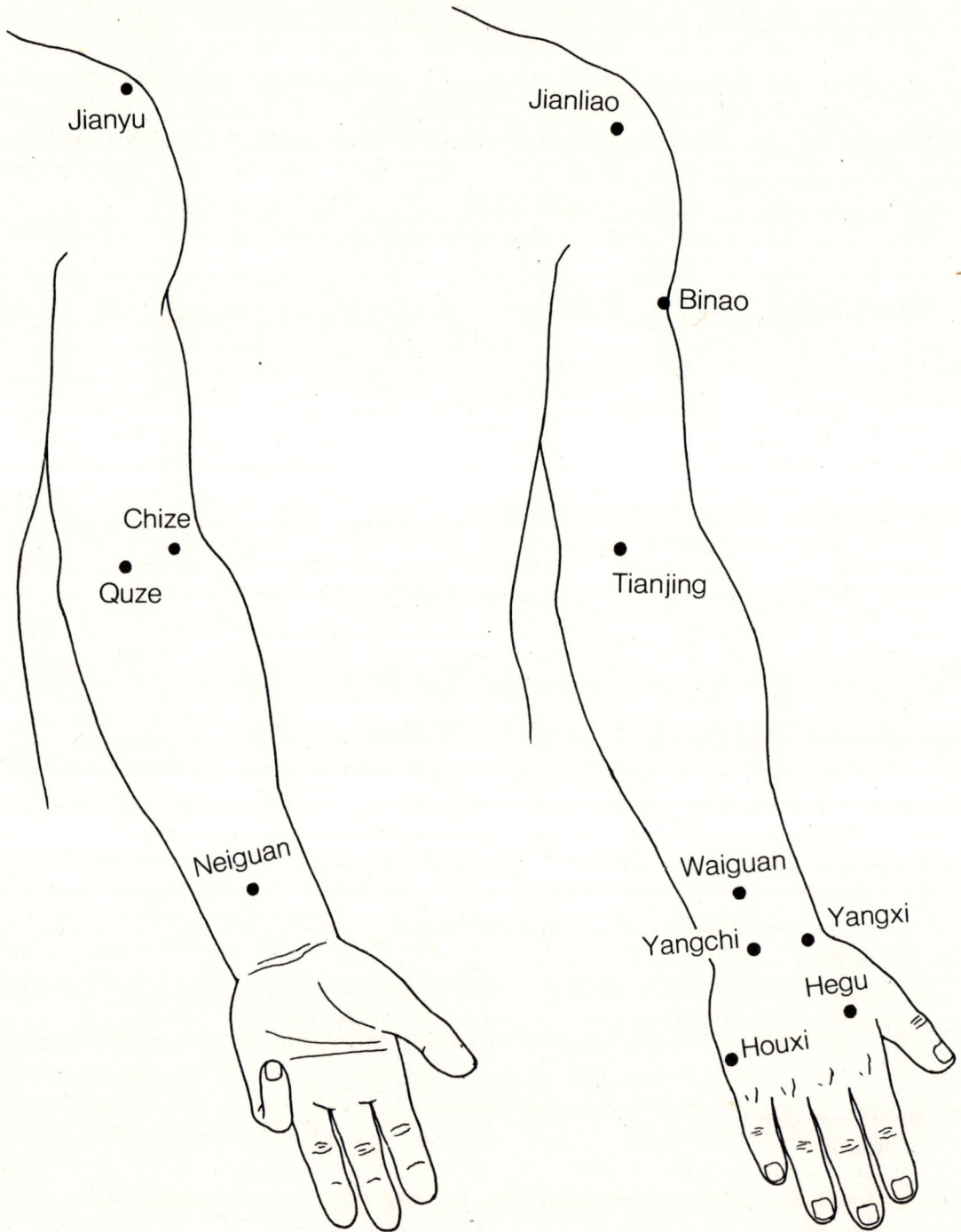

Figs. 13-14   Commonly Used Points on the Upper Limbs

inal emission and gastrointestinal dysfunction.

Manipulations: Digital hitting, pressing and kneading.

(4) Tianshu (ST 25): About 6 cm. lateral to the umbilicus. Beneath spread the inferior epigastric artery and vein.

Indications: Sprain of abdominal muscles, constipation, abdominal distension, enteritis and irregular menstruation.

Manipulations: Pressing and kneading. (See Fig. 15)

4) Commonly Used Points on the Lumbodorsal Area

(1) Dazhui (DU 14): Below the spinous process of the seventh cervical vertebra. Under Dazhui are the supraspinal ligament, the interspinal ligament, the interior interspinal venous plexus and the branch of the eighth cervical nerve.

Indications: Pain in shoulder and back, common cold with fever.

Manipulations: Digital pressing and kneading.

(2) Jianjing (GB 21): Midway between Dazhui (Du 14) and the acromion. Under it lie the trapezius muscle, and deep down between the levator muscle of scapula and the supraspinal muscle are the branches of the transverse cervical artery and vein, the accessory nerve and the suprascapular nerve.

Indications: Stiff neck, headache, pain in shoulder and back, difficulty in raising the hand and arm, and periarthritis of shoulder.

Manipulations: Digital pressing, grasping and kneading.

(3) Tianzong (SI 11): On the scapula, in the center of the subscapular fossa. Under it are the infraspinal muscle, the circumflex artery and vein of scapula and the suprascapular nerve.

Indications: Pain in shoulder and arm, distension and stuffiness in the chest and hypochondrium, difficulty in raising the upper limbs and pain in the lateral and posterior sides of elbow and arm.

Manipulations: Digital pressing and press-kneading.

(4) Fengmen (BL 12): On the back, below the spinous process of the second thoracic vertebra, about 4.5 cm beside the posterior midline. Posterosuperior musculus serratus; deep down are the longissimus muscle, and branches of the second intercostal artery and vein, and nerves.

Indications: Stiff neck, pain in waist and back.

Manipulations: Pressing, pushing and kneading.

(5) Mingmen (DU 4): Inferior to the spinous process of the second lumbar vertebra, at the level of the umbilicus. Beneath are the lumbodorsal fascia, the supraspinal ligament, the interspinal ligament, the lumbar arterial and venous branches, and nerve branches.

Indications: Lumbar muscle sprain, pain in waist and leg, lumbodorsal fascitis.

Manipulations: Digital pressing, press-kneading.

(6) Shenshu (BL 23): About 4.5 cm. lateral to the spinous process of the second lumbar vertebra, i.e., about 4.5 cm. lateral to Mingmen (DU 4). Beneath are the lumbodorsal fascia, the sacrospinal muscle, the second lumbar arterial and venous

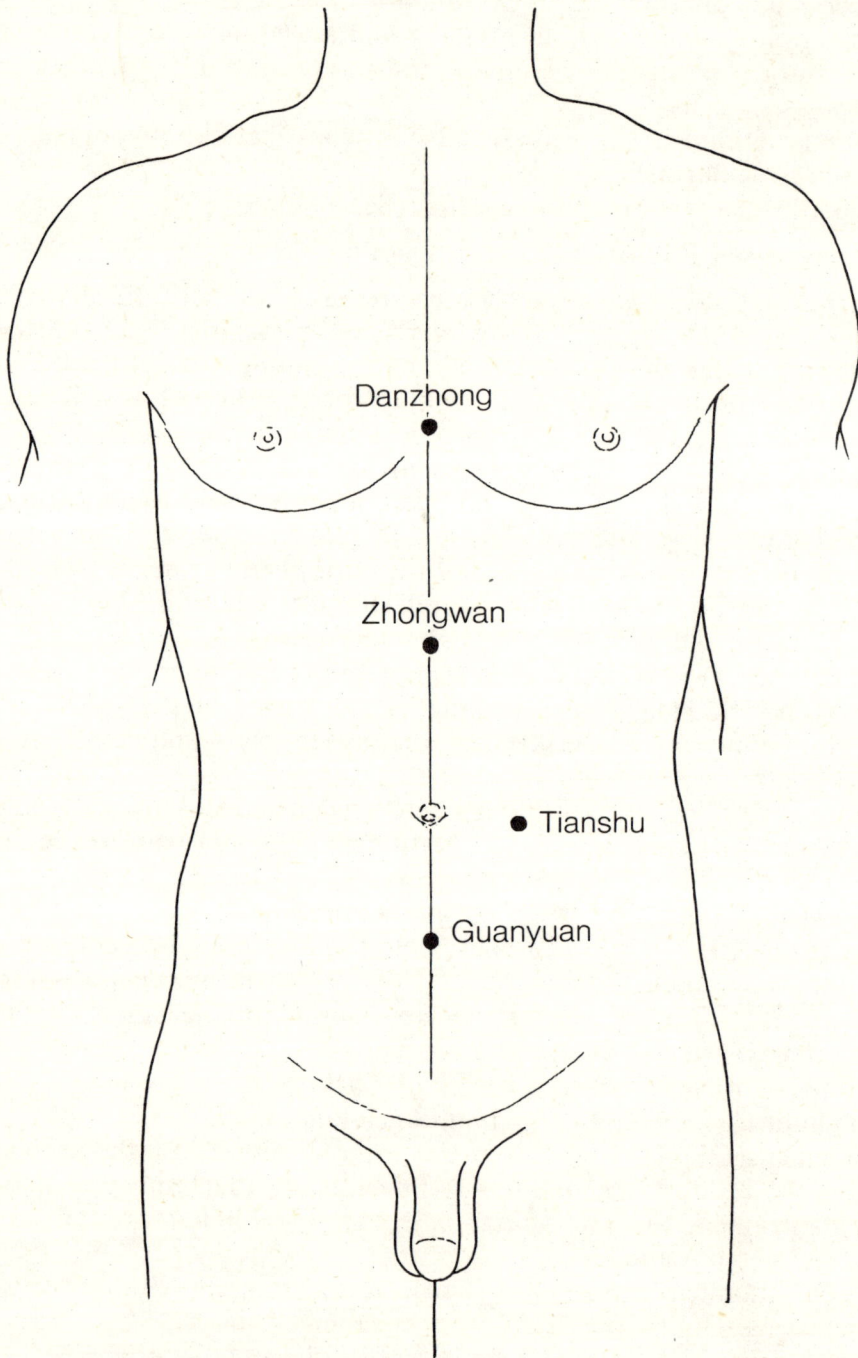

Fig. 15 Commonly Used Points on the Chest and Abdomen

branches and nerve branches, while deep down lies the lumbar nerve plexus.

Indications: Lumbago, lumbar muscle sprain, prolapse of lumbar intervertebral disc, soreness and flaccidity of waist and knee, irregular menstruation.

Manipulations: Digital pressing, scrubbing and foulage.

(7) Yaoyan (Extra Point): In the depression about 9-12 cm. lateral to the spinous process of the fourth lumbar vertebra. Beneath lies the broadest muscles of back, branches of the second lumbar artery and vein, and the superior clunial nerve.

Indications: Pain and soreness at the waist and leg, injury of lumbar soft tissues, injury of the superior clunial nerve.

Manipulations: Pressing and foulage. (See Fig. 16)

5) Commonly Used Points on the Lower Limbs

(1) Huantiao (GB 30): In the depression to the back of the great trochanter of femur. Beneath lies the major gluteal muscle, inferior border of the piriformis, the interior clunial nerves, the inferior gluteal artery and vein and, deep down, the sciatic nerve.

Indications: Sciatica, prolapse of lumbar intervertebral disc, injury of the piriformis, pain in the lumbosacral and hip joints.

Manipulations: Pressing, push-pressing and digital hitting.

(2) Chengfu (BL 36): In the middle of the cross gluteal striation inferior to the buttock, under which are the major gluteal muscle, the biceps muscle of thigh, the sciatic nerve, the inferior gluteal nerve and the ischial artery and vein.

Indications: All type of pain in the lumbosacral region, buttocks and thigh; sciatica; pain in waist and back; bursitis of ischial tuberosity, and injury of posterior thigh muscle.

Manipulations: Pressing and kneading, plus elbow-tip pressing if necessary. The strength should be deep and heavy.

(3) Fengshi (GB 31): On the lateral midline of thigh, about 21 cm. above the popliteal transverse striature. Beneath lie the fascia lata, the lateral muscle of thigh, and the muscular branches of the femoral nerve and lateral cutaneous nerve of thigh.

Indications: Pain in back and leg, gonarthrosis and injury of iliotibial tract.

Manipulations: Palm pressing, kneading and pushing.

(4) Yinmen (BL 37): At the cross point of the line connecting Chengfu (BL 36) and Weizhong (BL 40) points, about 18 cm. inferior to the midpoint of the gluteal fold. Under Yinmen are the semi-tendinous muscle, the biceps muscle of thigh, the third collateral branch of the deep femoral artery and vein, the posterior cutaneous nerve of thigh and, deep down, the sciatic nerve trunk.

Indications: Sciatica, pain in waist and leg, prolapse of lumbar intervertebral disc and sprain of posterior muscle group of thigh.

Manipulations: Palm-pressing, kneading and pushing.

(5) Xuehai (SP 10): About 6 cm. above the medial border of patella. Beneath spread the sartorius muscle, the great adductor of thigh, the musculus rectus

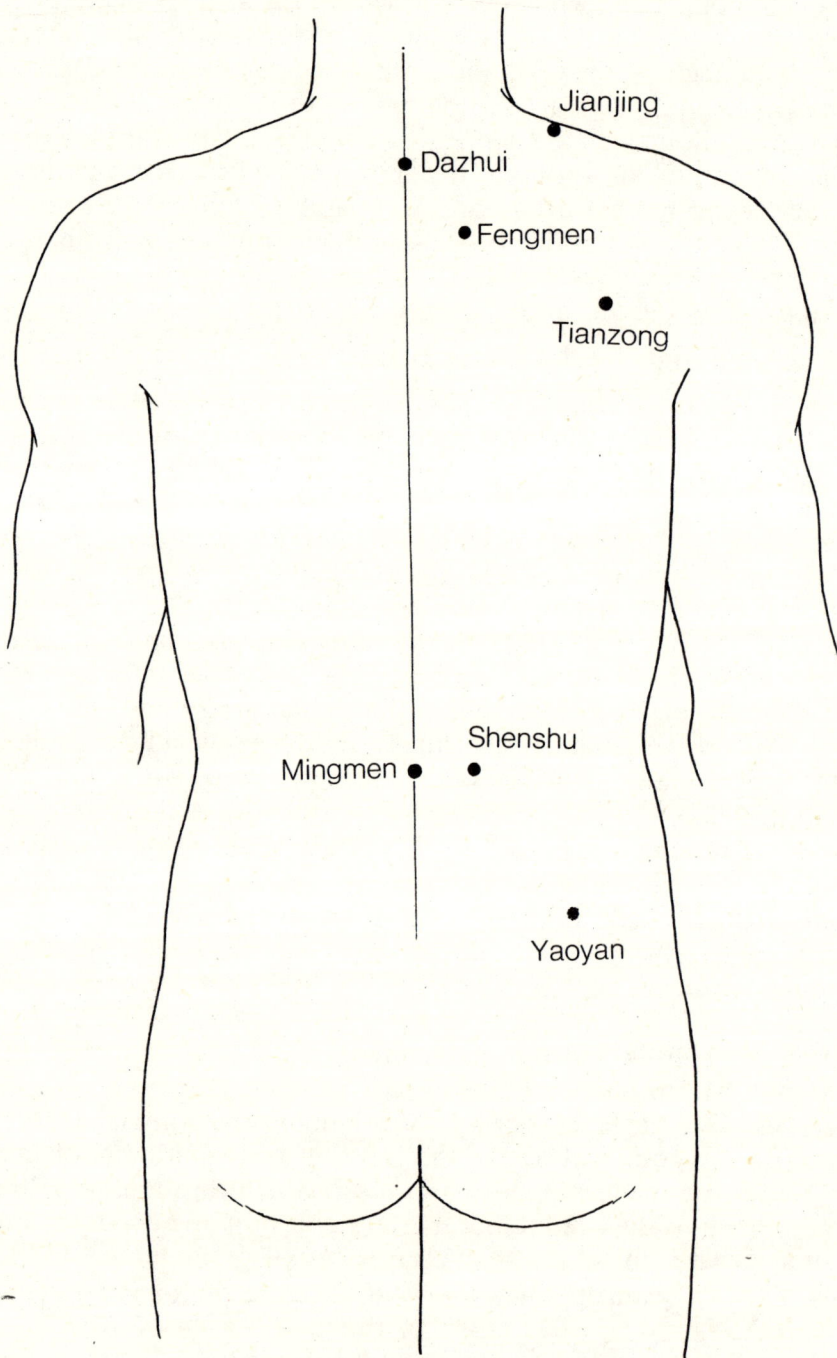

Fig. 16   Commonly Used Points on the Lumbodorsal Area

femoris, the medial cutaneous nerve of thigh and branches of femoral artery and vein.

Indications: Injury of the adductor muscle group of thigh, injury of meniscus, strain of patella and injury of knee fat pad.

Manipulations: Pressing, pushing, kneading and nipping.

(6) Heding (Extra Point): In the depression at the center of the upper border of patella. Beneath lie the quadriceps muscle of thigh, articular capsule of knee, the arterial and venous retia of knee joint and anterior cutaneous branches of the femoral nerve.

Indications: Arthritis of knee, bursitis of knee joint and enthesiopathy of the patellar tendon.

Manipulations: Finger-pressing and nipping.

(7) Weizhong (BL 40): At the exact midpoint of the popliteal transverse striacture. Under Weizhong spread the gastrocnemius, the popliteal muscle, the popliteal artery and the tibial nerve.

Indications: Lumbago, pain in the leg and knee joint, sciatica.

Manipulations: Pressing and kneading. Digital pressing to block blood flow and nerve conduction in order to promote blood circulation and on releasing the pressing and so removing blood stasis and relieving pain.

(8) Dubi (ST 35): On the knee, in the depression just below the patella, lateral to the patellar ligament. The lateral accessory ligament, the long extensor of toes, the articular branch of the peroneal nerve and the arterial and retia of the knee joint all lie beneath.

Indications: Chondromalacia of patella, enthesiopathy of patellar tendon and synovitis of knee.

Manipulations: Pressing and nipping.

(9) Xiyan (EX-LE 5): A pair of points on the two depressions medial and lateral to the patellar ligament which are located with the knee flexed. Beneath are the arterial and venous retia of knee joint, subpatellar branch of the saphenous nerve, fat pad, knee joint space and lateral cutaneous branch of thigh nerve.

Indications: Chondromalacia of patella, injury of fat pad and injury of meniscus.

Manipulations: Pressing and kneading.

(10) Zusanli (ST 36): About 9 cm. below Dubi, one finger-breadth from the anterior crest of the tibia. Beneath are distributed the anterotibial muscle, anterior tibial artery and vein, deep peroneal nerve, long extensor of toe, branches of the saphenous nerve and the lateral cutaneous nerve of gastrocnemius muscle.

Indications: Pain and soreness in the knee and leg, stomachache and abdominal distension.

Manipulations: Pressing, nipping and pushing.

(11) Xuanzhong (GB 39): About 9 cm. above the tip of the lateral malleolus, between the posterior border of the fibula and the long peroneal muscular tendon.

Beneath lie the long extensor of toe, the superficial peroneal nerve, the long peroneal muscle and the anterior tibial arterial and venous branches.

Indications: Sprain of lateral malleolus, pain in knee and leg, discomfort in the neck and pain in the chest and hypochondrium.

Manipulations: Pressing and kneading.

(12) Chengshan (BL 57): At the top of the depression between the two gastrocnemius muscles, which lie beneath, so do the peroneal nerve and the posterior tibial artery.

Indications: Systremma, pain in waist and leg, muscular cramp of leg.

Manipulations: Pressing, kneading, nipping and pushing.

(13) Qiuxu (GB 40): Anteroinferior to the external malleolus, in the depression lateral to the tendon of long extensor muscle of toe. Beneath are distributed the long extensor muscle of toe, the superficial peroneal nerve and the peroneal arterial branches.

Indications: Systremma, sprain of ankle joint, weakness of the lower limbs, sciatica, pain in neck, chest and hypochondrium.

Manipulations: Nipping and pushing.

(14) Jiexi (ST 41): On the midpoint of the dorsum of foot at the transverse malleolus crease, between the tendon of the musculus extensor digitorum longus and hallucis longus. Beneath are distributed the anterior tibial artery and vein, the superficial peroneal nerve and the deep peroneal nerve.

Indications: Sprain of ankle, tenosynovitis of foot.

Manipulations: Nipping and pushing.

(15) Shangqiu (SP 5): In the depression anteroinferior to the medial malleolus. Beneath lie the anterior tibial muscle, the tibial nerve, the anterior tibial artery and the great saphenous vein.

Indications: Sprain of ankle, injury of medial accessory malleolus ligament and injury of navicular bone.

Manipulations: Nipping and pushing.

(16) Kunlun (BL 60): In the depression between the posterior border of the lateral malleolus and the medial aspect of the tendon calcaneus. Beneath spread the long peroneal muscle, the superficial peroneal nerve, the peroneal artery and small saphenous vein.

Indications: Headache, pain in shoulder and back, pain at waist and leg, peritenonitis of Achilles tendon, pain in ankle joint and calcaneodynia.

Manipulations: Kneading and pushing.

(17) Taixi (KI 3): In the depression between the medial malleolus and the Achilles tendon. Under the point lie the posterior tibial artery and vein, the tibial nerve and the medial cutaneous nerve of leg.

Indications: Lumbago, peritenonitis of Achilles tendon, pain in ankle joint and calcaneodynia.

Manipulations: Kneading and pushing, placing the thumb and small finger at

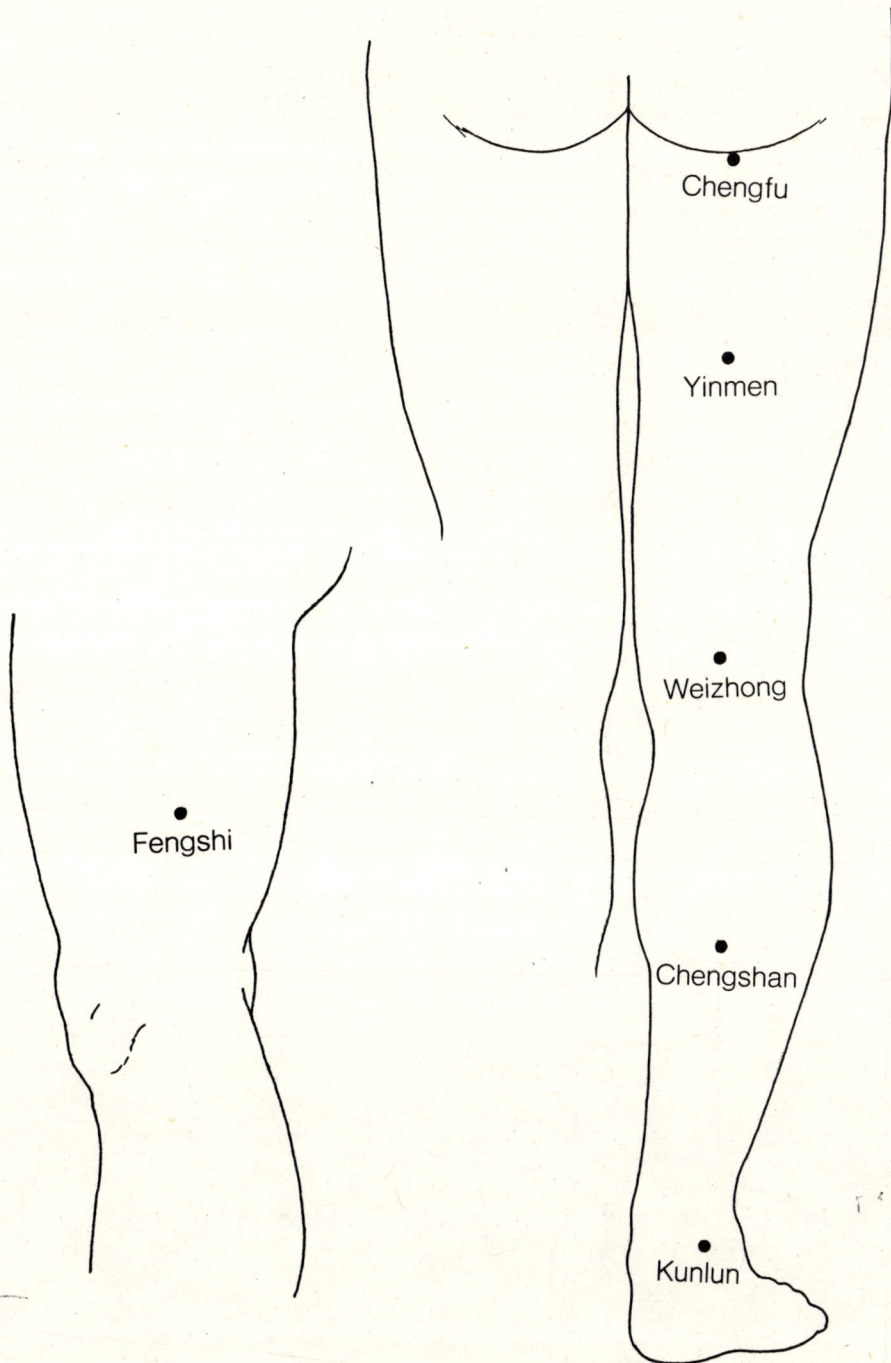

Fig. 17   Commonly Used Points on the Lower Limbs

Fengshi

Xuehai

Xiyan   Dubi

Heding

Dubi

Zusanli

Xuanzhong

Jiexi

Qiuxu   Kunlun

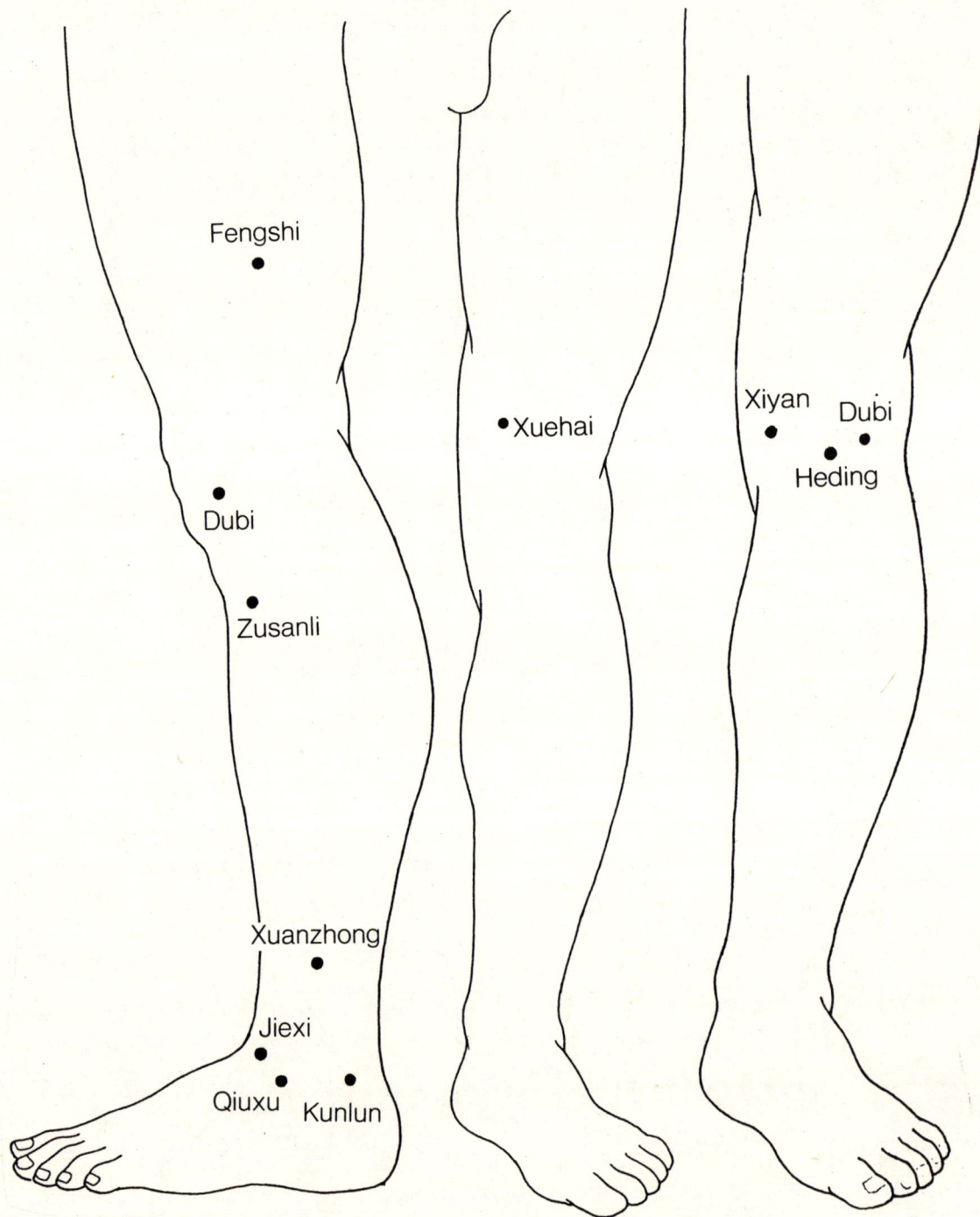

Fig. 18   Commonly Used Points on the Lower Limbs

Taixi and Kunlun respectively and knead-pressing them may relieve the pain in acute injury in the lumbodorsal region.

(18) Bafeng (Extra): At the ends of the spaces between the five toes, altogether 8 on both feet. Beneath these are the interosseous metatarsal muscles, the deep peroneal nerve and the superficial peroneal nerve.

Indications: Swelling and pain in metatarsus, disorder of ankle joint, pain in instep and contusion of metatarsophalangeal joints.

Manipulations: Kneading and pressing. (See Figs. 17 and 18)

Chapter 2
INJURY OF SHOULDER

1. Fracture of Clavicle

Injury Mechanism

1. Usually caused by such external force as collision in competition, hitting the ground with shoulder or palm when falling which causes impact on the clavicle and fracture.

2. The fracture often occurs at the intersection of the middle 1/3 or at the juncture of the middle and outer 1/3.

3. Fracture is often accompanied by overlapping displacement which is characterized by posterosuperior displacement of the medial section of the fracture due to pulling by the sternocleidomastoid and anteroinferior displacement of the lateral section due to the body weight and pulling by the greater pectoral muscle.

Symptoms and Diagnosis

1. There are pain, swelling and malformation at the clavicular region.

2. Local examination reveals swelling in incomplete fracture, with pain on pressure. In fracture of displacement, palpation may reveal the fracture and abnormal movement and the sensation of friction.

3. Motion of the upper limb is limited; the patient often supports the elbow of the affected side with the hand of the normal side.

4. X-ray examination is needed for a clear and exact picture of the fracture.

Treatment

1. Greenstick fracture: With no apparent fracture displacement apply triangular bandage suspensor to the shoulder and elbow for 2-3 weeks.

2. Manual reduction for fracture displacement:

a) Press acupoints Tianding (LI 17) and Quepen (ST 12) to relieve pain. (See Fig. 19)

b) Traction: With the patient in a sitting position, clasp the hands at the lumbar region, throwing out the chest with both shoulders stretching backward, an assistant, with one knee against the patient's back, performs posterior and superolateral traction on the shoulders with both hands.

c) Reduction: The massagist lifts and presses the fracture end to reduce the fracture.

d) Fixation: Make two rings with cotton and bandage, insert two cotton pads under the armpits for protection, and place the rings around both shoulders, tying them at the back area for strapping for four weeks.

e) Post-treatment observation: Self-sensation of numbness in the hand and weakening beat of the radial artery indicate that the axillary nerves and blood vessels are constricted and strapping must be adjusted promptly.

3. In case the above treatment is unsatisfactory, apply the following reduction methods:

a) Digital hitting on Tianding (LI 17) and Quepen (ST 12) to relieve pain, or use 1 percent procaine for local anaesthesia.

b) Making the patient in a sitting position, asking one assistant to hold the patient's body while another to perform posterolateral traction on the affected upper limb to remove the overlapping malformation.

c) The massagist pinches the fracture ends with both hands, push-pressing the protruding ends; in case of sunken fracture displacement lifts the fracture ends for reduction. Avoid forceful push-pressing or lifting to prevent injury to the subclavian artery and brachial plexus. (see Fig. 20)

d) Fixation: Instead of double-ring strapping, figure-8 strapping may be applied though it may loosen.

Post-treatment Functional Exercises

1. Clavicular fracture usually unites, and upper limb function is not impaired even if a unsatisfactory reduction or even a malformed union results.

2. The patient starts fist-making and palm-stretching movements the day after reduction and flexion-extension of elbow joint three days later.

3. Start daily manual treatment three days after the reduction, first by digital pressing on Quepen (ST 12), Binao (LI 14), Quchi (LI 11) and Shaohai (HT 3); (See Fig. 21) then apply gentle scrubbing and grasping of the muscles of the forearm and upper arm.

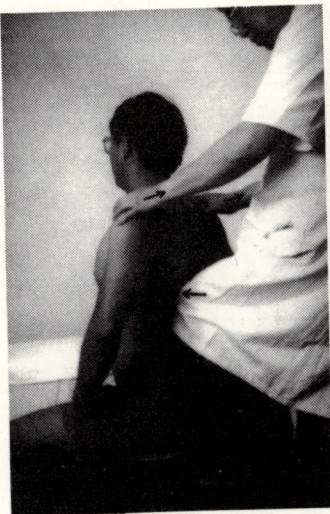

Fig. 19

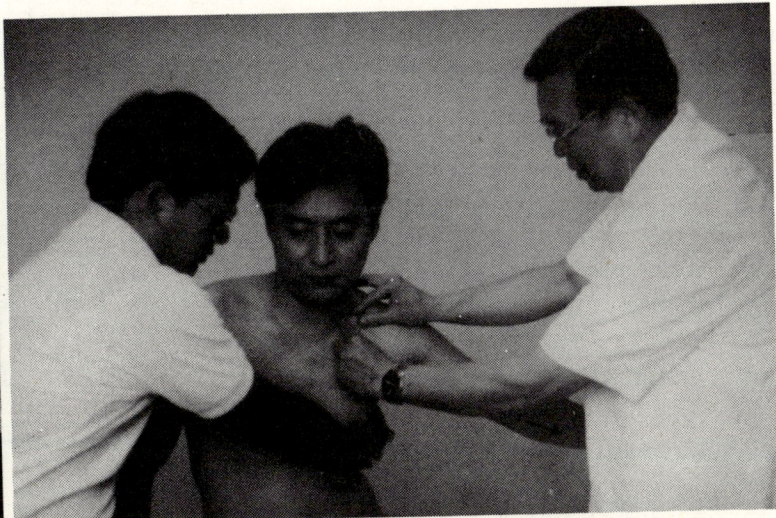

Fig. 20

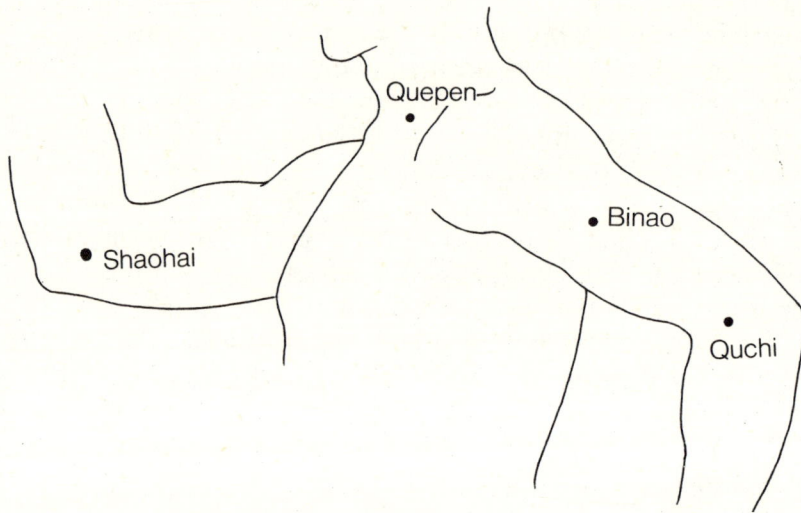

Fig. 21

4. Remove external strapping when pain in the fracture region has subsided and callus formed as shown by X-ray photograph three weeks after the reduction. Perform digital-hitting on Quepen (ST 12), Jianyu (LI 15) and Jianliao (SJ 14), plus gradual abduction and raising of the shoulder. Then perform giant circle movements of the shoulder; relax the stiffened deltoid muscle and the muscles around the shoulder with grasp-kneading manipulations from light to strong. Do not expect quick results.

2. Dislocation of Shoulder Joint

Injury Mechanism

1. Caused by external force. During a fall, when the upper limb rotates inward and stretches backward, the violent force of hitting the ground with the palm impacts forward along the longitudinal axis of the humerus, causing the head of the humerus penetrate the joint capsule ahead to result in forward dislocation.

2. The limb is abducted outward when the palm hits the ground, the tip of the acromion presses against the humerus so the lateral side of the surgical neck becomes the fulcrum and the head of humerus breaks through the lower border of the joint capsule to result in infraglenoid dislocation.

3. Continuous impact of the external force may cause the humerus to move beneath the coracoid process or the clavicle. This type of dislocation is called subcoracoid or subclavicular dislocation.

4. Complications of shoulder joint dislocation: Joint reduction is impaired when there are avulsion fracture of the greater tuberosity of humerus, tendon olisthy of

the long head of biceps brachii muscle, and out-slipping of the tendon from the intertubercular sulcus. Strong external force may cause fracture of the surgical neck of the humerus and pulling of the axillary nerve, which are manifested by paralysis of the deltoid muscle and numbness in the exterior shoulder skin. If dislocation of shoulder joint is not given prompt reduction or is not properly treated, frequent recurrence may lead to habitual dislocation.

Symptoms and Diagnosis

1. Pain, swelling and dysfunction of shoulder caused by trauma.

2. There is slight abduction of the affected limb, the hand of the normal limb supports the forearm of the affected limb, and the head and body incline toward the affected side.

3. Square-shoulder malformation: The shoulder joint region becomes empty and the acromion protrudes, eliminating the round appearance of the shoulder region.

4. Shoulder-reaching test (Duke's test): When reaching the hand of the affected side for the healthy shoulder, the elbow cannot press close to the chest wall; while trying to press the elbow close to the chest wall, the hand cannot reach the healthy shoulder.

5. X-ray examination may reveal the type of dislocation and show whether there are fracture complications.

Treatment

1. Digitally press acupoints Tianding (LI 17) and Quepen (ST 12).

2. Reduction by hand-traction and foot-propping: As the first choice manipulation of the reduction, this is performed in the following manner—the patient lies supine, the massagist props one foot against the armpit on the affected side, holds the wrist of the affected limb with both hands and performs traction gradually, forming a resistant traction with foot-propping. The outward force of foot-propping enables an outward moving the head of humerus. When a clear click is heard or a sudden sliding of the head of the humerus is felt, the shoulder resumes its round shape, indicating completion of the reduction. (See Fig. 22)

3. Three-person traction (performed in case the above manipulation is not successful).

a) With the patient in a sitting position, finger-press the above-said acupoints.

b) An assistant holds the patient's body firmly while another one clasps the wrist and performs persistent anteroinferior traction and shaking.

c) The massagist places both thumbs on the patient's shoulder with the fingers in the armpit. He lifts the head of the humerus outward with the thumb as the fixed point; an assistant performs outward rotation and then upward pushing of the affected limb until a click indicates the success of reduction.

d) The massagist carries the elbow of the affected side with one hand and kneads the shoulder to restore and regulate the muscles and tendons.

e) Apply triangular binder-strapping to the shoulder for three weeks. (See Fig. 23)

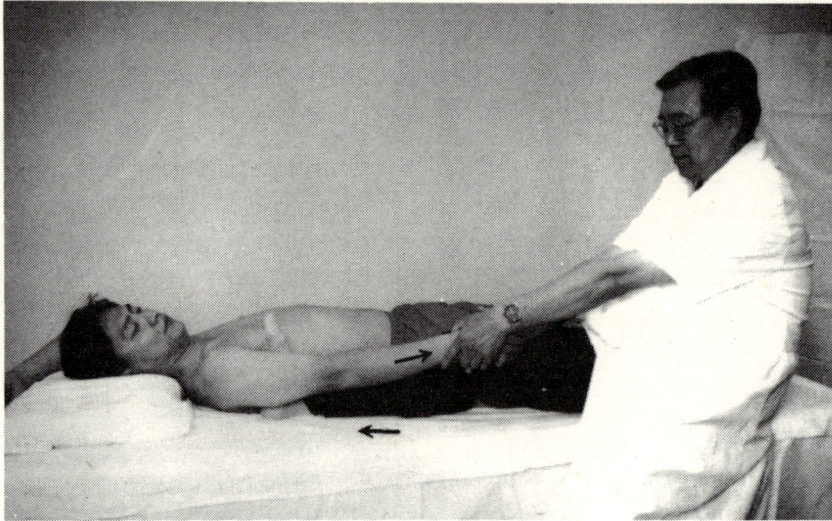

Fig. 22

Post-treatment Functional Exercise

1. Perform elbow and hand movement the day after treatment.

2. A week later press and knead muscles of shoulder and back to prevent amyotrophy and adhesion.

3. Remove the strapping 2-3 weeks later and practise shoulder movements gradually. Be careful not to remove the strapping or practise lifting movement of the shoulder too early. When the joint capsule is not fully repaired, shoulder activities may cause habitual joint dislocation.

Shoulder joint function will be impaired for some time after injury, so avoid by all means forceful traction and pulling, which could cause ossifying myositis. The training program needs to be worked out according to the degree of recovery of function and strength of the shoulder.

3. Contusion and Dislocation of Acromioclavicular Joint

The acromioclavicular joint consists of the articular surface of acromion of scapula and clavicle, which are linked by the acromioclavicular and coracoclavicular ligaments. Contusion and dislocation of this joint is a common sports injury.

Injury Mechanism

1. Contusion and dislocation of shoulder acromioclavicular joint is mainly caused by such direct external force as hitting the ground with anterior or posterior aspect of the shoulder during a fall, thus injuring the shoulder joint.

2. Caused by indirect external force, e.g., the movement of crucifix in the gymnastics rings, which may injure the acromioclavicular joint.

3. Classification:

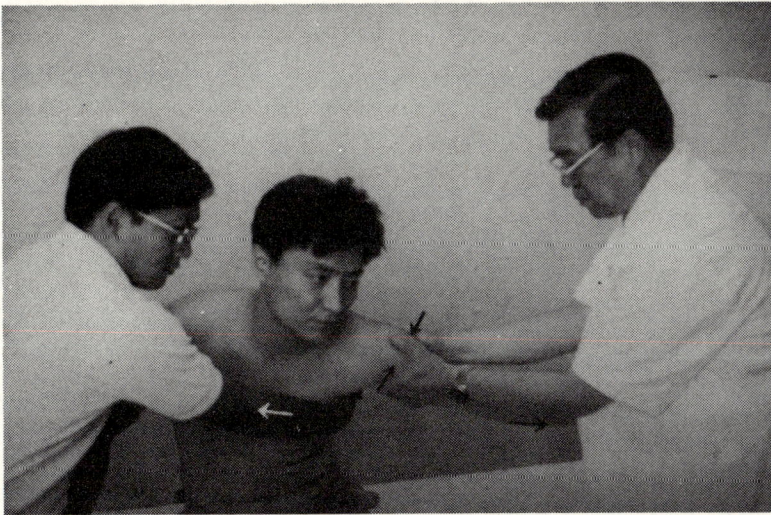

Fig. 23

a) Contusion of joint, referring to injury of the joint capsule or ligament only, without malformation.

b) Subluxation of joint, meaning partial tearing of joint capsule and ligament and slight upward displacement of the lateral border of clavicle, with slight malformation.

c) Dislocation of joint, referring to rupture of the acromioclavicular and coracoclavicular ligaments, complete separation of the clavicle and the acromion with obvious upward displacement.

Symptoms and Diagnosis

1. Aching and pain on pressure in the acromioclavicular region.

2. In dislocation of joint there is local swelling, protrusion of clavicle and, widening of the acromioclavicular joint space and abnormal movement of the clavicle end on pressure, i.e., the range of upward and downward movement of the clavicle is enlarged, showing sharp contrast to the normal shoulder on palpation.

3. Hanging down of the affected limb, abduction and raising are limited and local pain is sharp when lifting an object.

4. X-ray examination may rule out fracture of the lateral section of the clavicle but show the degree of dislocation. Front-view X-ray photograph of both acromioclavicular joints taken when pulling both upper limbs downward shows clearly the widened articular space on the semiluxated side.

Treatment

1. Treatment of contusion of joint:

a) With the patient in a sitting position, the massagist supports the elbow of the affected limb with one hand and with the other performs pinch-grasping manipulation on Jianjing (GB 21) and digital-kneading manipulation on the Jianyu (LI

15). Grasping and kneading manipulations on the shoulder and upper arm are also used to relax the muscles. (See Fig. 24)

b) The massagist places one hand at the acromioclavicular joint and with the other raises the arm on the affected side by holding the wrist, then applies slow traction and gentle rocking manipulation on the shoulder to reduce the slight movement.

c) Strap with triangular binder and resume training 1-2 weeks later.

2. Treatment of subluxation of joint:

a) With the patient in a sitting position and flexing the elbow, the massagist pushes the patient's elbow upward with one hand and presses the lateral border of the clavicle for reduction.

b) Fixation: Place cotton pads at the elbow and the lateral border of the clavicle respectively, when wind wide adhesive plaster from the back upward, passing the lateral border of the clavicle, forward to the anterior aspect of the upper arm and to the posterior aspect of the arm via the elbow. Then wind adhesive plaster from the posterior aspect of the shoulder, passing the lateral border of the clavicle and strap it downward obliquely at the chest region. Strap another two lengths of adhesive plaster in the same manner. Strap the upper limb with triangular binder or wrist-neck sling for 3-4 weeks.

c) Elastic tape strapping: Wind wide elastic tape past the elbow and clavicle longitudinally, giving the elbow upward support and pressing the clavicle downward to achieve the effects of reduction and strapping.

3. Treatment of dislocation of joint:

The manipulations for reduction and methods of strapping for dislocation of joint are the same as for subluxation though the period of strapping is longer, from

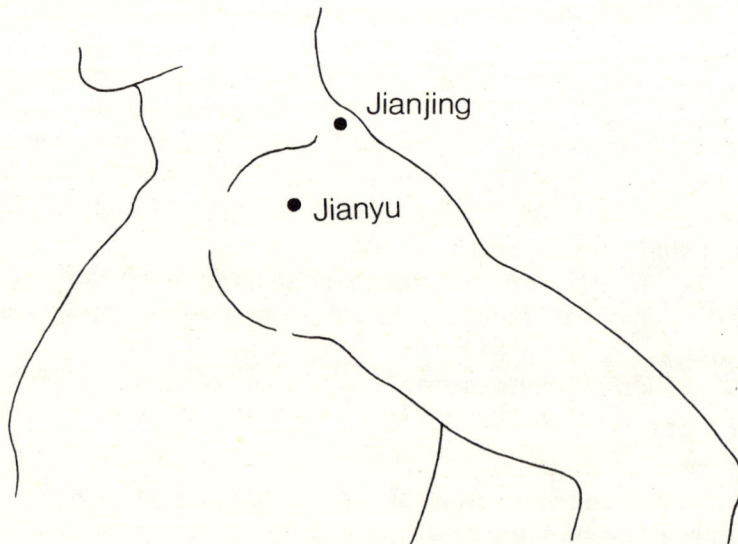

Fig. 24

six to eight weeks. Prematurely resuming activity, with insufficient union of the joint capsule and ligament, will cause habitual dislocation of the acromioclavicular joint and directly affect the function and strength of the shoulder.

Post-treatment Functional Exercise

The patient can start practising fist-making and palm-stretching the day after the injury, then receives treatment of the forearm and upper arm by gradual pressing and kneading manipulations three days later. Avoid any shoulder movement, especially upward and downward; sufficient strapping time is essential. Practise shoulder movement with light manipulations after removal of strapping, plus abduction and forward and backward swinging of the upper limb. Protracted strapping of the shoulder may cause scleromata, cords or large-area stiffness of muscles, which require manipulation by pressing, kneading, restoring and plucking to relax the muscles and tendon, and promote blood circulation by removing blood stasis for early recovery of functions.

4. Injury of Sternoclavicular Joint

The sternoclavicular joint consists of the sternal end of the clavicle and clavicular notch of the manubrium of sternum. The joint capsule is fixed by the sternoclavicular and interclavicular ligaments. The sternocleidomastoid originates from the anterior aspect of this joint, and some of the greater pectoral muscle also originates in the anteroinferior aspect of this joint. This injury has comparatively little effect on the upper limbs.

Injury Mechanism

Injury of the sternoclavicular joint is mostly caused by external force which, acting on the shoulder with the clavicle as the fulcrum, can injure the joint at the internal end of the clavicle. The injury is of two types: contusion of joint and dislocation of joint. Forward dislocation is more common than posterior dislocation.

Symptoms and Diagnosis

1. Sprain of joint: Pain in the sternoclavicular joint on one side, local swelling and pain on pressure which may be aggravated by movement of the sternoclavicular joint.

2. Dislocation of joint: Local pain, forward protrusion of the medial end of clavicle, the pain is worse than in sprain, and sternoclavicular joint movement is abnormal.

3. X-ray examination: Front-view photograph of both sternoclavicular joints taken when pulling both upper arms downward reveals the affected joint space widened, with the medial end of clavicle at a distance from the manubrium of sternum.

Treatment

1. Manual reduction: With the patient in a sitting position, an assistant stands

behind, supporting the patient's back with a knee and holding the patient's both shoulders tightly with hands and pulling toward the posteroinferior direction to fully separate the sternoclavicular joint. The massagist presses the medial end of the clavicle to reduce the dislocation. This is not difficult using manual treatment, but it is difficult to strap because any movement of shoulder and upper limb may cause recurrence of the sternoclavicular joint dislocation.

2. Fixation: Place cotton pads and pagoda-shaped paper pads on the sternoclavicular joint and strap with long and wide adhesive plaster tapes from the back to the chest obliquely via the joint, followed by pressure strapping with short wide adhesive plaster tapes along the same route. Or, apply figure-8 bandage to both shoulders to strap them at posterior extended position for 3-4 weeks.

Functional Exercises

At the early stage the patient moves the unstrapped joint but does not do any upward-downward or forward-backward movements of the shoulder, such as lifting objects, shrugging, or expanding the chest. Perform gentle pressing manipulation on the upper arm and forearm as well as muscles of shoulders for relaxing the muscles and tendons and activating the flow of qi and blood in the meridians and collaterals so as to prevent muscle stiffness and atrophy and achieve early resumption of functions.

5. Rotator Cuff Injury

The rotator cuff is a tendon plate consisting of the four muscular tendons of the infraspinal, the supraspinal, the teres minor and the subscapular muscles.

The medial aspect of the rotator cuff is linked with the joint capsule and at its lateral aspect is the subdeltoid bursa.

The rotator cuff functions in three ways: To ensure firm contact between the head of humerus and the glenoid cavity to stabilize the joint; to ensure that the head of humerus is not pulled to the acromion when the deltoid contracts to help with abduction of shoulder joint, and to ensure the shoulder rotation function of the supraspinal, infraspinal, the teres minor and the subscapular muscles.

Injury Mechanism

Strong supporting force of the upper limb against the ground and shoulder turning during a fall may cause acute injury to the rotator cuff. Such repeated over-range sprain of humerus as abduction and inward rotation of shoulder may cause injury due to squeezing, friction or repeated traction of the rotator cuff and synovial bursa by the greater tuberosity of humerus, acromion and the coracoacromial ligament, with the supraspinal muscle often being injured. This type of injury is chronic and may be myotenositis of supraspinal muscle, bursitis of deltoid muscle, or subacromial bursitis. However, since clinical diagnosis can scarcely distinguish between them and the treatment methods are the same, it is appropriate to refer to all of them as rotator cuff injury. If not given timely treatment or not cured, the chronic injury may lead to local denaturation of bone, cartilage, ligament, joint capsule and muscle, and the condition may affect physical training and competition.

Symptoms and Diagnosis

1. Shoulder pain: This pain is deep and aggravated by pulling or turning the shoulder. It may radiate to the upper arm.

2. Weakness of shoulder: The shoulder is of little help in movement and limited in abduction.

3. Pain on pressure in the shoulder: Pain is felt under the acromion and at the greater tuberosity of humerus, tenderness may also occur at the anterior or posterior aspect of shoulder.

4. Resistive test: Pain is felt in the shoulder when it is abducted at an angle of 80-90 degrees, becoming more severe during resistive abduction of the shoulder joint at this time. The pain is eased when the abduction angle is within 80 degrees or exceeds 120 degrees, or when tracting the shoulder for abduction.

Treatment

1. Acute injury:

a) With the patient in a sitting position, the massagist presses and kneads acupoints Jianyu (LI 15), Jianjing (GB 21) and Tianzong (SI 11). (See Fig. 25)

b) Apply light and gentle press-kneading manipulation on the deltoid muscle, accompanied by light and gentle pull-grasping manipulation on the back and upper arm to promote local blood circulation, and finally apply scrubbing on the deltoid and adjacent tissues until a sensation of heat runs deep. Keep the shoulder warm after treatment.

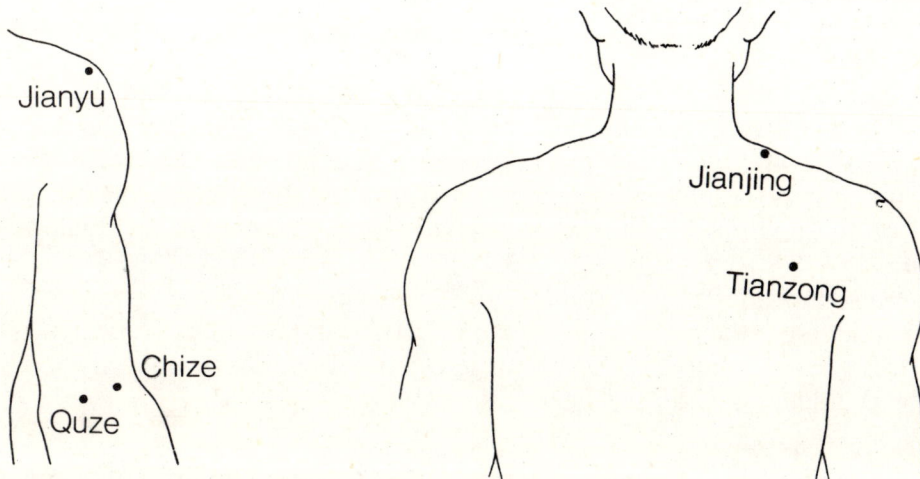

Fig. 25

2. Chronic sprain:

a) With the patient in a sitting position, the massagist performs digital pressing on acupoints Quepen (ST 12), Jianyu (LI 15), Jianjing (GB 21) and Tianzong (SI 11).

b) Perform gentle pressing and grasping manipulation on muscles of shoulder and scapular regions, with stress on the subacromial region and the deltoid muscle. Then apply flick-poking on the deltoid, the supraspinal, the subscapular and the teres minor muscles respectively with deep and strong force. Passively adduct, abduct and rotate the upper limb. Perform scraping and pushing manipulations on the tender area with the shoulder in abduction position to ensure strong stimulation to the pathological changes and promote local restoration. To finish off, manipulate by foulage, shaking and rocking at the shoulder to relax local adhesion.

c) Keep the shoulder warm after treatment, perform such strength and tenacity exercises as shoulder turning, shoulder pressing and strength exercise of the deltoid muscle.

Example: Mr. Li, male, gymnast, winner in many world competitions, suffered chronic rotator cuff injury of right shoulder which lacked force in movement, physical training and competition; nerve block with cortisone had little effect. Then, after receiving manual treatment during training, satisfactory curative effect was achieved.

6. Tenosynovitis of Long Head of Biceps Brachii

The tendon of long head of biceps brachii starts from the upper tuberosity of glenoid cavity, passes the head of humerus downward and enters the intertubercular sulcus via the articular cavity. The tendon in the sulcus is 5 cm. long and encircled by the tendon-sheath.

Injury Mechanism

The extent of muscular tendon movement of brachial biceps is the largest during abduction and outward rotation of shoulder. Repeated abduction and outward rotation of the shoulder and friction between the tendon and its tendon-sheath may cause traumatic inflammation in the synovium of the tendon-sheath, causing stricture of the tendon-sheath and limitation of movement of the tendon in its tendon-sheath.

Over-range movement of shoulder joint leads to excessive movement of the muscular tendon of brachial biceps in the intertubercular sulcus; repeated friction may also cause tenosynovitis. Some athletes may experience this after a single pulling of shoulder.

Symptoms and Diagnosis

1. There is pain in the shoulder which gradually aggravates after injury and radiates to the deltoid muscle and the upper arm.

2. The pain is exacerbated during abduction, backward extension and lifting of

the upper arm.

3. Local pain on pressure: The tendon feels thick and stiff when the intertubercular sulcus of humerus is palpated.

Treatment

1. With the patient in a sitting position, press acupoints Jianyu (LI 15), Tianding (LI 17) and Quepen (ST 12). (See Fig. 26)

2. Relax muscles of the shoulder, chest and back by pressing and grasping.

3. Relax the belly of arm biceps muscle and the end-point of the elbow by pressing and grasping.

4. The massagist supports the elbow of the affected side with one hand, and with the other, performs flick-poking manipulation along the muscular tendon of brachial biceps up and down in the intertubercular sulcus of the humerus. The manipulating strength for a new injury should be light and gentle, and heavy for a chronic case. When the shoulder is in backward stretching position, the tendon is more superficial, so it is easy to apply manual treatment to diminish inflammation and relax adhesion. Repeated push-pressing along the tendon may regulate and restore the muscles and tendons.

5. The massagist places both hands at the anterior and posterior sides of the diseased shoulder respectively to squeeze the should with both palms to restore tissues.

6. Apply both-hand foulage on the affected shoulder and upper arm, and palm-scrubbing on the intertubercular sulcus until a warm sensation runs deep, so as to promote local blood circulation. Keep the shoulder warm after treatment, protecting against invasion by cold and dampness.

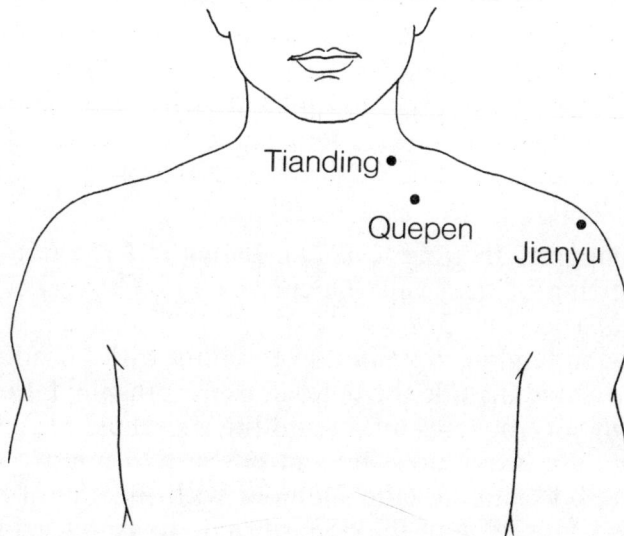

Fig. 26

7. Rheumatic Omalgia and Notalgia

Rheumatic omalgia and notalgia are not an independent disease but a syndrome. As it is not caused by injury it is apt to be neglected clinically.

Onset Mechanism

1. This disease occurs mostly after physical training or when the shoulder is exposed to wind and cold during sleep.

2. When the exogenous cold wind and dampness attacking the shoulders intrude into the shoulder-dorsal region and block the meridians and collaterals, pain will ensue. This is called *bi zheng* (arthralgia syndrome) in traditional Chinese medicine.

3. Exogenous cold and wind attacking the shoulder and back lead to dysfunction of nerve endings, micrangiums and muscular fascia in the tissues. Stimulation of the nerve endings may cause reflexive and wide-spread pain. Spasm of micrangiums may cause local ischemia and anoxia, also evoking pain. Inflammation may result at muscular fasciae. Pathological changes at the nerves, blood vessels, fasciae and muscles and the mutual influence among them aggravate the symptoms of omalgia and notalgia.

Symptoms and Diagnosis

1. There is no history of trauma in the shoulder-dorsal region, but a history of exposure to exogenous cold and dampness.

2. Aversion to cold, weakness, soreness and stiffness in the shoulder-dorsal region. The pain, which may be eased by heat, may radiate to the cervical area and the upper limbs.

3. Examination may reveal slight tension or muscles at the shoulder-dorsal region with movement slightly impaired and with apparent pain on pressure.

4. Long-term sprain and chilling in the shoulder-dorsal region may gradually lead to periarthritis of shoulder and muscular atrophy. Though in most cases the symptoms disappear without treatment, long-standing disease will hinder physical training.

Treatment

1. Pinch-grasp acupoints Jianjing (GB 21), Jianyu (LI 15) and Tianzong (SI 11) along with digit-pressing of acupoints Quchi (LI 11), Quze (PC 3), Hegu (LI 4) and the A Shi points. (See Fig. 27)

2. Relax muscles and tendons up and down mainly with kneading and pinching. Muscles to be manipulated include the deltoid, the supraspinal, the infraspinal, the trapezius, the teres major, the teres minor and the rhomboid muscles. For stiffened tissues and scleroma, use heavy pressing and pushing to remove spasm.

3. Perform passive adduction of the shoulder with the aim of making the hand reach the shoulder-dorsal region of the opposite side so as to tract the back muscles of the affected side. Tract and shake the shoulder joint.

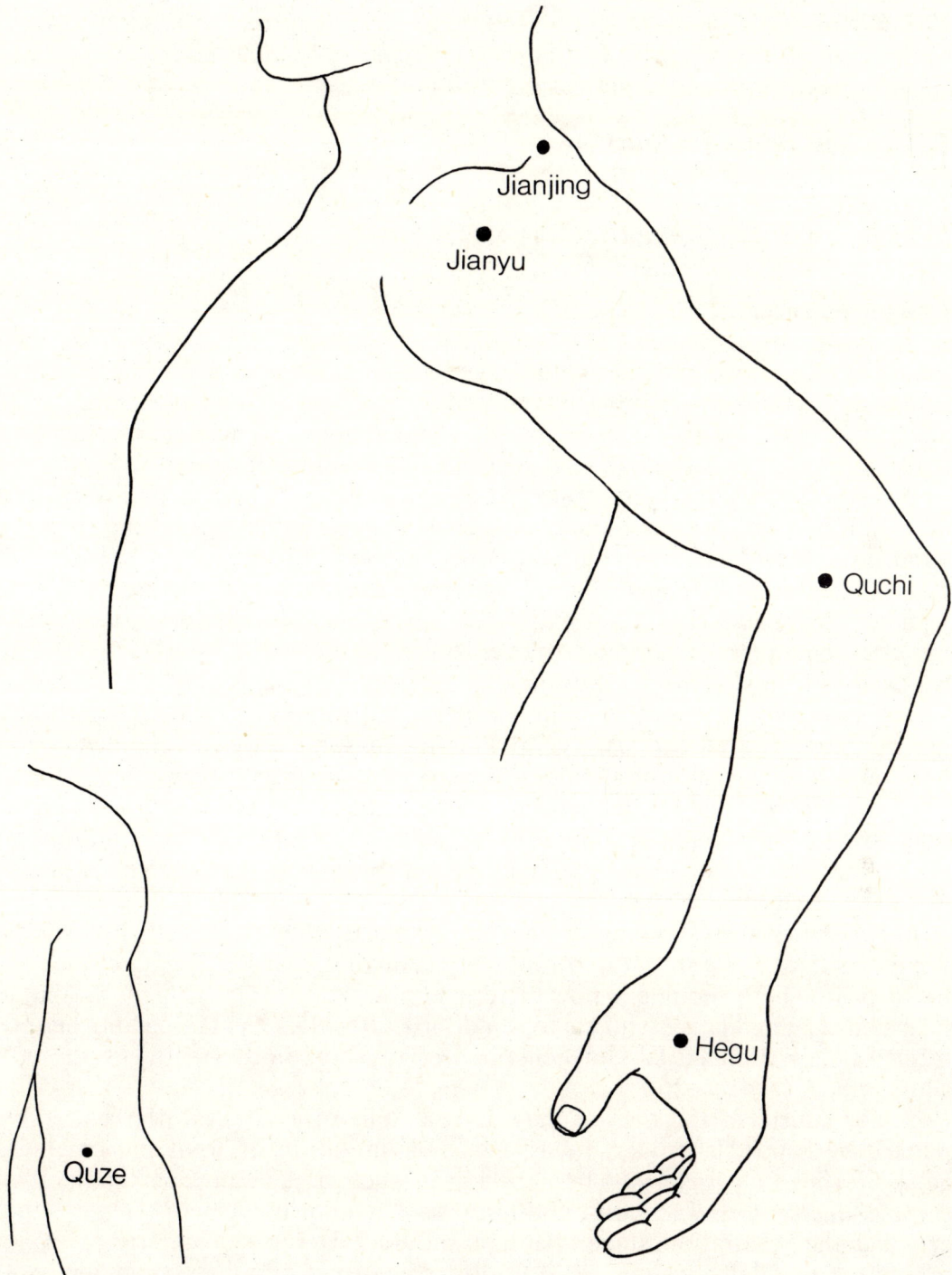

Fig. 27

4. Perform swift foulage and scrubbing to generate heat in the shoulder region until the skin turns slightly red to expel wind and relieve pain. Keep the shoulder-dorsal region warm and avoid further chilling.

8. Periarthritis of Shoulder

This disease is called *lou jian feng* (omalgia) and *dong jie jian* (frozen shoulder) in traditional Chinese medicine, and because it often occurs in people around the age of fifty it is also called "omalgia at fifty."

Onset Mechanism

1. Caused by pathogenic wind and cold: At about the age of fifty, people gradually experience general debility. Qi and blood become insufficient and vital energy is less, allowing pathogenic chill and dampness to lead to stagnation of qi and blood, poor nourishment of muscles and tendons as well as meridians and collaterals, causing pathological changes in the shoulder region.

2. Caused by trauma and strain: Excessive activity or repeated chronic injury of shoulder and local metabolic disturbance may block blood and lymphatic circulation, then cause hyperplasia, thickening, reduced elasticity and tissue adhesion in the fibrous tissues of joint capsule, coracohumeral ligament, muscular tendon of brachial biceps, teres major and minor muscles, rotator cuff and deltoid muscle. The range of shoulder movement is reduced by various factors until complete stiffness of the joint occurs.

3. Periarthritis of shoulder is in a way related to cervical spondylopathy: The nerve-ending type of cervical spondylopathy in some cases is characterized by omalgia and impairment of shoulder movement, and simply treating as periarthritis of shoulder is often unsatisfactory. However, the symptoms may be considerably relieved if the treatment is applied in combination with such manipulations for treating cervical spondylopathy as traction and rotation of the head and restoration of cervical tissues.

4. Periarthritis of shoulder is also referrable to rheumatic arthritis, shoulder symptoms may be local manifestations of rheumatic arthritis, e.g., constant alternative pain in both shoulders, now better and now worse, occurring more frequently in cold weather. This is similar to wandering arthralgia. As taking antirheumatic medicine may produce certain beneficial effect, combined treatment should be adopted.

5. The course of the disease may divided into three stages—the acute stage: marked by painful shoulder, myospasm and limitation of joint movement; the adhesion stage: characterized by adhesion of such tissue fibres as shoulder joint capsule, ligaments and tendons, and limitation of joint movement (frozen shoulder); and the restoration stage: Pain in shoulder is relaxed and range of joint movement gradually widens. Restoration of normal shoulder function can be expected in most cases.

Symptoms and Diagnosis

1. Pain in the shoulder: At the initial stage there is usually aching which gradually aggravates to dull pain and then a twinge which may awaken the patient during sleep. Some patients experience sudden onset of the disease with intolerable pain which may be aggravated by cold and eased by heat.

2. Restriction of shoulder movement: At the early stage the pain causes restriction to spasmodic protective movement, while at the late stage tissue adhesion may limit abduction, outward rotation and lifting of the shoulder; the patient may find it difficult to lift the arms, wash face, comb hair, dress, put hands into pockets and fasten a belt, until all shoulder movements are restricted. If both shoulders are affected, the patient will require care in daily life.

3. Tender area: Tenderness on pressure is widespread in the shoulder-dorsal region, being more marked in some areas. Beneath the tender area at the anterior aspect of shoulder are the tendon of humerus. Beneath the tender area at the lateral aspect of shoulder are the deltoid muscle, joint capsule and rotator cuff. The deltoid tender area covers three parts, i.e., the anterior, middle and posterior areas, with tenderness at the middle part being especially apparent. Beneath the tender area the posterior aspect of shoulder are the brachial triceps muscle and the teres major and minor muscles. Tension on the teres major and minor muscles may hinder abduction and outward rotation of shoulder. Beneath the tender area at the scapula are the supraspinal and infraspinal muscles. Beneath the tender area at the superior aspect of shoulder is the trapezius. Beneath the tender area at the medial aspect and inferior angle of scapula are the trapezius, the rhomboid muscle and the levator muscle of scapula. At the early stage of pathological changes there are only apparent tender areas, while at the late stage the tender areas may become widespread, assuming strip-like or a fanning-out tenderness. Thorough examination of tender locations and fine recording of the angle of movement range of shoulder joint in all directions are very important in treating periarthritis of shoulder and in appraising curative effects.

4. Changes in muscles: Stiffness of muscles, especially in the deltoid muscle, may be palpated on inspection; the brachial biceps tendon feels like a cord. Signs of amyotrophy appear at the shoulder-dorsal region at the late stage.

5. X-ray examination: The late stage shows osteoporosis at the humerus; calcification shadow in the soft tissues is seen in some patients. To prevent fracture, the strength of manual treatment in obvious osteoporosis should not be too heavy.

Treatment

Principles of manual treatment for this disease are promoting blood circulation, relieving pain and rigidity of muscles, separating adhesions, and activating meridians and collaterals.

1. Treatment in acute stage: Pain at this stage is severe and manipulation should be gentle.

47

a) Acupoint massage: Digitally press and knead acupoints Tianding (LI 17), Quepen (ST 12), Tianzong (SI 11), Jianyu (LI 15) and Jianjing (GB 21) 1-2 minutes each to relieve pain. (See Fig. 28)

b) With the patient in a sitting position, massage muscles around the shoulder by pressing, kneading and grasping. Muscles to be manipulated include the deltoid, the supraspinal, the infraspinal, the teres major and minor muscles, and the superior border of the trapezius. Or, with the patient in prone position, the massagist performs palm-pressing manipulations to relax the shoulder-dorsal muscles, including the trapezius, the rhomboid, the supraspinal, the infraspinal and the teres major and minor muscles.

c) Perform scrape-poking manipulation on the tender area: Use fairly strong scraping and flick-poking on the tender area with the thumb, stressing areas with cords and scleromata with pushing to dispel them. As a key procedure of the treatment this manipulation requires 20 minutes.

d) Pulling and traction of shoulder: The massagist presses the affected shoulder with one hand, holds the wrist of the affected side with other and exerts downward traction of the shoulder, then lifts the arm. Lifting the arm from the anterior side of the body is easy but difficult lifting it from the abduction position, so forced pulling should be avoided to prevent injuring the soft tissues and increasing pain.

e) Shaking manipulation: The massagist presses the affected shoulder with one hand and holds the wrist of the affected side with the other and performs loop-shaking of the upper arm, or shakes the shoulder by holding the wrist of the affected side with both hands to loosen the joint, accompanied by shaking the upper arm.

f) Squeezing the shoulder: The massagist places both hands at front and back

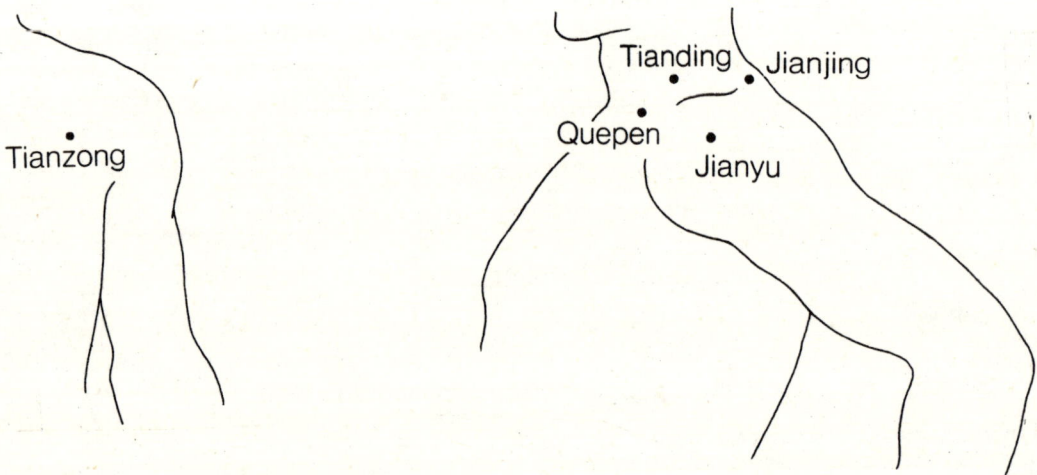

Fig. 28

of the affected shoulder respectively and squeezes the shoulder with palms facing each other to restore the tissues, then presses both hands on the shoulder-dorsal region to carry out scrubbing and foulage until the skin feels hot. Keep the shoulder-dorsal region warm after treatment.

2. Treatment in the chronic stage: Strong manipulations are often done to loose the joint and relax adhesion

a) Press acupoints Jianjing (GB 21), Jianyu (LI 15), Tianzong (SI 11), Quchi (LI 11), Qizhe (PC 3), Hegu (LI 4) and A Shi point.

b) Apply press-kneading manipulation to relax muscles of the shoulder-dorsal region.

c) Flick-poking and regulate-restoring manipulations: Apply flick-poking manipulation to restore shoulder-dorsal muscles. First flick-poke the brachial biceps tendon, the deltoid muscle, and the teres major and minor muscles; then flick-poke the supraspinal, the infraspinal and the trapezius muscles. To push and press along the direction of muscle fibres which have tendon is called regulate-restoring manipulation, of which there are six manipulating locations: the anterior aspect of shoulder (long head of biceps brachii), the lateral aspect of shoulder (for deltoid muscle, with stress on the central fibre), the posterior wall of armpit (the teres major and minor muscles), the superior aspect of shoulder (upper border of the trapezius muscle), the medial aspect and the inferior angle of scapula (the supraspinal, the infraspinal and the trapezius muscles). The force applied should be deep and penetrating so as to soften the stiffened muscles and separate adhesion. (See Fig. 29)

d) Traction manipulation: The massagist holds the elbow and lower arm of the affected side and tracts upward to lift the arm; hold for one minute before letting the upper arm down gently. Avoid sudden dropping of the arm so as not to cause pain to the shoulder. Inquire while pulling about the site where arm-lifting is impaired and perform repeated flick-poking and traction alternately at that site. (See Fig. 30)

e) Rotating manipulation: The massagist holds the patient's wrist and forearm firmly and rotates the upper arm to expand the movement range of the shoulder joint. This may be accompanied by shaking the shoulder to separate adhesion. The traction and rotating should be done gradually, avoiding abrupt exertion to avert fracture at the possibly decalcified humerus. (See Fig. 31)

f) Adduction and backward stretching of shoulder joint: The massagist presses the shoulder with one hand and holds the elbow of the affected side with the other for passive adduction of the shoulder by pushing the upper arm toward the central line, ensure traction of the dorsal muscles by trying to make the hand of the affected side reach the shoulder of the healthy side. In the same manner, stretch the shoulder backward, place the hand of the affected side at the back to try to make it reach the healthy side of the back. (See Fig. 32)

g) Shoulder pressing-foulage manipulation: The massagist holds the shoulder

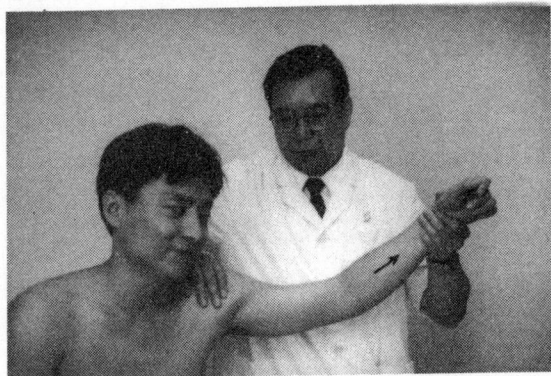

Fig. 29

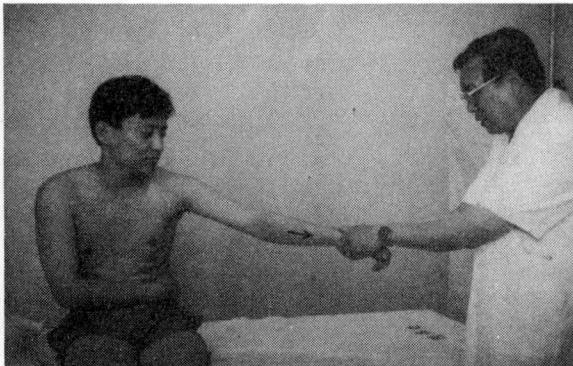

Fig. 30

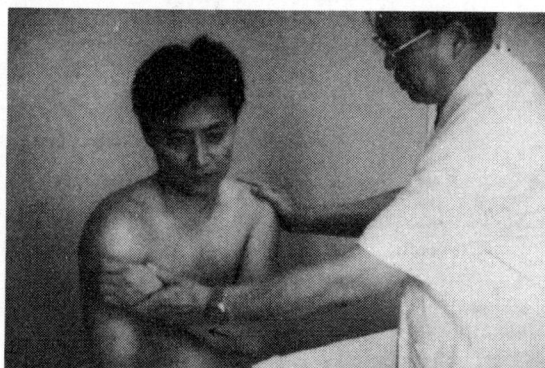

Fig. 31

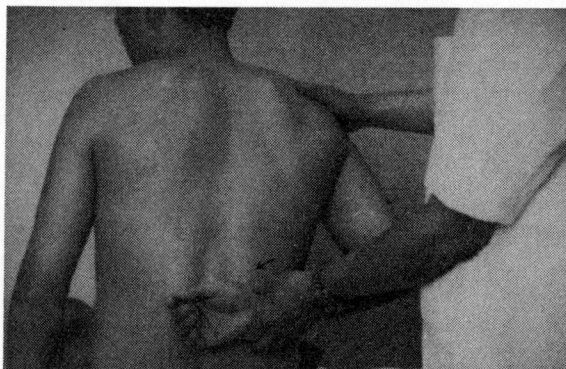

Fig. 32

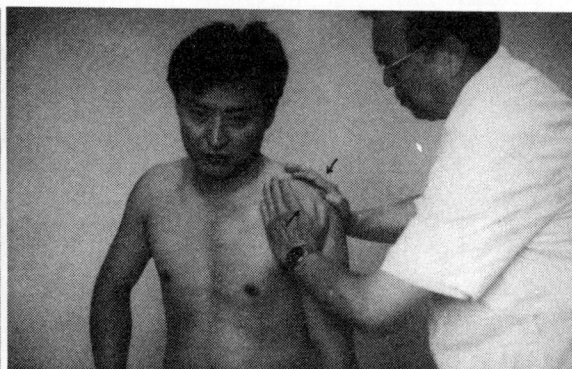

Fig. 33

with both hands and forcibly and repeatedly squeezes to restore shoulder tissues. Foulage-scrupling manipulation may also be applied to generate heat at the shoulder and upper arm. Keep shoulder warm after treatment or apply thermo-therapy. (See Fig. 33)

3. Functional exercises at restoration stage: Pinch-knead the affected shoulder and arm with the hand of the healthy side to first relax the muscles, then practise the following exercises:

a) Shoulder lifting: The patient stands facing a wall, with both hands climbing upward to raise the upper arms to the limit; or raise the affected side either with the hand of the healthy side or with this hand through a loop. The raising may start either from forward flexing position or from abduction position of the upper arm.

b) Behind-the-body hand shaking: Place both hands behind the back, carry the wrist of the affected side with the hand of the healthy side and perform traction of the wrist upward or downward the healthy side; and shake hands behind the head.

c) Inward and outward rotation of shoulder: Both hands make fists and flex elbows; adduct and outwardly flex the forearm to enable inward and outward rotation of shoulder.

d) Circling movement of shoulder: The patient bends forward with both upper arms hanging naturally to achieve traction of the shoulder by body weight and practises clockwise and counter-clockwise circling movement of the shoulder, swinging the upper arms to and fro.

Chapter 3
INJURY OF FOREARM AND UPPER ARM

1. Fracture of Humeral Shaft

Injury Mechanism

Fracture of humeral shaft is mainly caused by throwing. When practising throwing, due to the violent contraction of muscles, the throwing object produces a reacting force on the humerus and the strong torsional force exerted on the humerus causes oblique or spiral fracture of the humerus, with the location usually being at the junction of the medium and lower thirds. Because the radial nerve is located in the radial groove at the mid-section of the humerus, firmly linked with the humeral shaft by surrounding tissues, fracture at the middle and lower sections of the humerus is often complicated by radial nerve injury.

Symptoms and Diagnosis

1. The patient must have a history of trauma.

2. Acute pain and swelling in the upper arm and loss of function.

3. Malformation, abnormal movement and bone crepitation of upper arm.

4. When complicated by radial nerve injury, there may appear such symptoms as wrist dropping, inability to straighten metacarpophalangeal joints and dorsiflex and abduct the thumb, and slowing of sensation in the part of the hand between the thumb and index finger.

5. X-ray may enable a definite diagnosis and show the type of fracture and degree of displacement.

Treatment

1. Manual reduction: the massagist performs the following procedures:

a) Finger-pressing Tianding (LI 17), Quepen (ST 12), Zhongfu (LU 1) and Jiquan (HT 1) for 1-2 minutes each to relieve pain and cause numbness in the hand. (See Fig. 34)

b) Local Anaesthesia: If the effect of stopping pain by finger-pressing is not satisfactory, inject 10-20 ml. of 2 percent procaine into the fracture end and adjacent soft tissues.

c) With one assistant holding the shoulder of the affected side and another pulling the elbow and upper arm, the massagist re-positions the angulation deformity with both hands. For spiral fracture, the massagist must ascertain if the fracture is caused by inward or outward violent force. In re-positioning lateral rotation displacement, hold the distant limb and rotate in the opposite direction to the force. The manipulating force should be gentle in re-positioning the fracture,

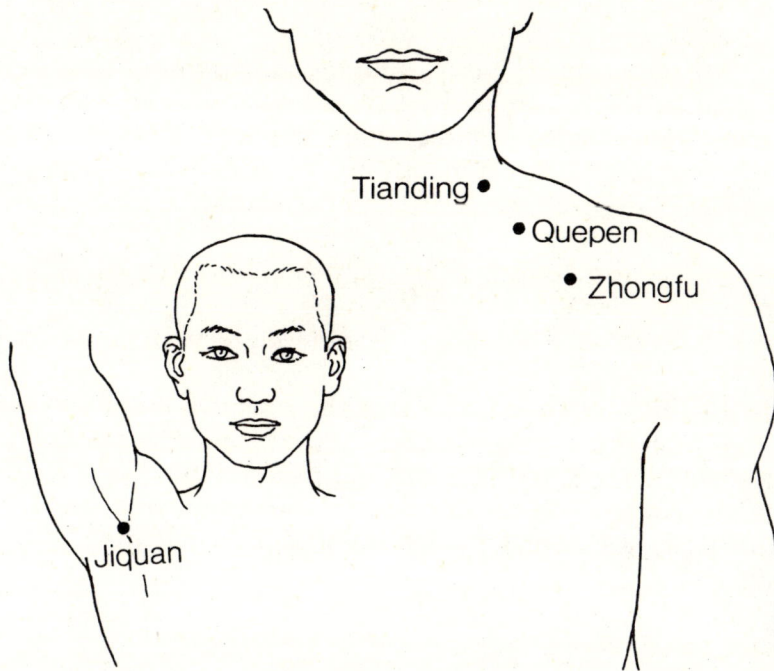

Fig. 34

then press the fracture end with the sensation of the hand. Avoid inverse bending method by all means in case the radial nerve may be injured.

2. Fixation: For fracture occurring at the lower one-third of the humerus, apply upper-arm over-the-elbow splint to fix. Place bone depressor at the fracture end. In order to prevent outward angulation displacement of the distant section due to inward adduction of limb caused by placing the forearm at the chest, three bone depressors need to be inserted in the splints at the medial and lateral aspects for strapping the upper arm. Four splints are required. The tightness of the ligature should be appropriate, as nerves and blood vessels would be pressed if too tight, while fracture displacement may occur if too loose. Appropriate tightness is achieved when strapping ligature moves within a margin of 1 cm. up and down when pulled by hand. Finally, suspend the strapping in front of the chest with elbow-flexion strapping for 6-8 weeks.

Functional Exercises

1. Early period: Start isotonic contraction of muscles of the affected limb the day after the reduction to speed union of the fracture; practise fist-making and palmar-extension movements to relax muscles and tendons and promote blood circulation. Avoid rotation movement of the upper arm to prevent recurrence of

fracture displacement.

2. Middle period: Begin to practise shoulder and elbow joint movement 2-3 weeks after injury.

a) Flexion and extension of elbow and shoulder joint. Hold the wrist of the affected side with hand of the healthy side for forward and backward motion of shoulder on the affected limb, then flex and extend elbow joint.

b) Raising both arms: Clasp the hands and use that of the healthy side to raise that of the affected side over the head, then make circling movements with both hands.

c) Massage the forearm and shoulder to prevent amyotrophy and adhesion with light and gentle force; avoid forced flexion and extension of joint.

3. Late period: Remove the splint strapping eight weeks after the fracture is united.

a) Massage the shoulder-dorsal region of the affected limb with punch-grasping manipulation; in case of scleromata and cords in the muscles, perform flick-poking manipulation to dispel them and regulate and restore the tissues. Assist the patient to expand the range of movement of shoulder and elbow joint.

b) The patient raises his arm to touch the head to make abduction and outward rotation of shoulder.

c) Practise throwing movement with the force gradually increased to promote the union of the fracture and increase muscle strength. However, attention should be made to avoid excessive rotation of the upper arm to prevent recurrence of fracture.

2. Supracondylar Fracture of Humerus

Supracondylar fracture of humerus is more often seen in teenagers, particularly in secondary school students and primary school pupils. The supracondylar portion is the weakest part of the humerus during childhood. The joint capsule of elbow and the accessory ligament are comparatively firm. So instead of elbow dislocation, supracondylar fracture is more likely in an elbow injury for teenagers.

Injury Mechanism

1. Indirect external force: Hitting the ground with hand when falling causes the elbow to bear the impact, hence the fracture. Most commonly seen is backward displacement of the distal end of the fracture, called fracture of the extension type.

2. Direct external force: The external force acts directly on the part directly to the back of the elbow, causing forward displacement of the distal end of fracture. This fairly rare type is called fracture of the flexion type.

Symptoms and Diagnosis

1. The patient has an obvious history of trauma and suffers from severe pain in the elbow and functional impairment.

2. Swelling and deformity of elbow: When the displacement caused by extension-

type supracondylar fracture of humerus is obvious, it looks similar to posterior dislocation of elbow joint. However, the post-elbow bone triangular relation of the former does not change, while that of the latter changes and, when moving the forearm, a sensation of bone fracture and abnormal activity may be felt and bone crepitation heard. Repeated forced test of bone friction sensation may aggravate tissue injury, so try to minimize movement of the upper limb.

3. Injury of blood vessels and nerves: The proximal fracture end may constrict or cause damage to the humeral artery and the median nerve in the cubital fossa, leading to weakening of pulse, dropping of skin temperature, cyanosis or paleness in skin colour, impairment of hand activity and slowness in feeling.

4. A definite diagnosis may be made by X-ray examination.

Treatment

The example cited here is supracondylar fracture of humerus of the extension type.

1. Strapping at elbow-flexed position. For incomplete fracture, apply elbow-flexion strapping with splint and triangular bandage wrapping for three weeks, then remove the strapping and resume elbow activity.

2. Manual reduction and strapping: If the fracture displacement is distinct, reduction and restoration are necessary.

a) Anaesthesia: Pressing acupoints Tianding (LI 17), Quepen (ST 12) and Jiquan (HT 1) to relieve pain, or use 2 percent procaine for local anaesthesia.

b) Manual reduction: Ask one assistant to hold the patient's upper arm and another to hold his wrist to effect slow traction along the direction of elbow malformation. To correct leftward or rightward displacement of the fracture end, the massagist presses and pushes both sides of the elbow hard with both hands. To correct forward or backward fracture displacement, the massagist pinches the proximal end of fracture to the front of the elbow with the four fingers of both hands and pushes the olecranon forward with both thumbs. While the assistants perform the traction and flex elbow slowly to a 90-degree position, the massagist should test whether the fracture is precisely reduced by hand sensation. If hand sensation cannot ascertain the degree of reduction, he should resort to roentgeno-scope or X-ray photograph for a satisfactory reduction. (See Fig. 35)

c) Splint fixation: Four splints are used. The splints for the lateral and medial aspects can extend beyond the elbow joint; the post-elbow splint should have a curvature to support the olecranon, and the ante-elbow splint should not be so long as to constrict the cubital fossa. To prevent lateral displacement of fracture, bone depressors need to be inserted at the lateral and medial aspects of the elbow in line with the direction of leftward or rightward fracture displacement. The tightness of strapping bandage should be moderate. Remove the splint after four weeks.

3. Attention should be paid to the following points in manual reduction and fixation:

a) The pulse of radial artery, motion of hand and sensation of skin must be

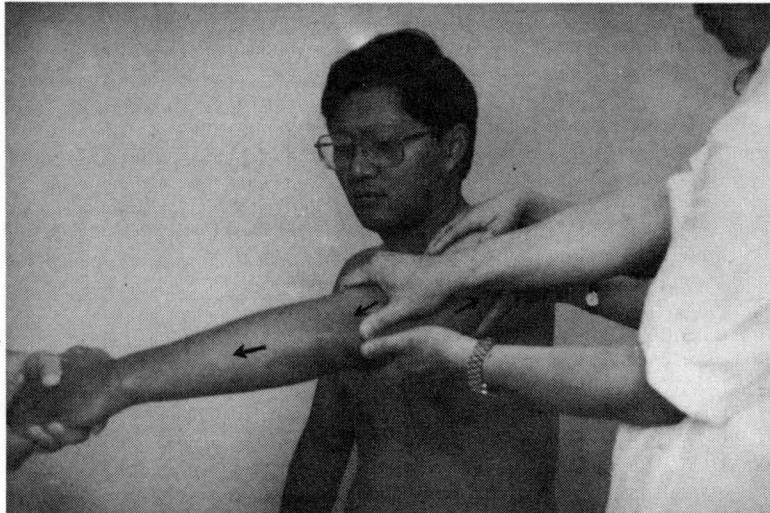

Fig. 35

examined before and after treatment. If the pulse of the radial artery is weak, the hand feels numb and painful and the skin feels cool and appears cyanotic after treatment, the elbow joint must be straightened from the flexed position or the strapping belt loosened. In case the symptoms persist, surgical examination of the radial artery is required. Long-term ischemia of limbs may cause ischemic spasm of forearm.

b) Prevent inversion of elbow: Inversion of elbow is the most commonly seen complication of supracondylar fracture of humerus.

c) Prevent eversion of elbow: If the fracture unites at eversion posture of elbow, the ulnar nerve is pulled at eversion position, thus causing ulnar neuritis.

Functional Exercises

1. In the first week, practise only extension and flexion of fingers and wrist, isotonic contraction of upper arm muscles and shoulder-lifting movements.

2. Practise various beginning functional exercises of shoulder joint one week later.

3. Practise flexion and extension movements of elbow joint after three weeks.

4. Remove splints after four weeks and practise elbow activity. Do not lift heavy objects with the affected side and avoid forced flexion and extension of elbow joint, as heavy manipulations may cause local hyperaemia or haematoma, which may lead to ossifying myositis of elbow and seriously hamper the functions of the elbow joint. Main manual treatment for rehabilitation is to massage the muscles of the fore and upper arm and help the patient with flexion and extension of the elbow joint with strength comfortable for the patient. In most cases elbow function can be restored to normal, but time is required.

3. Fracture of Lateral Epicondyle of Humerus and Epiphysiolysis

This disorder is more often seen in teenager athletes as well as secondary students and primary pupils.

Injury Mechanism

Fracture of lateral epicondyle of humerus is caused by indirect external force. When hitting the ground with the elbow joint slightly bent during a fall, the impact produced by the force will act on the lateral epicondyle along the radius, thus causing a fracture. The separated sclerites include parts of the lateral epicondyle, epiphysis of capitulum of humerus and trochlear epiphysis. If the fracture occurs only at the epiphysis of the capitulum of humerus, it is called epiphysiolysis of capitellum. The extensor muscle group of forearm adheres to the lateral epicondyle of humerus, so the sclerites may be displaced due to traction by the extensor muscle group after fracture. According to the degree of displacement, the fracture may be of a non-displacement type, lateral displacement, or eversion displacement fracture.

Symptoms and Diagnosis

1. There are swelling and pain at the lateral aspect of elbow and motor impairment and the joint is in semi-flexed position after the trauma.

2. There is tenderness on pressure at the lateral epicondyle of humerus and moving sclerites may be palpated locally.

3. X-ray examination can help make a definite diagnosis and show the situation of fracture displacement.

Treatment

1. Non-displacement fracture: Apply suspensory bandage strapping to the upper limb for 2-3 weeks.

2. Manual reduction: Manual reduction is necessary in case of displacement.

a) Anaesthesia: Use 2 percent procaine for local anaesthesia.

b) For serious swelling of the elbow, apply repeated push-pressing from the centre of the swelling to all directions with the thumb for detumescence. The force should be gentle so as not to aggravate the pain. Relieving swelling may help in palpating the fracture and reducing it.

c) The massagist holds the wrist of the affected arm to set the elbow in a slightly bent position with the forearm flat, pushing the sclerites backward hard and reducing the everted sclerites with the thumb and index finger.

d) Make the elbow flex so as to enable the sclerites contact the proximal fracture face, push and press the sclerites inward and upward to close the fracture faces.

e) Push and press the sclerites with the thumb and straighten the elbow joint gradually.

3. Fixation: Place bone depressors at the lateral condyle and the upper border of the medial epicondyle of humerus respectively; strap with four splints protrud-

ing beyond the elbow for three weeks. (See Fig. 36)

Functional Exercises

1. Practise shoulder and finger movements, mild finger- and wrist-extension movements in the first week to relax the traction by the extensor muscle group on the sclerites. From the second week, practise gradual flexion and extension movements of elbow and forceful extension of wrist.

2. Remove the strapping after three weeks and practise flexion and extension movements of elbow, adding pronation and supination of the forearm. Perform massage on the forearm, with stress on the extensor, to relax the tightened muscles and help the affected elbow to expand the range of movement.

4. Fracture of Medial Epicondyle of Humerus and Epiphysiolysis

This injury is mostly seen in teenager athletes, secondary school students and primary pupils as well as gymnasts.

Injury Mechanism

When falling with the elbow straight and the hand hitting the ground, the external force may cause violent eversion of the elbow joint, violent contraction of the flexor group of forearm, avulsion of the medial epicondyle of humerus and anterointerior displacement of bone fragments due to the traction by muscles, and even the complication of elbow joint dislocation. In light of degree of displacement of bone fragments or the epiphysis, this disorder may fall into four types: (a) Mere fracture or epiphysiolysis, with slight displacement of fractured bone fragments; (b) displacement of fractured bone fragments; (c) displacement of fractured bone

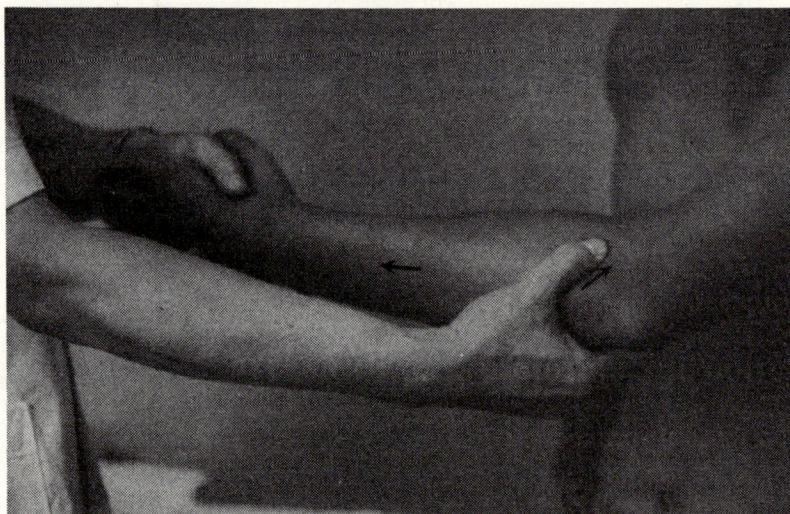

Fig. 36

fragments into the articular cavity complicated by subluxation of joint; and (d) fracture complicated by elbow joint dislocation, which is rare.

Symptoms and Diagnosis

1. Swelling and pain at the medial aspect of elbow after trauma.

2. Apparent pressure tenderness at the medial humeral epicondyle, while moving sclerites and bone friction can be felt.

3. Motor impairment of elbow joint.

4. X-ray examination can produce a definite diagnosis and confirm the degree of fracture displacement.

Treatment

1. Manual reduction:

a) Anaesthesia: Use 2 percent procaine for local anaesthesia.

b) With regard to types (a) and (b), that is, fracture or epiphysiolysis with slight displacement of fractured bone fragments, and displacement of fractured bone fragments, first flex the affected elbow at a 90-degree position, pronate the forearm and flex the wrist to relax the flexor group and pronator of forearm; push and press the fractured bone upwards with the thumb; and place a bone depressor pad at the medial epicondyle of humerus and strap with small splints extending beyond the elbow.

c) For type (c), that is, displacement of fractured bone fragments into the articular cavity complicated by subluxation of joint, straighten the affected elbow and forcefully abduct the elbow to increase the medial space of joint, supinate the forearm and forcefully extend the wrist and fingers, and pull the sclerite out of the joint using the pulling force of the flexor of the forearm. If the sclerite still cannot be pulled out, feel out the border of the sclerite with the thumb and prize it out with a thick needle. If the border of the sclerite cannot be palpated clearly, prize and pluck it out with the help of a roentgenoscope. Having the fractured sclerite pulled out from the articular cavity, continue the treatment using the procedure for displacement of fractured bone fragments.

d) For type (d), that is, fracture complicated by elbow joint dislocation, ask an assistant to perform traction of the elbow joint, supinates the forearm and keep the wrist and fingers extended so as to help the flexor of the forearm maintain tension and prevent the medial epicondyle from being incarcerated into the articular cavity, while the massagist pushes the humerus outward with one hand and pulls the radius and ulna inward with the other to reduce the joint. Then, continue the treatment as for the displacement of fractured bone fragments.

2. Duration of fracture fixation: Three weeks for types (a) and (b), and four weeks for types (c) and (d) since there is widespread tearing of soft tissue.

Functional Exercises

During the first week avoid rotation of the forearm as well as flexion and extension of the wrist in case the fractured bone may displace; begin practising shoulder and wrist movements after one week and gradual elbow flexion after two weeks. Start doing exercises of flexion and extension of elbow and rotation of forearm after the strapping is removed.

Elbow functions may be restored to normal in most patients. In the process, massage treatment should be continued by pressing and kneading the muscle groups of the upper arm and forearm so as to make them relaxed. To prevent ossifying myositis of joint, avoid forceful flexion and extension of the elbow.

5. Dislocation of Elbow Joint

Injury Mechanism

1. Posterior dislocation of elbow joint: When falling, the upper arm abducts with the palm hitting the ground. The external force transmits along the ulna upwards to fix the elbow joint in overextended position and makes the olecranal end of ulna the fulcrum in the olecranon, and eventually the semilunar incisure separates from the humeral trochlear and displaces in a backward position. As a result, both the ulna and the small head of the radius slip in the posterosuperior direction, forming posterior dislocation of elbow joint. The elbow articular capsule, the collateral ligaments, the periosteum and muscular tendons are all injured to different degrees.

2. Dislocation complicated by fracture: In posterolateral dislocation of elbow joint due to external force, fracture may occur at the medial epicondyle of humerus, which is the type (d) of fracture of medial epicondyle of humerus, discussed in the previous section. Sometimes, the coracoid process of ulna may collide with the humerus trochlear, causing fracture of the coracoid process of ulna or injury of humeral cartilage.

3. Anterior dislocation of elbow joint: Impact of external force on the posterior aspect of elbow may cause the ulnar olecranon to move to the front aspect of the elbow. This type of dislocation is rare.

Symptoms and Diagnosis

1. Severe pain, swelling in elbow and loss of function.

2. Obvious malformation of elbow and loss of the post-elbow triangular bony relation (normally, the medial and lateral epicondyles and the olecranon form an isosceles triangle when flexing the elbow and the three bony processes form a straight line when extending the elbow).

3. The forearm appears to be shorter than normal and firth of the elbow joint turns thick, the lower border of humerus may be felt at the anterior side of elbow while the dislocated ulnar olecranon may be felt at the posterior side.

4. X-ray photograph may produce a definite diagnosis, show the degree of displacement and reveal if there is fracture.

Treatment

1. Anaesthesia

a) Acupressure point anaesthesia: Press acupoints Quepen (ST 12) and Jiquan (HT 1) for 1-2 minutes each. (See Fig. 37)

b) Local anaesthesia: Inject 4 ml. of 2 percent procaine into the articulation and 8-10 ml. into the peripheral tissues of the articulation.

c) Brachial plexus anaesthesia: To be used in serious injury or when the methods recommended above are not effective.

2. Manual reduction

a) With an assistant performing traction of the upper arm, the massagist holds the wrist on the affected side and performs traction along the original trend of malformation with one hand, and pushes and presses the lower end of the humerus backward at the anterior aspect of the elbow with the thumb of the other hand, and pulls the olecranon forward from the rear of the elbow with the other four fingers. A click heard indicates success of the reduction.

b) Traction by two assistants: The traction should be performed along the original trend of malformation and not with the elbow joint in extended position because when the elbow joint in an extended position the coracoid process of ulna is in the olecranon fossa and the joint cannot be separated however strong the force may be. Traction by two assistants is more effective. The massagist may press and push the humerus and the ulna with both hands from the anterior and posterior aspects of the elbow respectively. After the reduction, the pain should be relieved, the joint should be able to flex and extend, and the bony triangular relation should resume. (See Fig. 38)

The strength used for manual reduction should not be too strong so as not to aggravate the injury of the elbow soft tissues.

Example: Miss Ren, gymnast, fell from the uneven bar during a national championship with the right hand hitting the ground, causing posterior dislocation of the right elbow. The massagist first pressed Quepen (ST 12) and Jiquan (HT 1) to relieve pain. Then, with two assistants performing traction along the trend of the dislocation, the massagist succeeded in reducing the elbow joint with only one treatment. A follow-up visit half a year later showed no undesirable sequelae.

3. Fixation: In order to prevent local edema and exudate, it is necessary to reduce the elbow temperature, and a simple way to do this is with cold running water, then apply pressure dressing with thick cotton pads and strap with suspensory triangular bandage. If blood circulation and nerve sensation of the hand are normal after treatment, the pressure dressing can be removed after two days while keeping the triangular bandage in place.

Functional Exercises and Rehabilitation Treatment

1. Practise isometric contraction of muscles of the upper arm and forearm, flexion and extension of wrist, fist making and palmar extension as well as shoulder movement the day after the reduction treatment.

2. Press and grasp the distal end of shoulder and forearm to promote blood circulation and prevent atrophy and stiffness of muscles. Soft tissues around the

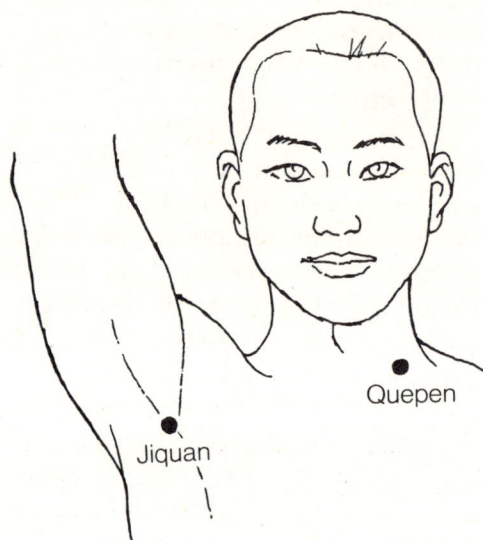

Fig. 37

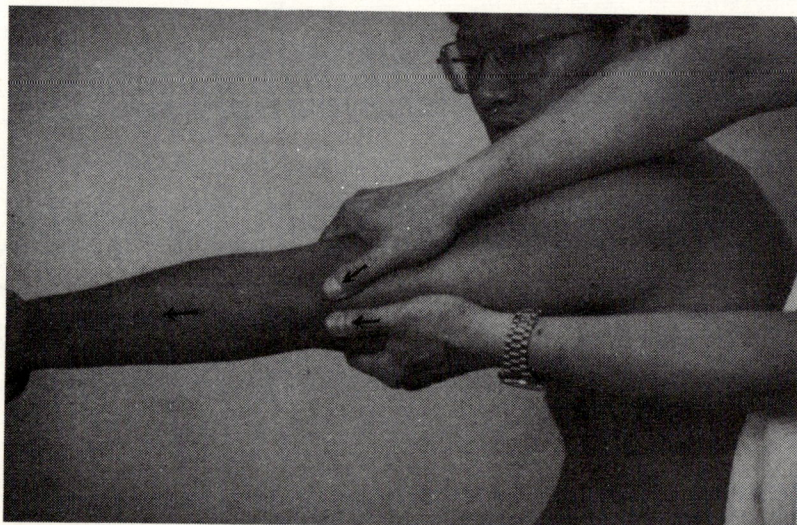

Fig. 38

elbow should not be massaged.

3. Remove the strapping after three weeks, and the patient may practise appropriate flexion and extension of elbow joint. Massage Quchi (LI 11), Chizhe (LU 5), Quzhe (PC 3), Shaohai (HT 3) and Jianyu (LI 15) to stimulate blood circulation and relax muscles and tendons. Massage forearm and upper arm muscle groups along with flexion and extension of elbow joint.

Initial exercise and manual rehabilitation usually restore elbow functions in most patients. However, forced flexion and extension of elbow joint or heavy massage around the elbow are forbidden in manual treatment. Otherwise, swelling may occur again in the elbow in a light case which may even lead to, in a serious case, anconal myositis ossificans which may seriously hamper the joint functions and cause the patient unnecessary pain.

6. Subluxation of Capitulum Radii

This disorder mostly happens in children under six years old and in such juvenile athletes as gymnasts.

Injury Mechanism

1. Pulling of forearm. The caput radii of young children is not fully developed, and the caput and neck of caput radii are almost equal, while the annular ligament is rather flaccid. So, when pulled by external force, the caput radii is liable to slip downward from the annular ligament or be incarcerated in the folds of the annular ligament and cannot reduce spontaneously, causing subluxation. Subluxation of this type is fairly common.

2. For juvenile athletes, especially gymnasts, due to long-term support with the elbow, the range of movement of capitulum radii is enlarged and the annual ligament is relatively flaccid, so sudden pulling of the elbow or supporting and rotating movements with the elbow may cause subluxation of capitulum radii.

Symptoms and Diagnosis

1. The elbow is painful and cannot be moved freely when it is pulled and rotated.

2. With the elbow joint in semi-flexed position, the forearm can pronate but not supinate, and the hand cannot be raised.

3. There is no apparent local swelling and the appearance looks normal; there is tenderness on pressure at the capitulum radii; transverse cords or thickening may be palpated.

4. The patient feels weakness of the elbow, slight pain when rotating the forearm, and movements of elbow are affected.

Treatment

1. Digitally press acupoints Quchi (LI 11). (See Fig. 39)

2. The massagist holds the affected wrist, tracts downward and rotates the forearm repeatedly with one hand while pressing and pushing the capitulum radii

with the thumb of the other. When a snap is heard, the pain disappears immediately and elbow activity returns to normal. No fixation is needed.

3. Perform soft and gentle flick-plucking manipulation at the external aspect of elbow for restoring the soft tissues. (See Fig. 40)

7. Olecranal Fracture

Injury Mechanism

1. Fracture caused by indirect external force: This is the type most often seen. Under the olecranon is the end-point of the brachial triceps muscle, violent contraction of which may cause avulsion fracture of the olecranon and upward displacement of fractured bone. Hitting the ground with the palm during a falling results in contraction of the brachial triceps muscle and extension of elbow because of the effect of body weight. This may also cause olecranal fracture.

2. Fracture caused by direct external force: Touching the ground with elbow directly produces impact on the ulnar olecranon, thus causing fracture that is often comminuted and without obvious displacement.

Symptoms and Diagnosis

1. Swelling, pain and tenderness occur at the ulnar olecranon posterior to the elbow joint; in case of local haemorrhage, subcutaneous cyst may be felt at the back of the elbow.

2. Extension of elbow joint is affected.

3. Fracture space may be felt at the olecranon.

4. X-ray may produce a definite diagnosis. But the incomplete union of olecranal epiphysis of teenagers should not be diagnosed as olecranal fracture, rather the

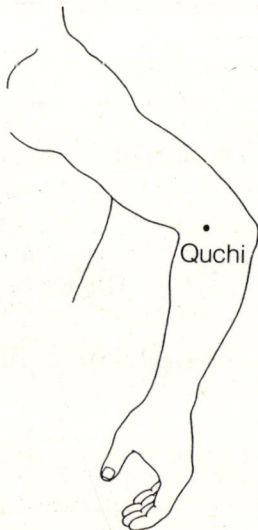

Fig. 39

Quchi

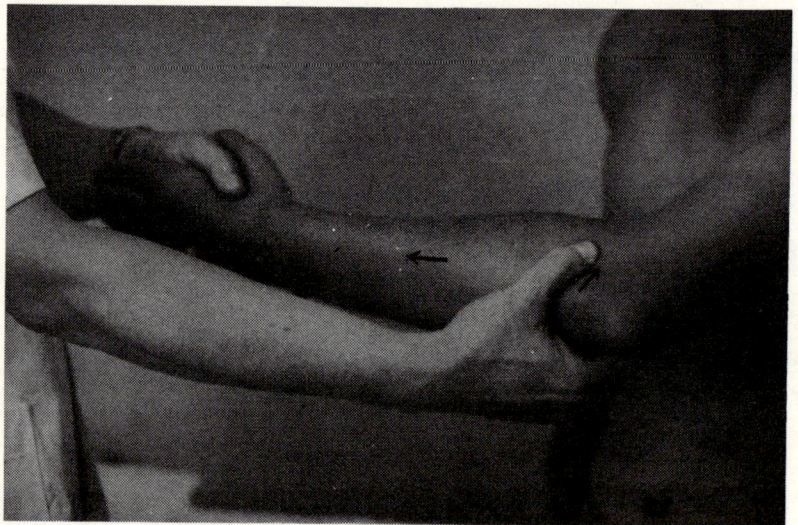

Fig. 40

olecranon of the healthy side should be X-rayed, if necessary, for comparison.

Treatment

1. Strap with triangular bandage for 2-3 weeks for fracture without displacement.

2. Manual reduction should be performed for fracture with displacement.

a) Press acupoints Quepen (ST 12) and Jiquan (HT 1) for acupoint anaesthesia or use 2 percent procaine for local anaesthesia.

b) While asking the patient to hold the elbow joint straight out, the massagist pushes the fractured bone downward with the thumb and the index finger to reduce it toward the proximal end of the bone. In case of obvious swelling at the rear aspect of the elbow, first perform gentle pushing manipulation toward the periphery for detumescence to attain a better hand sensation and better reduction. For most patients, a desirable reduction can be expected. After reduction, flex the elbow joint to 20 degrees, i.e., at the semi-extended position, and strap the ulnar olecranon region with a round or crescent bone-rejoining pad to prevent recurrence of displacement of the fractured bone. Then strap by placing splints at the front and rear aspects of the elbow, with the one at the rear aspect protruding beyond the elbow. Long-arm plastic support, which better conforms to the configuration of the posterior aspect of elbow, may be used. Either method should last for three weeks.

Functional Exercises

Practise fist-making, palmar flexion and shoulder activity after reduction. After the removal of strapping three weeks later, practise active exercises of elbow joint, massage muscles of the upper arm and forearm to avoid adhesion and atrophy of muscles.

8. Fracture of Capitulum Radii

This disorder is liable to be misdiagnosed, and if not given timely treatment, patients could suffer from impairment of the rotating function of arm after a malformed union of the fracture.

Injury Mechanism

Hitting the ground with the palm when the elbow joint is extended and forearm pronates during falling may result in upward conduction of the violent force and cause the capitulum radii to impact on the capitulum of humerus, thus resulting in fracture of the capitulum radii. This fracture may be divided into the following types:

a) Fracture of the neck of radius or epiphysiolysis: The capitulum radii displaces laterally, usually assuming the appearance of "having a cap on askew."

b) Fissured fracture (with cracks on the bone).

c) Compression fracture or impacted fracture.

d) Comminuted fracture.

Symptoms and Diagnosis

1. The patient must have a history of trauma.

2. Obvious swelling and tenderness at the lower aspect of elbow; the displaced fracture end may be palpated. For diagnosis, a comparison can be made with the unaffected elbow.

3. Impairment of rotation of forearm; pain while trying to rotate it. The pain will be particularly sharp when the forearm is supinated.

4. X-ray examination produces a definite diagnosis. The upper leg of the radius may be X-rayed, if necessary, with the forearm in pronated or supinated position.

Treatment

1. Acupoint pressing: Press acupoints Quepen (ST 12), Jianyu (LI 15), Binao (LI 14) and Quchi (LI 11). Be sure to avoid strong pressing and pushing on the capitulum radii when pressing Quchi (LI 11). (See Fig. 41)

2. For a patient without obvious fracture displacement, the massagist carries the wrist with one hand and gently regulates and restores the soft tissues of the capitulum radii along the longitudinal axis with the other, then applies triangular bandage strapping.

3. For a patient with obvious fracture displacement, ask one assistant to hold the patient's upper arm and another to hold the wrist to exert traction, repeated rotation of the forearm to set the elbow joint at adduction position so as to widen the external space of articulation, while the massagist pushes and squeezes the displaced capitulum radii toward the medial aspect. In most cases the fracture can be reduced.

In case the reduction is not satisfactory, insert a thick syringe needle or Kirschner pin into the skin to correct the posture of the inclined bone fragment (this called the needle-poking method), then apply strapping with bandage or forearm plastic support for 3-4 weeks.

Functional Exercises

Start hand activity as early as possible and stop rotation movement of forearm for two weeks. Begin to practise flexion and extension of elbow joint and rotation of the forearm when strapping is removed after three weeks. Exercises of supporting movement can start after 1-2 months.

9. Osteochondral Injury of Capitellum

Injury Mechanism

During rotation of forearm and forced supporting movement of elbow, mutual collision between the capitulum radii and the capitulum of humerus, either one strong collision or repeated collisions, may cause osteochondral fracture of the capitellum. Fragments of bone and cartilage from bone fracture, osteochondral

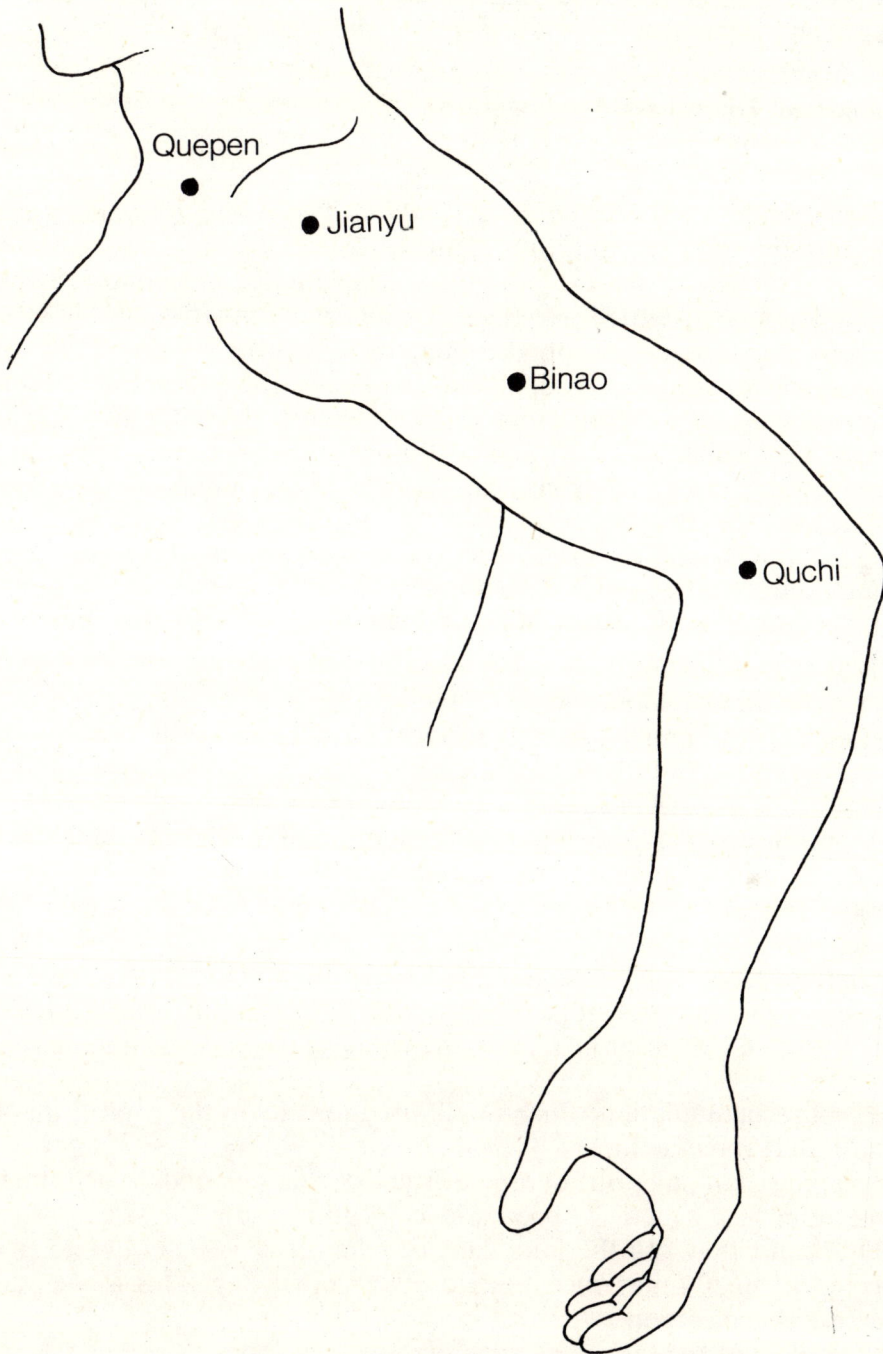

Fig. 41

fracture or avulsion osteochondritis may enter the articulation and form joint bodies; hyperplasia of new bone appears at the fractured surface of bone, causing osteoarthropathy.

Symptoms and Diagnosis

1. The patient has a medical history of acute trauma or of chronic strain of elbow.

2. Local tenderness, swelling and synovial hypertrophy of elbow occur at the capitulum radii and the capitulum of humerus.

3. Pain when flexing and extending the elbow joint. The pain is less serious when doing supporting movement. Extension of elbow is hindered, and in a serious case locked joint appears and joint bodies may be felt at the border of the articulation.

4. X-ray examination: No particular changes will be found at the initial stage. However, it must be differentiated from traumatic synovitis at this stage. At the late stage, the surface of capitulum of humerus becomes rough, or there appears damage or defect; free bodies may be found in the articulation, the articular space changes little, and this needs to be differentiated from bone joint tuberculosis which is characterized by the symptoms of swelling in the joint, thickening of synovium, amyotrophy assuming rhombic swelling; the festered abscess forms a fistula; damage of substance of bone and narrowing of articular space can be seen.

Treatment

Manual treatment alone is not directly effective. However, it can dilate the capillaries, improve nutrient supply to local muscles and skin, prevent amyotrophy and promote recovery of cartilage tissues.

1. Treatment at early stage:

a) As this disorder shows no particular symptoms at the early stage, it is difficult to make a correct diagnose. When initial symptoms manifest at the elbow region, the patient should cut the frequency of supporting or rotating movements with the upper limbs.

b) Digitally press acupoints Jianyu (LI 15), Binao (LI 14) and Quchi (LI 11).

c) Press-knead and flick-poke the arm biceps muscle, the brachial triceps muscle and the flexor and extensor groups of the forearm to relax the muscles at the elbow region.

d) Pushing manipulation: Push in all directions from the capitulum of humerus to reduce local tumefaction.

e) Scraping manipulation: Scrape at the external epicondyle of humerus, capitulum of humerus, articular space and capitulum radii by turn to stimulate the lateral bone of elbow and the joint capsule; the force used should go from light to strong; repeat 10-20 times once a day or every other day. This is the main method for treating this disorder.

2. Treatment at the late stage with obvious symptoms:

a) Stop training involving supporting and rotation movements with elbow. If X-ray examination reveals changes in the bone substance, triangular-bandage or plastic supporting strapping should be applied for 6-8 weeks for short-term strapping will not help repair the cartilage. When X-ray photograph shows improvement of the situation, remove the strapping and practise strength exercises of elbow joint.

b) The strapping can be removed from time to time for flexion and extension of elbow joint and massage treatment of muscles of the upper limbs to prevent stiffness of joint and atrophy of muscles.

c) Manual treatment is the same as for disorders at the early stage.

3. Manual reduction for locked joint:

a) Press acupoints Binao (LI 14) and Quchi (LI 11).

b) Asking one assistant to hold the patient's upper arm with the elbow slightly bent, the massagist tracts the wrist and rotates the forearm with one hand while feeling out the borders of free bodies and press-pushing them into the joint with the thumb and index finger of the other hand. If the press-pushing fails to reposition them, set the elbow joint at adduction position to widen the lateral articular space and press-push the free bodies again. If the free bodies lie at the medial aspect of elbow, set the elbow at eversion position to widen the medial articular space and press-push again. If the free bodies lies posterior or anterior to the elbow, extend or semi-flex the elbow while performing traction of the articular joint and press-push the free bodies. If the borders of the free bodies are not clearly felt, they should be felt out by pressing the tender spot. Once the free bodies are re-positioned, the locked joint will be released, the pain relieved and the flexion and extension of the elbow return to normal.

c) Gently press along the joint space to regulate and restore the joint capsule and peripheral soft tissues.

d) For repeated recurrence of locked joint, surgical excision of the free bodies in joint is necessary.

Example: Miss Xu, 16 years old, was a gymnast. She suffered from osteochondritis in both elbows accompanied by free bodies in joint and locked joint. Through manual treatment, she was able to take part in training and competitions. However, because of repeated locked joint, surgical excision was finally resorted to.

10. Tennis Elbow

A frequently occurring disorder, tennis elbow is also called external humeral epicondylitis, humeroradial articulation synovitis and syndrome of external epicondyle of humerus. Aside from often being seen in players of badminton, tennis, table tennis and fencing, it is also common in workers who repeatedly rotate the forearm, such as in tilers, fitters, cooks and massagists.

Injury Mechanism

1. Attached to the external epicondyle of humerus are the extensor carpi muscle and the extensor of fingers. Contraction and pulling of these muscles can cause

stress on the general extensor tendon, and excessive contraction and pulling of these muscles may injure it and even other structures such as the humeroradial articular synovium and the annular ligament.

2. Repeated strenuous contraction and pulling of extensor muscle groups caused by repeated flexion and extension of wrist and pronation and supination of forearm may lead to pathological changes in the external epicondyle of humerus itself and the surrounding tissues.

3. Local myospasm may constrict the nerve and blood vessel tracts and cause pain.

4. Local symptoms may arise from the unstable position of the capitulum radii due to synovial incarceration of elbow joint and flaccidity of annular ligament.

Symptoms and Diagnosis

1. Slow onset, and pain at the lateral aspect of elbow joint which possibly radiates to the lateral aspect of forearm.

2. Weakness in grasping things, easy dropping of things, and pain which is particularly serious when making a fist or wringing out a towel.

3. Tender area: Mainly at the dorsum of the external epicondyle of humerus, posterior aspect of the humeroradial articulation, the capitulum radii or the dorsal aspect of the neck of radius. There may be tissue thickening.

4. Extensor tendon-traction test: Flex the elbow, wrist and fingers, then pronate the forearm and extend the elbow. Pain will felt at the external epicondyle of humerus. Resistive test: Pain may also be felt when straightening the elbow, pronating the forearm and flexing the dorsal aspect of the wrist.

Treatment

1. Press acupoints Quepen (ST 12), Zhongji (RN 3), Quchi (LI 11), Chize (LU 15) and Shaohai (HT 3). (See Fig. 42)

2. Making the patient to sit, the massagist holds the patient's wrist with one hand and performs petrissage with the other, using palm-rubbing and grasping from the middle part of the upper arm downward along the elbow to relax the muscles and activate the meridians and collaterals. (See Fig. 43)

3. The massagist holds the patient's elbow with one hand, holds the wrist with the other and does flexion and extension movements of elbow, followed by over-flexion and over-extension movements of the elbow to 5-10 times to relax the elbow joint.

4. With the elbow and wrist of the affected limb flexing and the forearm pronating, the massagist straightens the elbow joint with force, i.e., performs extensor tendon-traction test 5-10 times. The force applied for elbow extension should not be too strong so as not to exacerbate the pathological changes.

5. Tender spot manipulation: Perform heavy scraping at the external joint space of elbow of the external epicondyle of humerus, capitulum radii, the neck of radius and areas with apparent tender on pressure, then flick-poke these spots with the thumb for five times. This is the main method of manual treatment for this

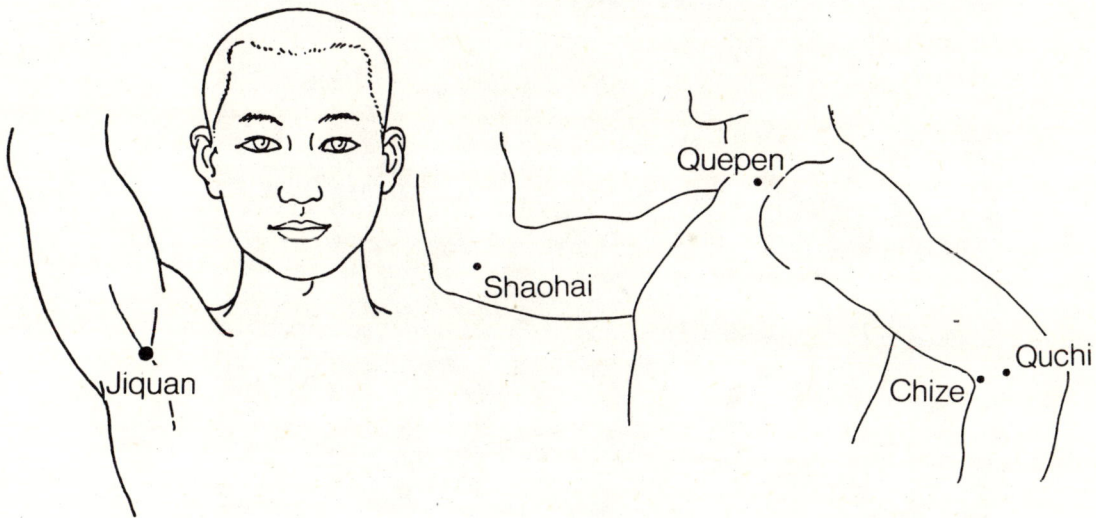

Fig. 42

disorder. In some patients the symptoms become worse and this is only a reaction to the manual treatment. In such a situation, the treatment should be temporarily stop and resume one or two days later. The patients should stop strenuous elbow movement and rotation of forearm, and use hot compress or hot bath to help eliminate the inflammation.

11. Injury of Collateral Ulnar Ligament of Elbow Joint

Among the tissues inside the elbow are joint capsule, synovium, collateral ulnar ligament, common flexor tendons and round pronator muscle of forearm as well as the internal epicondyle of humerus. For all the tissues inside the elbow, injury of the ulnar ligament is the most important.

Injury Mechanism

1. Acute injury: Sudden abduction of elbow joint, as in javelin throwing, may cause pulling of soft tissues of the internal aspect of elbow. Injury of the collateral ligament may be divided into partial laceration of fibrae, incomplete rupture and complete rupture.

2. Sudden violent contraction of flexor and round pronator muscle of forearm produces a strong impact on the common muscular tendons, thus causes injury to their points of attachment.

3. Chronic strain: Repeated pulling or medial aspect of elbow, as in crucifix in the rings, javelin throwing and soft spiking in volleyball, may gradually result in flaccidity of the medial joint capsule of elbow and of the medial collateral ligament.

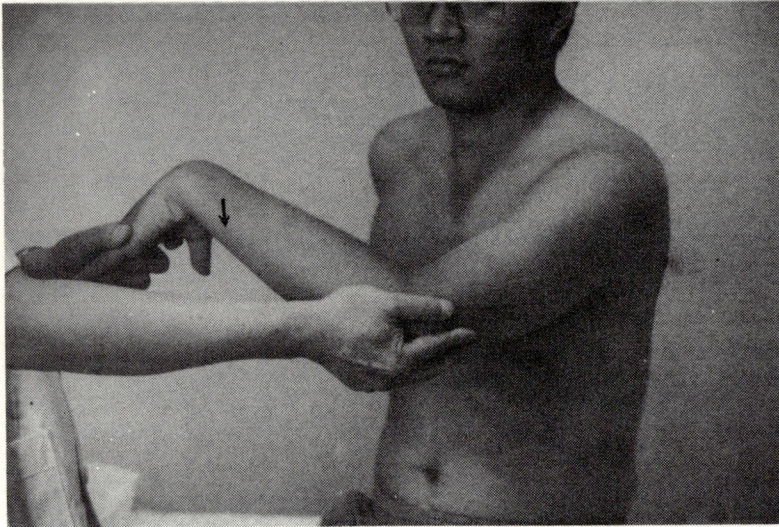

Fig. 43

At the advanced stage, such pathological changes as calcification of soft tissues and hyperplasia of medial epicondyle of humerus may occur.

Symptoms and Diagnosis

1. Acute injury: Pain, swelling and local tenderness on pressure after sudden abduction of the elbow joint. Tender spot often occurs at the joint space and may be aggravated by eversion of elbow. Lateral pulling of elbow joint may enlarge the medial joint space and an "opening" may be felt , indicating complete rupture of the medial collateral ligament. Flexion and extension of the elbow joint are hindered.

2. Chronic strain: The elbow feels week and painful, the pain radiates to the medial aspect of forearm with local tenderness; medial tissues of the joint are swollen and thickened.

3. Resistive pain is felt when flexing the wrist and pronating the forearm. Over-extension test of elbow and wrist is positive: Straightening the affected elbow and over-extending the wrist joint pull the common tendon of flexor, thus causing pain at the medial aspect of elbow.

Treatment

1. Press acupoints Jiquan (HT 1), Shaohai (HT 3) and Quchi LI 11). (See Fig. 44)

2. Acute injury: For a case of incomplete rupture of the medial collateral ligament, first press-knead the flexor group of the forearm and the upper arm to relax the muscles, then push-press the medial aspect of the elbow joint to regulate and restore the disordered ligament fibrae and reposition the articular synovium. The manipulation should not be too strong. For a light case, first use strapping for

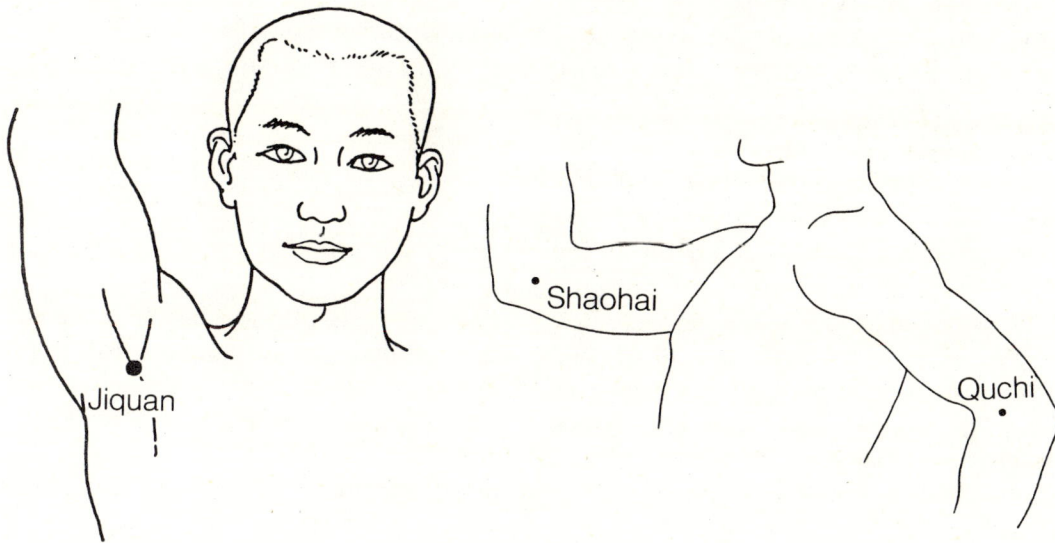

Fig. 44

three days, then practise flexion and extension of elbow joint. For a serious case, apply pressure dressing for two days to prevent exudate, then replace the pressure dressing with triangular bandage for a week. For complete rupture of ligament, surgical suturing is needed.

3. Chronic strain: First press-knead the flexor group of upper arm and forearm to relax the muscles with gentle manipulation; at the same time flex and extend passively the wrist joint to relax the tense and spasmodic flexor group of wrist. Then perform flick-poking at tender spots around the medial epicondyle of humerus and the medial joint space of elbow, then along the ulnar flexor of wrist for 5-10 times. Regulate and restore the above muscles and tissues along the longitudinal axis of the upper limb. This manipulation is the key method for treating chronic strain. Also, perform foulage and scrubbing manipulations at the elbow and forearm until a sensation of heat runs deep to promote blood circulation and disperse blood stasis.

12. Anconal Traumatic Synovitis

Anconal traumatic synovitis may be caused by any type of elbow injury.

Injury Mechanism

1. Acute injury: May be caused by sudden over-flexion and over-extension of elbow joint, strenuous supporting movement, impact on the bone, squeezing of synovium and incarceration of synovium in the joint. Other acute elbow injuries may also be complicated by acute traumatic synovitis. Hyperaemia, edema and exudation at the diseased synovium may cause tumefaction and hydropsy in the joint.

73

2. Chronic injury: Caused by elbow movement with overload and repeated friction and squeezing of the synovium by the joint. Osteoarthropathy, due to repeated stimulation by spur, may also occur along with traumatic synovitis.

Symptoms and Diagnosis

1. Acute injury: pain in elbow, restriction of elbow joint movement, elbow being locked in a semi-flexed position and serious pain when flexing or extending the elbow.

2. Tender area: Most occurring at the posterior and lateral aspects of elbow, tender area helps define the whereabouts of the injury.

3. Hydrarthrosis: In acute period, sudden hydrarthrosis may occur, which may disappear when local pushing and pressing is performed and whose location may change with the change of body postures. It is necessary to differentiate it from edema in the peripheral soft tissues of elbow, whose location does not change when body posture changes. In some cases of chronic synovitis there may be no hydropsy, which occurs only along with increase of elbow work and will diminish after rest.

4. Thickening of synovium: Unlike normal synovium, an inflamed synovium feels thickened, especially at the edge. There is also a squeezing pain in the thickened synovium.

Treatment

1. Press acupoints Shaohai (HT 3), Quchi (LI 11) and Quzhe (PC 3). (See Fig. 45)

2. Acute period: The massagist holds the wrist and pulls and at the same time rotates the forearm with the elbow as the center to relax the joint and reduce

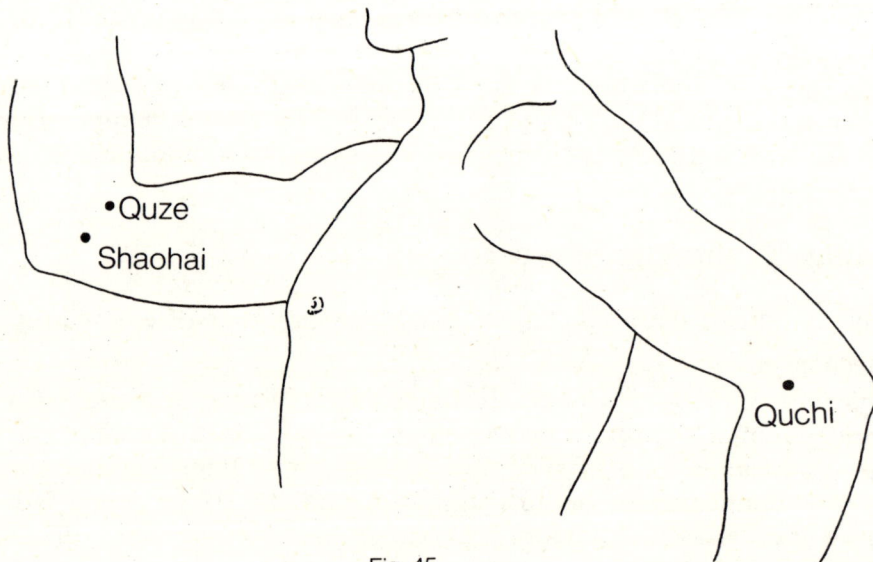

Fig. 45

squeezing on the articular synovium; then pushes and presses 4-5 times gently toward the adjacent tissues from the tender area. The force applied should be light so as not to aggravate the swelling. Apply pressure dressing with elastic bandage or cotton pads and suspend the elbow with triangular binder; remove the dressing after two days.

3. Chronic period: Perform press-kneading at the elbow centering on the tender area. Use scraping method at the thickened synovium with strong stimulation to improve blood circulation, and promote subsidence of swelling and absorption of hydrarthrosis. Hydrarthrosis may be relieved temporarily by puncture, and it will soon reoccur. Manual treatment, however, may remove the hydropsy gradually. As the last step, the massagist carries the elbow in both hands to squeeze and reduce the joint. The patient may receive treatment while continuing training. The patient should not expect immediate results.

13. Olecranal Bursitis

There are two bursae at the olecranon, one between the olecranon and tendon, called the inferior synovial bursa of the brachial triceps muscle, and the other is between the olecranon and a site under the skin, called the subcutaneous bursa. Normal bursae have the functions of lubricating tendons and cushioning local impact.

Injury Mechanism

1. Acute injury: Acute bursitis may be induced by impact on the posterior aspect of elbow, manifested as local hydropsy or haematoma. If not given timely or correct treatment, it will become chronic.

2. Chronic injury: Repeated exertion of the brachial triceps muscle or repeated friction of the posterior aspect of elbow may stimulate the post-elbow bursa, inducing chronic inflammation with the symptoms of synovial thickening and accumulation of synovial fluid, hence cyst. Olecranal bursitis may also be induced by repeated friction of the posterior aspect of elbow due to pressing with elbow tip during treatment by the massagist.

Symptoms and Diagnosis

1. Acute bursitis: Pain, swelling and tenderness appear at the posterior aspect of elbow following injury, the diseased area feels undulant, while the joint movement does not appear to be affected. Acute bursitis should be differentiated from olecranal fracture and rupture of tendon of the brachial triceps muscle. In case of olecranal fracture, fracture fissures may be felt and X-ray examination may verify it. Rupture of the tendon of the brachial triceps muscle can be correctly diagnosed by resistive or gravity test of the brachial triceps muscle (the elbow cannot be stretched straight when bending the waist or stretching the arm).

2. Chronic bursitis: There is discomfort at the posterior aspect of the elbow; synovial bursa becomes thickened, forming a round or oval cyst with smooth

surface and elasticity, undulant feeling but without apparent tenderness on pressure. The cyst may move but not disappear when push-squeezed from the lateral aspect.

Treatment

1. Press acupoints Shaohai (HT 3), Quchi (LI 11) and Quzhe (PC 3).

2. Acute injury: Apply pressure dressing with thick cotton pads or elastic bandage to prevent bleeding and edema of elbow. Remove the dressing the next day and perform gentle grasping manipulation on the posterior muscles of upper arm, focusing on the tendon of the brachial triceps muscle; then perform scrubbing manipulation along the olecranon upward until a warm feeling runs deep to promote the detumescence. If swelling or hydropsy occurs at the posterior aspect of elbow, it should be removed by push-kneading manipulation from the olecranon toward the surrounding area gently so as to avoid increasing the swelling. For a serious case of acute injury of olecranal bursa, let the elbow rest for 1-2 weeks.

3. Chronic bursitis: Pull and rotate the elbow to relax the joint, then scrapes and push-press the thickened bursae, applying more forceful manipulation to the diseased areas to promote blood flow and subsidence of inflammation and hydropsy.

4. Manual treatment of post-elbow cyst: At the initial stage, the cyst wall is very thin and the patient can flex the elbow forcefully to increase the pressure within the cyst while the massagist pushes and squeezes the cyst with both thumbs to rupture the cyst wall and discharge the fluid, then push to all directions to disperse the remaining fluid under the skin and be absorbed gradually. If the cyst wall is thick and cannot be ruptured by pushing and squeezing, the massagist may disinfect the elbow with tincture of iodine alcohol, followed by puncturing the cyst at various sites with a sterilized triangular needle, then pushes and presses to squeeze the remaining fluid in the cyst into the subcutaneous part for absorption. The elbow should rest for two days after the puncturing.

14. Traumatic Osteoarthritis

A common disease, this is also called osteoarthropathy of the elbow joint. It involves a series of pathological changes, such as denaturation of cartilage, hyperosteogeny, chronic synovitis, thickening of joint capsule and hydrarthrosis.

Injury Mechanism

1. Chronic injury: Repeated squeezing, collision and abrading between capitulum of humerus and capitulum radii as well as between the ulnar olecranon and the olecranal fossa of humerus, such as repeated impact caused on the elbow in vaulting horse, may cause denaturation and malacia of cartilage surface, and rupture and falling off of cartilage and exposure of bony tissues, resulting in avulsion osteochondritis. Hyperosteogeny occurs later at the border of the bone and at the point of attachment of joint capsule; the bone surface turns rough,

forming spur. Falling off of ruptured cartilage and hyperplastic sclerites form free bodies in the articulation, clinically manifested as locked joint. Long-term stimulation to the articular synovium induces hyperplastic thickening, resulting in chronic synovitis.

2. Prolonged abnormal elbow joint activity with a load may induce malposition of joint and injury of joint surface, causing hyperosteogeny.

3. Fracture in the joint: Owing to faulty reduction of fracture, even though the fracture unites, the joint surface is rough, and prolonged friction hurts the joint, expose the bony tissues and gradually form hyperosteogeny.

Symptoms and Diagnosis

1. Early symptoms include aching and impaired movement of the joint, and the joint cannot flex or extend fully or move freely. Active motion may improve the range of its movement and ease the pain, which, however, may be aggravated again with increasing amount of exercise. At the late stage, a snap may heard or locked joint found on movement.

2. Local tenderness: Pain on passive flexion or extension of joint, occasionally a sensation of friction. Thickening of articular synovium or hydrarthrosis may be palpated.

3. X-ray may reveal rough articular surface, hyperosteogeny and, occasionally, free bone fragments.

Treatment

For early cases with light pathological manifestations, manual treatment may yield a remarkable curative effect. For cases with obvious hyperosteogeny, the symptoms may also be eased somewhat.

1. Press acupoints Tianding (SJ 10), Quchi (LI 11), Quzhe (PC 3) and Shaohai (HT 3) to clear and activate the meridians and collaterals. (See Fig. 46)

2. The massagist performs grasping manipulation on muscles groups of the upper arm and forearm for 3-5 times to relax myospasm caused by osteoarthropathy. The relaxed muscles in turn can ease the pulling force on the joint and the pressure on the articular surface. Rotating the elbow by holding the wrist may also loosen the joint. Then, the massagist performs thumb-scraping or pushing manipulations at the painful point at the elbow for 5-10 times to stimulate the diseased area for relieving pain in the elbow. When there are cords or scleromata in the elbow tissues, dispel them by plucking manipulation. The above manipulations may help relax the symptoms and improve functions to prevent further worsening of the conditions. When the elbow joint pain intensifies, reduce or stop training involving the elbow to reduce load on the joint.

3. Manual treatment for locked joint: When one assistant holds the upper arm of the affected limb and effects reverse traction, the massagist holds and tracts the wrist with one hand and puts the other hand at the joint body or tender area of the elbow to perform elbow traction, flexion, extension and rotation to widen the joint surface. Press and push the joint body to reposition it in the articular cavity.

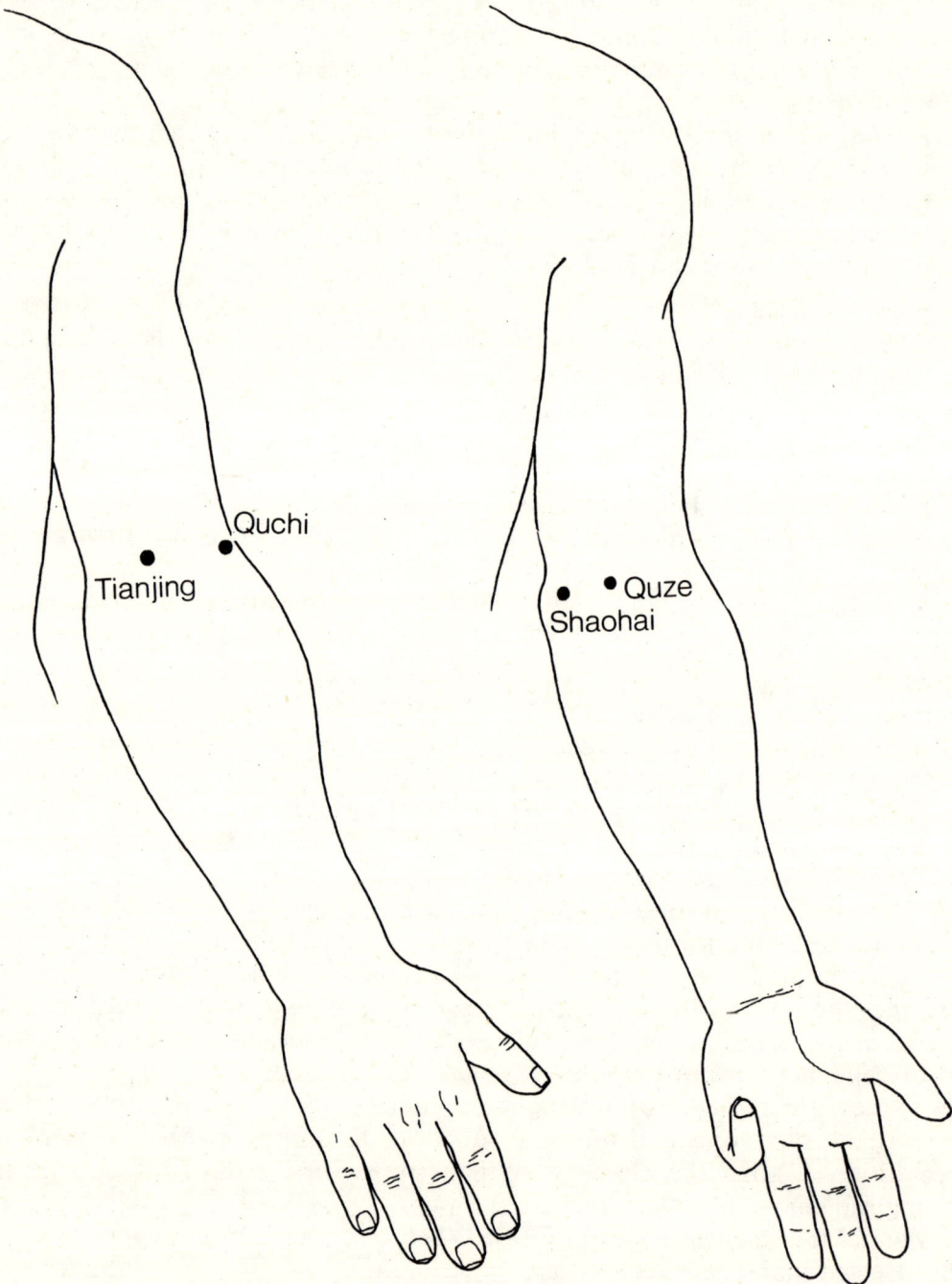

Fig. 46

In cases with distinct spur that hinders elbow function, surgical removal of it is recommended.

15. Myositis Ossificans of Elbow

Though this sports injury is rare, an improperly handled elbow injury may induce myositis ossificans and once it occurs, elbow function is serious hindered.

Injury Mechanism

Myositis ossificans is a sequela of dislocation, fracture and ligamental injury of elbow joint. Laceration, stripping and displacement of the injured periosteum and the haematoma formed beneath the periosteum may cause periosteal proliferation, such as organization, calcification and ossification of the haematoma, and finally forming new bone around the elbow joint, which is a late-stage complication of elbow injury.

This disease, often results from elbow fracture and dislocation in children and teenagers, such as epicondylar fracture humerus. Repeated manual treatment of improper manipulation by the massagist may aggravate the injury of periosteum and soft tissues. For limitation of joint movement caused by elbow injury, the massagist often treats the elbow with strong manual force to widen the range of movement of the joint. Repeated forced flexion and extension of the joint may seem to widen the outward movement range, yet each round of treatment may cause laceration and bleeding of joint capsule, ligament and periosteum, resulting in small haematoma and even ossification. When the ossification develops, it will lead to stiffness of the joint.

Symptoms and Diagnosis

1. Early stage symptoms are joint pain, swelling and restricted movement, while at the late stage the joint becomes stiff.

2. X-ray examination provides the main basis for diagnosis. At the early stage, mist-like shadow is found around the joint which later becomes a lumpish calcification shadow. In some cases it forms larger bone fragments which may or may not link with bony tissues. After several months, the calcification shadow may partially disappear and the ossification border becomes smooth and clearly out-lined.

Treatment

Prevention is of first importance as no satisfactory therapy is known.

1. For fracture dislocation after elbow trauma, timely manual reduction with gentle force is necessary. Improper forceful manipulation should be avoided.

2. Recovery of elbow functions must proceed step by step; haste may not bring success. For most cases of elbow joint trauma in teenagers, normal joint functions can be restored after active elbow movements. The situation will deteriorate, even with myositis ossificans occurring, if forceful flexion and extension of the elbow

joint are practised to increase the joint's range of movement. Gentle manipulation is desirable in treating elbow trauma in teenagers during the recovery period to promote the recovery of functions. If the massagist finds it difficult to master the manipulation, allow natural recovery.

3. At the initial stage of myositis ossificans, massage muscle groups of upper arm and forearm gently to promote absorption of calcificio, and assist the affected side to flex and extend. Make a powder from 9 grams of safflower, 30 grams of frankincense, 30 grams of myrrh, 15 grams of hyacinth bletilla, 15 grams of capejasmine, 30 grams of goldthread root, 30 grams of yellow corktree bark and 30 grams of flavescent sophora root and mix the powder with honey for external application every other day.

4. At the advanced stage of myositis ossificans, as the ossifying scope stabilizes and the elbow function is hindered by the ossified bone fragments, surgery is required to resect the bone.

16. Injury of Ulnar Nerve

The ulnar nerve passes through its groove. Pathological changes at the elbow joint may constrict the ulnar nerve, which runs downward between the ulnar flexor muscle of wrist and the deep flexor digitorum and between the superficial flexor digitorum and the ulnar flexor muscle of wrist to enter the palm at the transverse carpal ligament.

Injury Mechanism

1. Acute injury: Direct pulling on the ulnar nerve due to fracture displacement caused by dislocation of elbow joint or fracture of medial epicondyle of humerus.

2. Constriction of the ulnar nerve: Thickening of fascia of the wrist ulnar flexor muscle and hypcrosteogeny at the ulnar nerve groove may all constrict and abrade the ulnar nerve and cause ulnar neuritis. This is common in weight-lifting and throwing events.

3. Constriction on the ulnar nerve due to special body postures required in certain sports, such as cycling. Forward moving of the center of body gravity may constrict the ulnar nerve around the pisiform bone by the bicycle bar.

Symptoms and Diagnosis

1. In a light case of ulnar nerve injury there is aching and weakness in the fingers and the hand is subject to fatigue.

2. In a serious case, the ulnar aspect of the little and index fingers is slow in feeling, abduction and adduction of fingers are limited, and the strength in grasping paper with straight fingers weakens or is lost.

3. Myotrophy: Manifested as atrophy of the interosseous muscle and the lesser thenar muscle. Serious injury to the ulnar nerve may cause a paw-like malformation of the hand, particularly serious for the little and index fingers.

Treatment

1. Correct wrong movements, remove pathogenic factors, adjust amount of exercise and training method and strengthen muscle training of the upper arm. Prevent osteoarthritis of elbow, especially hyperosteogeny at the groove of the ulnar nerve or humerus.

2. Press acupoints Quepen (ST 12), Jiquan (HT 1), Shaohai (HT 3) and Houxi (SI 3). (See Fig. 47)

3. Press and knead muscles of the ulnar aspect of upper arm and forearm, focusing on the ulnar flexor muscle of wrist, repeat 4-5 times to relax the spasmodic muscle and promote the flow of qi and blood.

4. Stimulate the ulnar nerve in the groove of the ulnar nerve at the medial aspect of elbow with nipping or flick-poking manipulation. The nerve in this area becomes round and cord-like. Its stimulation may produce tingling pain as that caused by a shock from the forearm to the little finger. Also stimulate the ulnar nerve at the ulnar aspect of the wrist cross striation and around the pisiform bone. This is a key method in treating injury to the ulnar nerve. The stimulation may help excite the nerve, promote its conductive function and restore muscular strength and feeling in hand. Such stimulation should be performed once a day or every other day.

17. Fracture of Radius and Ulna

Injury Mechanism

1. Direct external force: The injury is caused by hitting or squashing by heavy object. The fracture lines of the radius and ulnar break are almost at the same

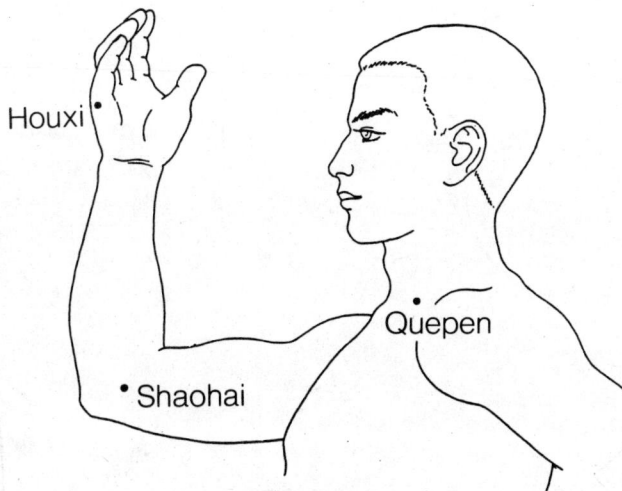

Fig. 47

level, giving it the name transverse or comminuted fracture.

2. External conductance: Hitting the ground with the palm when falling, the reacting force causes fracture at the middle section or the upper 1/3 of the radius and at the lower part of the ulna, so the two fracture lines are not at the same level.

3. External torsion: Over-twisting of forearm may cause fracture, usually spiral fracture.

Symptoms and Diagnosis

1. Obvious history of trauma. Usually when the forearm is struck, squeezed or over-twisted when hitting the ground with palm in falling.

2. Severe pain, local swelling and ecchymoma in forearm and forearm dysfunction.

3. Malformation and abnormal movement of forearm, bone crepitation or sensation of friction of the bone.

4. X-ray examination helps confirm the type and degree of the fracture. The photograph should include the superior and inferior radius and ulnar articulations to see it there is dislocation of them.

Treatment

1. Anaesthesia: Sufficient local or brachial plexus anaesthesia. Or acupressure point anaesthesia: Press acupoints Tianding (LI 17), Quepen (ST 12) and Jiquan (HT 1) for 2-3 minutes each. (See Fig. 48)

2. Fracture reduction:

 a) Making the patient lying supine with the shoulder abducting to 90 degrees, the elbow flexing to 70 degrees and the forearm in natural position, the massagist feels out the location of the four fracture ends of the radius and ulna.

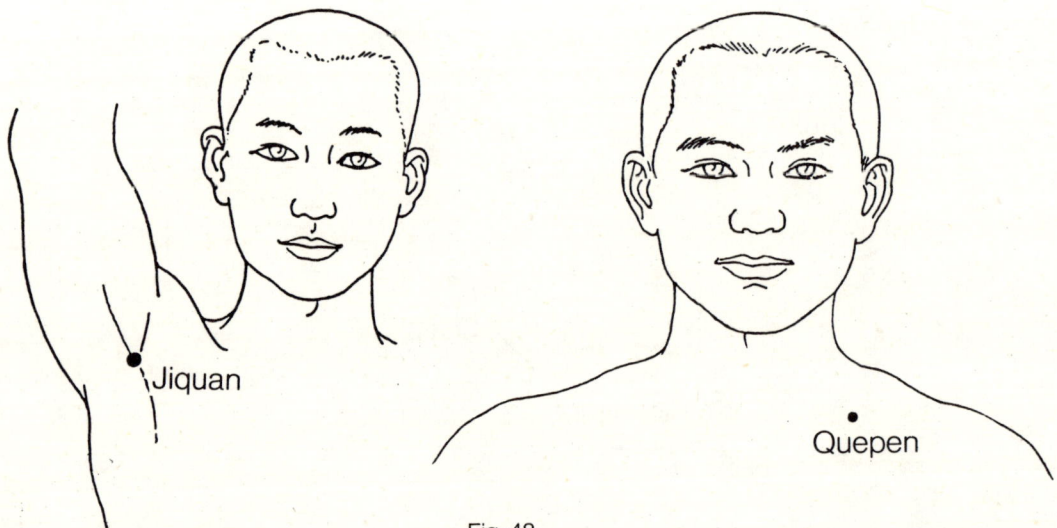

Fig. 48

b) One assistant holds the patient's elbow, another holds the wrist of the affected limb and performs traction for 5 minutes using slow and sustained force while avoiding rough traction or a force varying in strength until the overlapping teratism or angulated malformation is reduced.

c) Separation of fractured ends of radius and ulna: The massagist squeezes the bone space from the palmar and dorsal aspects of the fracture with the thumb and the index, middle and little fingers to separate the fractured ends of radius and ulna and tighten periosteum so as to facilitate the reduction and fixation of the fracture.

d) Lifting and pressing manipulations: The massagist holds the upper and lower sections of the fracture of the radius and ulna with both hands respectively, supports and presses the protruded fracture end downward with the other four fingers. This manipulation is repeated several times. If the fractures are not at the same level, first reduce the comparatively stable fracture using the same lift-pressing method, then reduce the other.

e) Reverse bending manipulation: If lifting and pressing manipulations do not achieve a reduction, the massagist enlarges the original angulated malformation to a certain degree under traction. When the massagist feels that the protruded and the sunken ends meet, he performs reverse bending with the fracture ends as fulcrum for a reduction. After reduction, the massagist holds the fracture part tightly with one hand and strokes the bone along the longitudinal axis to achieve better reduction and restore the dislocated soft tissues along the longitudinal axis. For better accuracy, reduce the fracture under X-ray roentgenoscopy. (See Fig. 49)

3. Fracture fixation:

a) Placement of bone-separating pads: When the fracture lines of radius and ulna occur at the same level, place a long bone-separating pad at the palmar and dorsal aspects of the forearm respectively with the fracture line as the center to tighten the periosteum and so help fix the fracture ends. When the two fracture lines are not at the same level, place a bone-separating pad the lower section of the palmar and dorsal aspects of the forearm respectively, though it is not advisable to place the pads at the palmar aspect of the upper third section of the forearm for it may constrict the branch of the brachial artery. (See Fig. 50)

b) With the help of an assistant and in accordance with the trend of angulation displacement and lateral displacement of fracture, place two more small bone-pressure pads, apply strapping to the forearm with four short splints and four bandages. The short splints at the ulnar aspect should be long enough to extend beyond the wrist joint to prevent ulnar deviation of the hand, which could cause angulation displacement of the fracture toward the humeral aspect. Finally, bend the elbow joint at an angle of 90 degrees, rest the forearm on a supporting board and suspend with bandage before the chest.

Manual Treatment for Rehabilitation

1. After treatment, attention should be paid to the blood circulation of fingers

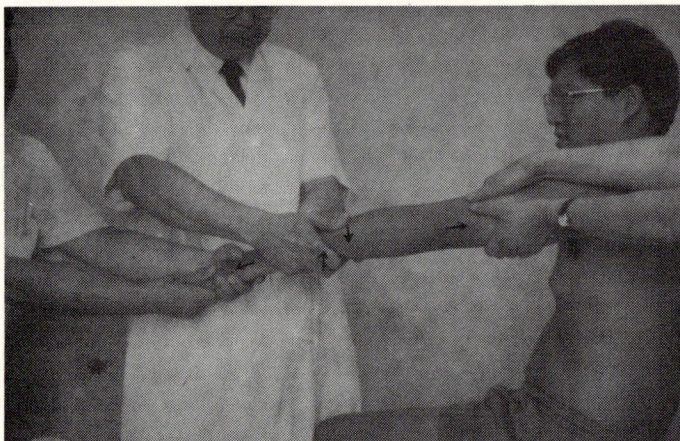

Fig. 49

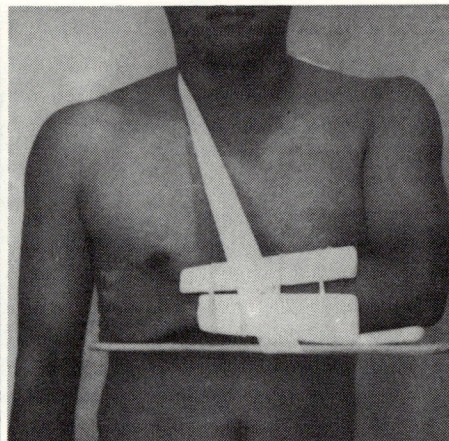

Fig. 50

and feeling of nerves and make timely adjustment of the bandage tightness to avoid ischemic contracture. Examine by roentgenoscopy once every 3-4 days for possible fracture displacement which would require prompt correction.

2. Start fist-making and palm-stretching exercises the day after treatment and resume shoulder- and elbow-joint movements a week later, supplemented by press-kneading of shoulder and upper arm muscles. Relax spasmodic cords, maintain muscle elasticity, promote union of the fracture and avoid spasm. Forearm rotation is not allowed at this stage. Such movements may start gradually only 4-6 weeks later. After eight weeks, the splint strapping may be removed, since the fracture has clinically united and callus formed as shown by X-ray picture.

3. Perform press-kneading manipulation on forearm muscle groups to soften the muscles stiffened by prolonged strapping. The massagist holds the fractured part with one hand to protect this part and grasps the hand on the affected side with the other to help the patient perform daily pronation and supination movements of the forearm.

Chapter 4
INJURY OF WRIST AND HAND

1. Distal Fracture and Epiphysiolysis of Radius

Injury Mechanism

Composed of loose bony matters, the lower end of radius is its weakest part. Touching the ground abruptly with palm when falling may cause fracture at the point 2-3 cm. above the wrist articular surface due to body gravity and the reacting force of the ground. It is manifested in children as epiphysiolysis, which is a straight type of distal fracture of radius, also called Colles' fracture, while hitting the ground with the back of hand causes a bending type of distal fracture of radius, which is also called Smith's fracture. More often found is the straight type, which is dealt with here. This type of fracture is usually complicated by fracture of styloid process of ulna while the triangular cartilage disk of the inferior radioulnar joint moves to the dorsal aspect of the radius. This is referred to as complication by injury of the triangular cartilage of wrist. When there is obvious displacement of the distal fracture end, the palmar flexor tendon and the dorsal extensor tendon are constricted, hampering the sliding of the tendons. There are a few cases of comminuted fracture in which the fracture end points toward the wrist joint and the function of wrist may be hampered after union of the fracture.

Symptoms and Diagnosis

1. Obvious pain, swelling and dysfunction.

2. Malformation: The distal fracture end displaces toward the dorsal and radial aspects while the proximal end displaces toward the palmar aspect, causing fork-like malformation of hand and wrist when viewed from one side as well as spear-like malformation and increase of wrist width when viewed from the front.

3. For a case without distinct displacement, there are local swelling, thickening and rough bony surface to the feel and obvious tenderness on pressure, while in a case with obvious displacement, crepitation of bone may be heard and a sensation of bone friction felt.

4. X-ray photograph should reveal the specific situation of the fracture.

Treatment

1. Manual reduction:

a) Anaesthesia: Digitally press acupoints Quepen (ST 12), Jiquan (HT 1) and Quchi (LI 11), or use 2 percent procaine for local anaesthesia.

b) Making the patient sit or lie down, one assistant grasps the elbow for traction and another pulls at the five fingers; the massagist puts both his thumbs against the dorsal aspect of the distal fracture section and places the other four fingers at the palmar aspect of the proximal fracture section. Then, both assistants perform traction simultaneously while the massagist push-presses from the distal end toward the palmar end with force and lifts the proximal section toward the dorsal aspect so as to feel the move of the fracture ends, and finally bends the wrist joint to make it lean toward the ulnar aspect to reduce the lateral displacement of the fracture. It is easy to achieve manual reduction, and even an anatomic reduction in most cases of distal fracture and epiphysiolysis of radius.

c) The massagist performs gentle massage along the forearm and wrist to restore the muscles, tendons and ligaments so as to promote the repair of the soft tissues. (See Fig. 51)

2. Splint fixation: Use four splints for fixation after reduction. Splints for the dorsal and radial aspects should extend beyond the wrist joint, while those for the ulnar aspect should not press the styloid process of ulna. Bind them with three bandages. Rest the forearm on a supporting board with vertical column, with the hand gripping the column. Suspend the triangular binder at the chest.

Rehabilitation Treatment and Functional Exercises

1. Begin practising fist-making and palm-stretching movements the day after treatment but avoid wrist activity and forearm rotation. Start flexion and extension movements on the second day.

2. At the initial stage, massage treatment may be carried out on the forearm and elbow. Digitally press acupoints Quepen (ST 12) and Jiquan (HT 1) one minute each. When the pressing suddenly stops, there may be a sensation of numbness and warm feeling in the hand. This is a method to promote blood circulation by removing blood stasis.

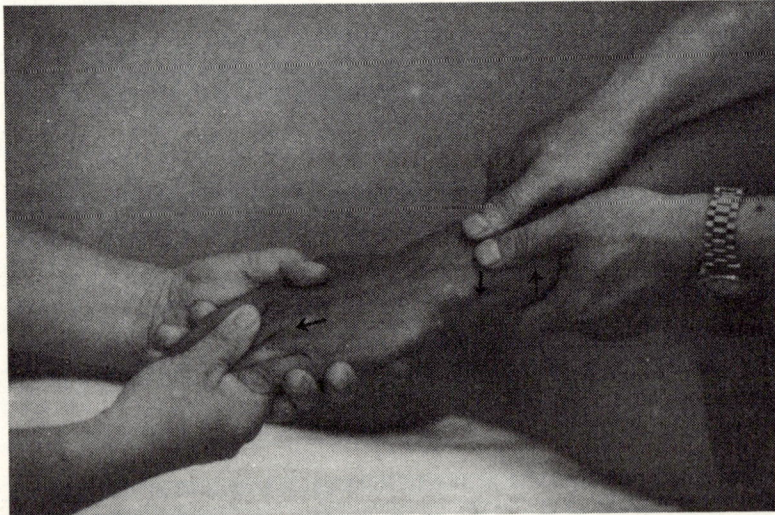

Fig. 51

3. Remove the splints after four weeks and gradually resume wrist activity and forearm rotation. The massagist may give help in the wrist activities, but the manipulation force must be gentle. Relax the muscles of the distal section of forearm by press-kneading, while focusing on masses of muscles with flick-poking manipulation to disperse them. The wrist functions may become basically normal after two months.

2. Fracture of Scaphoid Bone

Fracture of scaphoid bone is a very common sports injury, accounting for a big part of wrist fracture cases.

Injury Mechanism

Fracture of the scaphoid bone is caused mainly by indirect external force. When falling with the palm hitting the ground at a dorsiflexed position or with the radius at deviating position, the radius may pass the impact to the scaphoid bone and fracture it. Some cases are of fatigue fracture of wrist, such as those caused by repeated impact on the wrist in gymnastics and impact on the hands by water surface when diving into water.

The scaphoid bone of wrist is reinforced with surrounding ligaments. But, as there is no powerful muscle attached to it, displacement seldom occurs in an fracture. Yet, the fracture unites slowly because of poor supply of blood to the scaphoid bone and such sequelae as ischemic necrosis of scaphoid bone and osteoarthropathy of wrist are likely to occur.

According to the time of fracture, it can be divided into new or old fracture.

Symptoms and Diagnosis

1. When the injury is due to falling in a usual posture, there will be swelling, tenderness and haematocele at the wrist, with the swelling being particularly evident at the depression between the long extensor muscle of thumb and the tendon. There is always the possibility of fracture.

2. Limited function: The wrist feels weak and there is pain during dorsiflexion and rotation movements.

3. X-ray examination: Fracture line is visible in front-view X-ray photograph in a serious fracture, while in a slight fracture no fracture line is found during X-ray examination taken immediately after the injury and the diagnosis may be missed. The fracture line will be visible after two weeks when typical symptoms appear at the wrist after the bone substance at the fracture ends is absorbed. A second X-ray examination should then be taken for correct diagnosis and, if necessary, additional sideways X-ray photographs of the wrist are to be taken with the palm pronated at angles of 30, 45 and 60 degrees. When the long axis of scaphoid bone forms a 60-degree angle with the horizontal axis of the wrist, so the whole scaphoid bone, especially the fracture line, is more evidently visible. Ischemic necrosis of the scaphoid bone indicates increased bone density.

Treatment

1. Press acupoints Hegu (LI 4), Yangchi (SJ 4), and Yangxi (LI 5) which is in the depression between the tendons of short and long extensor muscles of thumb and should not be pressed too hard. (See Fig. 52).

2. If tumefaction at the wrist is serious, the massagist may perform push-pressing manipulation with both thumbs from distal to proximal end for detumescence, then relax the forearm muscles, particularly the extensor and flexor muscle groups at the radial aspect with press-kneading manipulation.

3. Fixation: Manual reduction is not necessary since fracture displacement is not evident. Mould wet common hard paper into the shape of forearm and wrist and wrap the forearm and the dorsal, palmar and radial aspects of the wrist with it so that the wrist joint rests at deviating position toward the palmar aspect. Place a cotton ball or paper pad at the site of Yangxi (LI 5), then bind the hard paper with bandages. Change the paper every 2-4 weeks and keep the strapping in place for 2-3 months. This method can also be applied to old fracture of the scaphoid bone. During the period of strapping, elbow and different phalangeal joints of hand, except the wrist joint, should be exercised. No supporting movement with wrist is allowed. Repeated impact on the scaphoid bone may lead to local ischemic necrosis. (See Fig. 53)

4. Perform stroking and petrissage manipulations on the affected hand, press-kneading on the muscles of forearm to relax the muscles and tendons and activate the flow of qi and blood in the meridians and collaterals once a day. After the removal of the strapping, gently massage the wrist part and nasopharyngeal fossa to promote the union of the fracture. The force should be very gentle to avoid shearing force acting on the scaphoid bone and affecting its union.

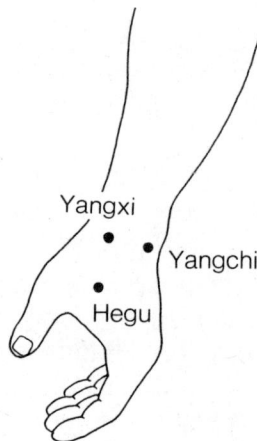

Fig. 52

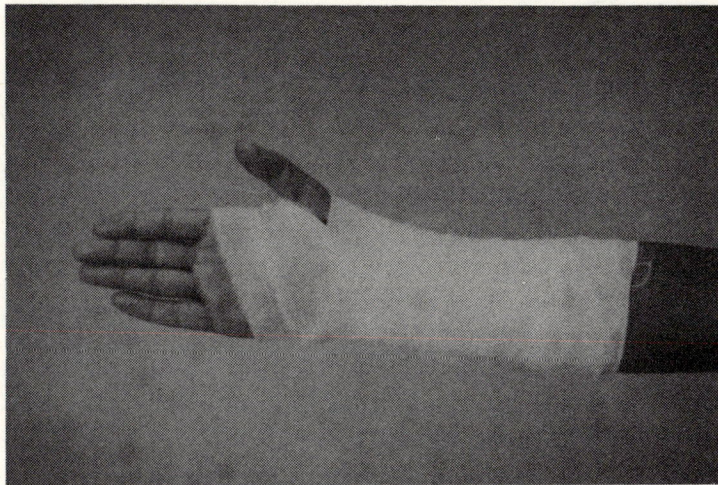

Fig. 53

3. Lunate Dislocation

The lunate is located at the middle of the proximal row of carpal bone. It is crescent in shape when viewed sideways. Its concavity forms a joint with the capitate bone and its convexity faces the distal end of radius. Lunate dislocation accounts for most carpal bone dislocations, with forward lunate dislocation being the most frequently seen.

Injury Mechanism

Forward lunate dislocation is caused by indirect violent force. When falling with palm hitting the ground at an extreme dorsiflexed posture, the lunate is squeezed between the lower end of radius and the capitate bone, so it displaces toward the palmar aspect and bursts the joint capsule.

Symptoms and Diagnosis

1. Distinct tumefaction and fierce pain at the palmar aspect of wrist, and flexion and extension of wrist joint are serious hampered.

2. Head of the third metacarpal bone appears obviously shortened when making a fist.

3. The dislocated lunate is squeezed into the carpal canal and constricts the flexor muscular tendons of fingers and the median nerve, so the fingers are semi-extended, the abducting force of the thumb becomes weak and the sensation of the thumb and index and middle fingers disappears.

4. X-ray examination: Front-view X-ray photo shows that the lunate turns triangular from its normal quadrilateral shape, while side-view photo shows the lunate concavity separates from the capitate bone, dislocates toward the palmar aspect and capitate bone approaches the joint surface of radius.

Treatment

1. Acupoint anaesthesia: Press acupoints Quchi (LI 11), Hegu (LI 4), Yangchi (SJ 4) and Yangxi (LI 5). (Fig. 54)

2. Manual reduction: The massagist palpates the site of the dislocated lunate. An assistant tracts the affected palm forward and sets the wrist joint at extreme dorsiflexed position to enlarge the space between the capitate bone and radius, while the massagist pushes back the lunate from the palmar aspect with the thumb or prizes the lunate with a thick syringe needle through the skin to reduce the lunate. After reduction, the wrist pain should soon subside and activities become basically normal. The massagist then squeezes the wrist from both dorsal and palm sides with both hands and restores tendons and soft tissues by press-kneading manipulation. Finally, the wrist joint is strapped in a slightly bending position for two weeks to promote repair of the tissues. (See Fig. 55)

Functional Exercises

Use of finger may start right after manual reduction but no wrist activity is allowed. After the removal of the strapping, practise and try to resume wrist functions with the help of the massagist, relieve tumescence in the wrist by flat pushing though at this juncture the patient should be advised not to make any over-extension or supporting movements with the wrist. Keep press-kneading the forearm muscles once a day. In this way, the function of the wrist will return to normal in a month's time.

4. Fracture of Metacarpal Bone

A traumatic injury that occurs frequently, it may be of three types according to

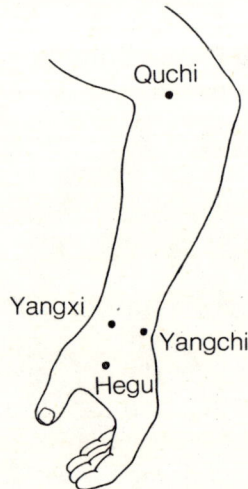

Fig. 54

the site of the fracture: (a) Fracture of metacarpal shaft; (b) pure fracture of the base of the first metacarpal bone or fracture and dislocation of the base of the first metacarpal bone, which is also called Bennett's fracture; and (c) cervix metacarpal fracture.

1) Fracture of Metacarpal Shaft

A commonly seen fracture, it is caused either by direct violent force or by indirect external force. Direct violent force, such as external impact on the dorsal aspect of hand, may in most cases cause transverse fracture or comminuted fracture. Indirect external force may cause oblique or spiral fracture. Pulling at the metacarpal bone by flexor muscle of fingers and interosseous muscle may cause angulation or lateral displacement of the fracture toward the dorsal aspect. In hand injury, there is local pain and failure to make fist, angulated malformation and sinking of the head of metacarpal bone may be seen at the back of hand; the pain becomes serious when pushing the head of the metacarpal bone. Use X-ray for detailed diagnosis of the fracture.

Treatment

1. The massagist holds the finger and tracts along the longitudinal axis of the metacarpal bone with one hand and presses the angulated fracture end from the back of the hand with the other to correct the angulated malformation. The massagist then presses and squeezes both aspects of the fractured metacarpal bone from the palmar side and the back of the hand with the thumb and index finger to correct lateral fracture displacement, and finally regulates and restores the soft tissues of the palm and back of the hand. Only precise reduction of the fracture will ensure the patient's ability to undergo normal physical training after the union of the fracture. (See Fig. 56)

2. Apply bandage and splint strapping to the palm and back of the hand for three weeks by placing a splint on each side.

3. Practise finger movement, limbering them up within a week. After removal of the splints, strong fist-making movement is not advisable soon. It is better to knead the finger and relax the muscle and tendon first.

Example: Miss Huang, gymnast, injured her hand while participating in a vaulting horse contest at the 1984 Shanghai International Gymnastics Invitational Tournament. X-ray diagnosis showed fracture of the second metacarpal bone which was reduced at a hospital. Later, X-ray examination showed that the fracture had been basically reduced. However, because some degree of fracture malformation remained that could disturb bar-gripping movement, a second manual reduction was performed five days later to fully reduce the fracture. After strapping for three weeks, the fracture was united and regular training was resumed.

2) Fracture of the First Metacarpal Bone

Simple fracture of the base of the first metacarpal bone is caused by external force exerted on the longitudinal axis of thumb or by forced passive flexion of

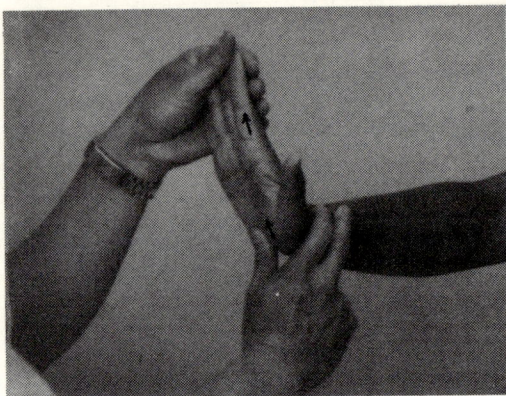

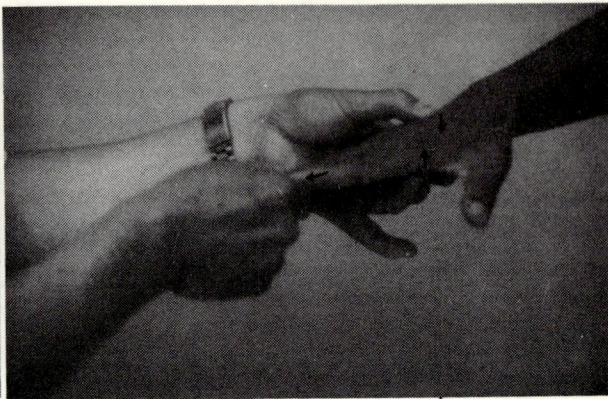

Fig. 55   Fig. 56

thumb. Examples are fracture caused by external force exerted directly on the tip of the thumb or by striking with the fist. Angulated malformation toward the dorsal aspect often occurs and in some cases incarceration of fracture end.

Treatment

1. Acupoint anaesthesia: Hegu (LI 4), Yangchi (SJ 4) and Yangxi (LI 5).

2. The massagist grips the thumb, tracts slowly and abducts the metacarpal bone with one hand while pushing and pressing the protruded fracture end with the thumb of the other hand; feels out the displacement of the fracture end until the surface of the first metacarpal bone feels smooth, this shows that the reduction is completed; and finally presses and restores the adjacent soft tissues with the thumb and index fingers.

3. Fixation: Put an aluminum tongue depressor or iron sheet from the radial aspect of forearm to the tip of the thumb to strap the thumb in abducted position for three weeks. Start functional exercises of the other four fingers and apply massage on muscles of the forearm the day after treatment, and be sure not to move the wrist.

If dislocation accompanies the fracture of the base of the first metacarpal bone, the fracture line starts at the basal part of the first metacarpal bone, extends to the outer area and leads to the wrist joint. The relation between the small bone fragments and the trapezium bone of the medial triangle does not change. The lateral fracture end, due to pulling by the long abductor muscle of thumb and contraction of its flexor muscle, displaces toward the lateral dorsal aspect.

Manual treatment of fracture of the base of the first metacarpal bone accompanied by dislocation is basically the same as that for simple fracture of the base of the first metacarpal bone. Strapping is applied by placing a bone-pressing pad at the base of the metacarpal bone. Because there is mutual incarceration between the fracture ends, the reduction is relatively easy, though because recurrence of dislocation is likely. Because of this, X-ray examination should be taken every few days for a check. If dislocation recurs, repeat the reduction. However, frequent recurring dislocation requires surgery and internal fixation with Kirschner pins.

3) Cervix Metacarpal Fracture

In this type of fracture, the head of the metacarpal bone is pulled by the interosseous muscle and the fracture part displaces toward the dorsal aspect. Major clinical manifestations include local swelling, limited flexion and extension of fingers and projected malformation at the back of the hand.

Treatment

The massagist tracts the affected finger, bends the metacarpophalangeal joint to a right angle, pushes the first phalange to the dorsal aspect and exerts pressure on the back of the hand at the proximal end of fracture. With the reduction completed, keep the metacarpophalangeal joint at 90 degrees and apply fixation with metal plates from the dorsum of finger to the wrist for 2-3 weeks.

5. Phalangeal Fracture

Phalangeal fracture is frequently encountered in sports injury. Though the fracture is not serious, function of the hand may be impaired if it is not treated properly.

Injury Mechanism

Phalangeal fracture is mostly caused by indirect sudden force, such as fingers being hit by volleyball in block, or caused by direct sudden force, such as in squash injury. The fracture may be divided into transverse, oblique, and comminuted fracture.

When fracture happens at the proximal section of phalange, due to the pulling by extensor muscle of finger and the lumbrical muscle, there may be angulated malformation toward the palmar aspect. In a fracture of the middle section of the phalange, pulling of the superficial flexor muscle of finger may cause bending toward either dorsal or palmar aspect, depending on the site of the fracture. Fracture of the distal section of phalange is often an avulsion fracture and that caused by crush injury is often a comminuted fracture.

Symptoms and Diagnosis

The injured finger is painful, with tenderness on pressure and tumefaction, and pressing the finger along the longitudinal axis intensifies the pain. The finger is malformed, and these symptoms may be complicated by abnormal movement of finger and sensation of friction of bone. Final diagnosis depends on X-ray examination.

Treatment

Finger functions are complicated and fine, so reduction of the fracture must be precise, especially for fracture of the thumb and index finger. So, attention should be taken against malformed union and serious impediment in hand functions.

1. With the patient in sitting or supine position, the massagist tracts the finger tip with one hand and with the thumb and index finger of the other pushes and squeezes the distal fracture end along the trend of fracture displacement and lifts the proximal end to correct the palmar or dorsal angulated malformation. This is followed by pressing and pushing the phalanx from the both sides of the affected finger toward the centre with the thumb and index finger to correct the lateral displacement. For comminuted fracture of the last section of phalange, simply squeeze toward the centre. For avulsion fracture, no special manual reduction is needed as long as the functional position of finger is fixed. The small bone sclerites will reduce naturally.

2. Repeatedly press-knead along the longitudinal axis of finger to regulate and restore soft tissues of the finger, which may greatly help the union of the fracture and the recovery of functions.

3. Fixation: Place metal plates at the palmar aspect of the finger and fix them at the functional position with adhesive tape. Avoid fixing the metacarpophalangeal joint and phalangeal joint at the extended position as it may result in stiff phalangeal and metacarpophalangeal joints and hinder finger flexion. For avulsion fracture of the last section of phalange, fix the finger at over-extended position of the distal interphalangeal joint and at flexed position of the proximal interphalangeal joint.

Rehabilitation Exercises

Fix the finger by strapping for 3-4 weeks. Start limbering up the unstrapped fingers and metacarpophalangeal joints the day after treatment. After removal of the fixation and gradual active flexion and extension of the phalangeal joint, the massagist presses and pinches both sides of the finger with thumb and index finger to relax the collateral ligament of phalangeal joint, then presses and pinches both the palmar and dorsal aspects of the finger to relax the interphalangeal joint capsule, the flexor and extensor muscular tendons and tendon sheath, and finally helps flexing and extending the finger to the limit without causing local pain.

Example: Mr. Wang, a volleyball player, had left index finger hit by volleyball in blocking, resulting in local pain. X-ray examination revealed fracture of proximal section of phalange of the left index finger. He continued training without adequate local strapping and two months later the fracture remained and the phalange joint became stiff. He participated in a world cup competition only by protecting the index finger with plastic finger cap.

6. Dislocation of Metacarpophalangeal Joint and Interphalangeal Joint

Most common among joint dislocations in sports injuries are dislocation of metacarpophalangeal joint and interphalangeal joint of hand.

Injury Mechanism

This injury is mostly caused by indirect external force, resulting in over-extension of finger such as in the finger tip being hit by a ball or falling from the horizontal bar with the finger hitting the bar which cause the finger to dislocate toward the dorsal aspect and assume an inverted angle of 90 degrees. If the finger is hit by sudden force on the lateral side, distinct lateral displacement of the finger will be evident and possibly been complicated by injury of the joint capsule and the collateral ligament.

Symptoms and Diagnosis

1. Apparent finger malformation, backward dislocation or local dislocation after trauma.

2. Dislocated bone ends may be felt beneath the skin.

Treatment

1. The massagist tracts the patient's injured finger with one hand while pushing and squeezing the dislocated bone ends with the other. A snap indicates the success of the reduction. Then, he straps the finger or metacarpophalangeal joint at a semi-flexed position for 1-2 weeks.

2. Manual reduction of dislocated metacarpophalangeal joint of the thumb is fairly difficult because the head of the metacarpal bone may lodge between the long and short flexor tendons of thumb, or the metacarpal cervix may be blocked by the burst joint capsule. The massagist must tract the thumb to enlarge the angle of dorsiflexed malformation and shake the thumb sideways to release the metacarpal cervix from the tendon, then flex and track the thumb with one hand and perform push-squeezing manipulation on the metacarpal cervix to reposition it.

Rehabilitation Exercises

Practise active flexion and extension of joint after removal of the strapping. The massagist applies gentle pinching manipulation around the joint to accelerate back flow of lymph and blood, relieve swelling and promote early union of joint capsule and collateral ligament.

7. Contusion of Phalangeal and Metacarpophalangeal Joints

Impact of external force on finger tips when the fingers are over-extended or are twisted may cause contusion of phalangeal and metacarpophalangeal joints, which includes mainly injury of joint capsules, collateral ligaments and cartilages of joint. This is a common sports injury.

Symptoms and Diagnosis

1. Pain, swelling, impairment of activity and local tenderness on pressure at the finger joint. If the collateral ligament is ruptured, lateral displacement of finger may occur.

2. Chronic joint contusion may result in thickening of and tenderness on pressure at the joint capsule. The chronic contusion may result from improper treatment of acute contusion, inappropriate fixation and repeated injury in physical training.

3. X-ray photograph may help rule out minor fracture.

Treatment

1. Acute contusion: Wash the wound with cold water to prevent edematous exudation of tissues. Then the massagist pulls at the finger with one hand and regulates and gently restores adjacent tissues of the joint with the other, avoiding press-kneading. Pressure dressing with cotton pad is then applied for one day.

2. Start massage the day after treatment mainly for restoring and treating the injured soft tissues. The massagist can tracts the finger with one hand and applies gentle kneading around the joint with the thumb and index finger of the other. If the finger joint is swollen, the massagist should push and press the finger from the distal to the proximal end, then flex and extend the joint to prevent adhesion. For an old contusion, the manipulation force should be stronger than in an acute one. The thickening of joint capsule, the massagist must perform local nipping as a supplementary treatment and help the patient flex and extend the joint.

3. Cut exercises of the diseased finger in training for 3-5 days after injury and bind the injured finger together with adjacent fingers with adhesive plaster to prevent further injury.

8. Stenosing Tenovaginitis of Styloid Process of Radius

Injury Mechanism

At the lower end of the radius, muscular tendons of the long abductor and short extensor of thumb pass through the tendon sheath and enters the dorsum of thumb. The styloid process of radius is at the medial aspect of the tendon sheath, its lateral and dorsal aspects being fixed by the common wrist ligament. The tendon groove is narrow and shallow, so when the thumb and wrist move, the tendon sheath is subject to friction, and mechanical stimulation due to long-term over-extension of excessive physical use of the thumb and wrist may cause edema at the tendon and tendon sheath which in turn results in thickening of tendon sheath, hence the stenosis.

Symptoms and Diagnosis

1. Onset is slow, with pain at the styloid process of radius, which may radiates to the forearm.

2. The thumb and wrist feel weak, especially when lifting heavy objects.

3. Local swelling, obvious tenderness, and in some cases palpable nodes.

4. Fist-making and palmar flexion test is positive: There will be pain at the styloid process of radius when the thumb is placed in the center of the palm, a fist

made and the wrist is flexed toward the ulnar aspect.

Treatment

1. Press acupoints Quchi (LI 11), Quze (PC 3), Hegu (LI 4), Yangxi (LI 5) and Waiguan (SJ 5). (See Fig. 57)

2. Gently press, knead and push along the dorsum of forearm to the first metacarpal bone to promote blood circulation by removing blood stasis.

3. Rest the affected thumb at the center of the palm and make a fist. The massagist helps with passive deviation of wrist toward the ulnar aspect, i.e., passively tracts the tendon and sheath. Apply heavy nipping manipulation at the styloid process of radius to relax the stenosing sheath, then apply pluck-poking manipulation along the long flexor of thumb and short extensor of thumb lateral to the forearm to the first metacarpal bone, with stress on the styloid process of radius. Finally press and restore the soft tissues along the long axis.

4. Scrap along the forearm to the first metacarpal bone until warmth is felt to promote blood circulation. This treatment may also be supplemented by infusion with traditional Chinese herbal medicine.

9. Thecal Cyst of Wrist

Referring to cyst near the articular capsule and tendon sheath, thecal cyst of wrist is filled with glue-like fluid. The cyst cavity may or may not link with the articular capsule or tendon sheath. It is often seen at the dorsum of wrist, palmar aspect of wrist joint, and dorsal and palmar aspects of fingers. Acute injury and chronic strain cause more and more fluid to be secreted from the sheath but as very little is absorbed, there is local retention of fluid which may become glue-like

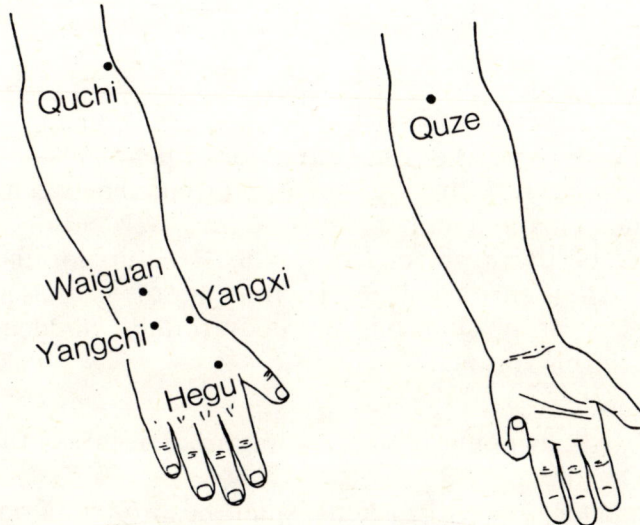

Fig. 57

or jelly-like. The cyst wall thickens and may adhere to adjacent tissues and last for a long time.

Symptoms and Mechanism

1. Slow-growing and painless swelling appears at the diseased site; in some cases wrist strength weakens.

2. Round swelling appears at the back of hand with a diameter under 2 cm. It feels soft and swollen, with no adhesion to skin.

Treatment

1. For a cyst at the dorsum of wrist, bend the wrist to the extreme to increase pressure in the cyst so it will become hard and stable. Then the massagist performs sudden squeezing with both thumbs in the direction of the sheath. In most cases the cyst is ruptured with fluid flowing out and the cyst disappearing.

2. Perform parting pushing manipulation at the dorsal aspect of wrist to push the fluid from the cyst into the adjacent tissues to promote early absorption. Then apply local pressure dressing for one day. If there is still swelling, apply gentle pushing for detumescence.

3. If manual pushing does not remove a cyst with a thick wall, the massagist may first disinfect the skin and pierce through the surface of the cyst at different sites with a three-edged needle to let the fluid flow into subcutaneous tissues. Finally, apply push-squeezing to remove the cyst. Apply pressure dressing for one day after treatment.

10. Separation of Distal Radioulnar Joint

Distal radioulnar joint is composed of ulnar notch at the lower end of the radius and annular articular surface of ulna.

Injury Mechanism

The main function of the distal radioulnar joint is to make pronation and supination motions. During rotation of forearm, when the palm is fixed and the forearm still rotates with force, the palmar and dorsal ligaments and the triangular cartilage will be lacerated, resulting in increased distance between the radius and ulna at the distal end. This may either be a one-time wrist injury or a secondary injury from fracture of the lower end of radius, fracture of the lower middle section of radius, or from chronic strain, such as in free exercises in gymnastics when the hand rests on an object while the body rotates. Sudden motion of the forearm may result in this trauma.

Symptoms and Diagnosis

1. Pain at wrist, weak gripping power, limitation of rotation function of wrist joint.

2. Transverse diameter of wrist thickens, small head of ulna bulges, the range of movement of radius and ulna enlarges when moving them to and fro.

3. A normal X-ray photo shows the radius and ulna overlapping; then they are separated, the space between them enlarges without overlapping. Side-view X-ray photo shows the lower end of the ulna displacing toward the dorsal aspect.

Treatment

1. Manual reduction of acute injury: The massagist tracts the palm of the diseased side with one hand to fully supinate the forearm and presses the dorsum of ulna with other hand until a snap is heard, indicating the success of reduction. This is followed by regulating and restoring the tissues of the forearm and wrist along the longitudinal axis. Apply pressure dressing with bandage for one week. When strapped, dorsiflexion of wrist is allowed but not rotation or supporting movements of wrist.

2. Treatment of chronic injury:

a) Press acupoints Neiguan (PC 6) and Waiguan (SJ 5). (See Fig. 58)

b) The massagist grasps the patient's wrist with both hands, holds it in slightly bending position while pulling and shaking to relax it.

c) Press-knead along the muscles of the forearm. The massagist places his thumb and index finger between the radius and ulna, and applies strong pinching and pressing to stimulate the interosseous membrane for better stability. Under traction, the massagist grips the wrist transversely and squeezes the lower ends of radius and ulna hard for better approximation.

d) After treatment, strap the wrist with bandage. In physical training, the patient needs to wear elastic wrist pad and strap the wrist with wide adhesive plaster tape. In case of definite pain at the wrist, reduce the amount of training or stop physical training.

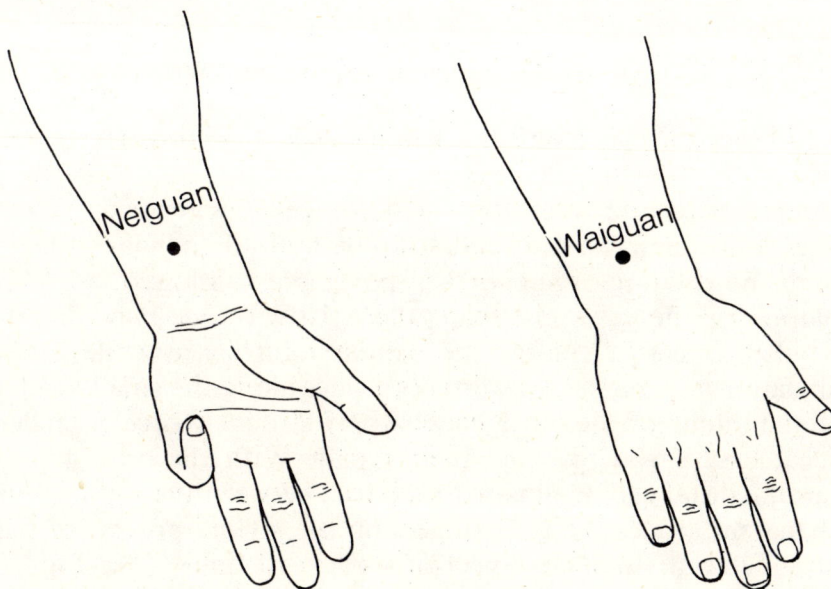

Fig. 58

11. Injury of Triangular Discoid Cartilage of Wrist

Triangular cartilage of wrist is located above the small head of ulna, assuming a triangular shape; its periphery is thick and the center thin. As its tip adheres to the base of the styloid process of ulna and its base to the border of ulnar notch at the distal end of radius, it separates the radiocarpal articulation from the distal radioulnar joint and, together with the dorsal and palmar ligaments, limits over-rotation of the forearm and maintains stability of the distal radioulnar joint.

Injury Mechanism

When falling down with the weight on the palm and the wrist in an over-extended position, the forearm pronates or deviates toward the ulnar aspect, so the triangular discoid cartilage is squeezed by the ulna and the triangular bone, causing injury. A light case is a crush injury at the triangular discoid cartilage, while a serious one means ruptured discoid cartilage. Chronic injury may be caused by repeated dorsiflexion and squeezing of wrist.

Symptoms and Diagnosis

1. Pain in wrist, exacerbated by rotating or supporting movements. In some cases, a snap can be heard.

2. Wrist strength and gripping power of hand fail.

3. Distal radioulnar joint becomes loose; there is intermittent tenderness on pressure on the articular space at the distal end of ulna. Friction pain may occur on deviating the wrist extremely toward the palmar aspect or rotating it to the dorsum.

Treatment

1. Press acupoints Yangxi (LI 5), Neiguan PC 6) and Waiguan (SJ 5). (See Fig. 59)

2. Press and knead muscles along the palmar aspect of forearm to relax the muscle group.

3. The massagist grips and tracts the wrist, shakes clockwise to relax it and restore its tissues. For a new wrist injury, strap with elastic bandage for 3-7 days during which time no rotating or supporting movement is allowed.

4. For an old injury, the massagist tracts the wrist with one hand and deviates it toward the radial aspect to enlarge the palmar joint space while performing scraping manipulation and massage toward both sides along the small head of ulna 5-10 times with the thumb of the other hand. Apply stronger force at tender areas to stimulate local tissues and promote their repair. With the wrist tracted, the massagist grasps the distal end of ulna with the part between the thumb and index finger of one hand and places the four fingers on the styloid process of radius to forcefully push-squeeze the palmar aspect of wrist 5-10 times. (See Figs. 60 and 61)

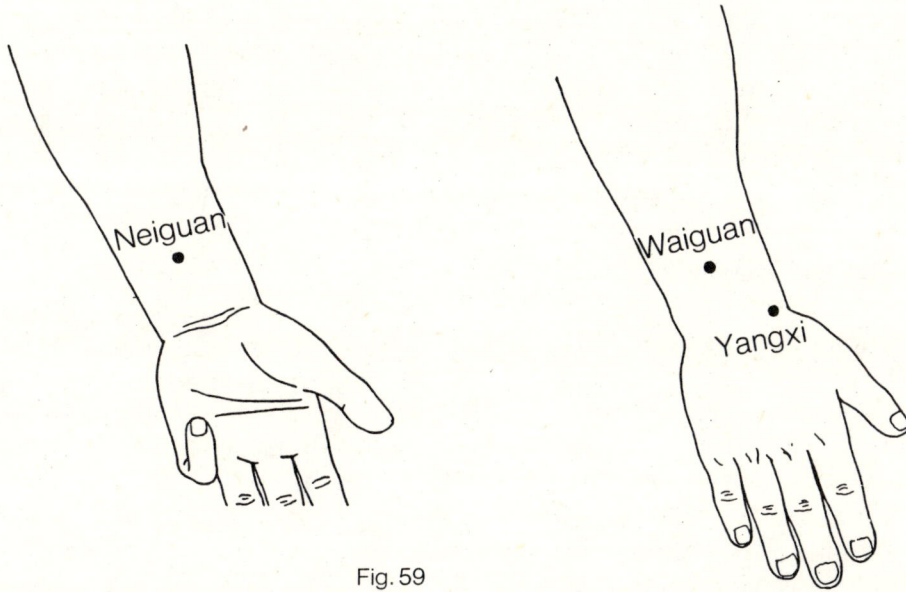

Fig. 59

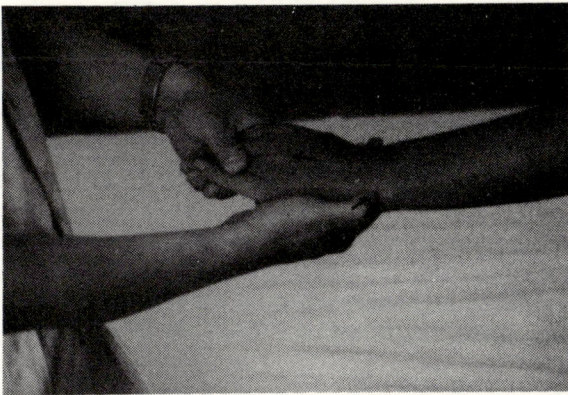

Fig. 60

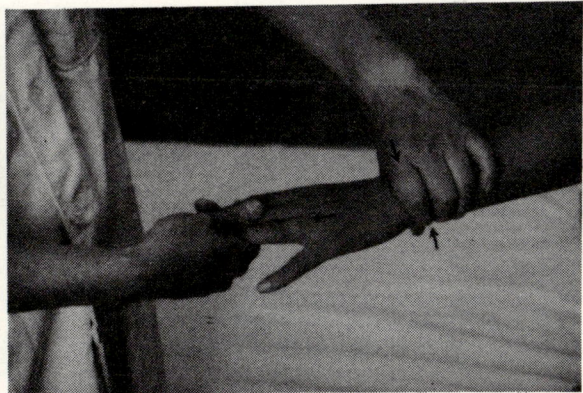

Fig. 61

12. Carpal Tunnel Syndrome

At the palmar aspect of carpal tunnel there is transverse ligament of wrist and at the other three aspects are the carpal bones. Passing through the carpal tunnel are the long flexor tendon of thumb, the deep flexor tendon of finger, the superficial flexor tendon of finger and the median nerve.

Injury Mechanism

Normally, the muscular tendons and the median nerve in the carpal tunnel are not squeezed; but when the carpal tunnel becomes comparatively stenosed, the

101

tendons and median nerve are squeezed, causing local symptoms. Reasons for stenosis of carpal tunnel include: a) The carpal tunnel is subject to external squeezing, such as athletes' palm pads constricting the wrist; when gripping with force, tendons and transverse ligament of wrist may repeatedly squeeze and constrict the median nerve; b) intrusion of hyperosteogeny, fracture or dislocation of carpal bone into the carpal tunnel; and c) thickening of transverse ligament of wrist and swelling of muscular tendon in the carpal tunnel.

Symptoms and Diagnosis

1. At the initial stage the fingers feel numb, especially the index finger, then the thumb, middle finger and ring finger. The pain is worsened at night or in the morning and may refer to elbow.

2. The thumb flexes outwardly, both palms feel weak in mutual confrontation, the radial aspect of thumb, index finger, middle finger and ring finger are slow in sensation.

3. Numbness and pain are aggravated when pressing the palmar aspect of wrist for 1-2 minutes. When stimulating the median nerve by percussing the carpal tunnel, there is a radiating twinge in the finger.

Treatment

1. Press acupoints Neiguan (PC 6) and Waiguan (SJ 5).

2. With the forearm resting and the wrist flat with the palm facing upward, the massagist press-kneads the muscles of the forearm along the flexor tendon of finger to relax the muscles.

3. Perform gentle press-kneading and scraping manipulations on the carpal tunnel, pull at the wrist to move it in all directions. Then press the carpal tunnel with thumb for 2-3 minutes.

4. Transversely flick-poke the tendons inside the carpal tunnel 5-10 times, perform scrubbing manipulation on the local site until a hot sensation is felt to stimulate the carpal tunnel area for promoting blood circulation and detumescence.

13. Sprain of Wrist Joint

The wrist joint can flex, extend, adduct, abduct and rotate. In physical training, its activity is more frequent and range of motion large, subjecting it to injury.

Injury Mechanism

1. Acute sprain: A number of factors may cause injury to the ligaments and synovium of wrist and they include sudden impact of external force on the wrist, hitting the ground with palm when falling, and squeezing and over-twisting of the wrist. Sprain at dorsiflexed position may injure the palmar ligament; over-flexion of wrist may injure the dorsal ligament; over-deviation to the ulnar aspect may injure the radial ligament; and over-deviation to the radial aspect may injure the ulnar collateral ligament. In some cases, several ligaments are injured simul-

taneously. Acute sprain of wrist may be accompanied by injury of muscular tendons, tendon sheath and articular capsule.

2. Chronic strain: Over-burdened activity of wrist may cause injury to soft tissues, cartilage and wrist bones, including traumatic synovitis of wrist joint and strain of ligaments.

Symptoms and Diagnosis

1. Pain, weakness and slight limitation of movement when the wrist is sprained.

2. Tumefaction at wrist area. During the acute period of sprain the tumefaction develops quickly and is accompanied by tenderness on pressure. In the chronic period tumefaction is not evident but the tissues feel thickened and masses may be felt.

3. There are tenderness on pressure and restrictive pain at the initial and end points of ligament on the injured side. Hydrarthrosis may appear in a serious case.

4. X-ray examination does not show any abnormality, and this may rule out fracture of the lower section of radius, fracture of the scaphoid bone and lunate dislocation.

Treatment

1. Press acupoints Hegu (LI 4), Lieque (LU 7), Yangchi (SJ 4), Neiguan (PC 6), Waiguan (SJ 5) and Quchi (LI 11). (See Fig. 62)

2. Acute wrist sprain:

a) First massage the forearm to relax its muscles and promote the flow of qi and blood in the meridians and collaterals. The massagist holds and tracts the hand on the affected side slowly with both hands and helps the wrist with palmar flexion, dorsiflexion and rotation movements, then regulates and restores the soft and bony

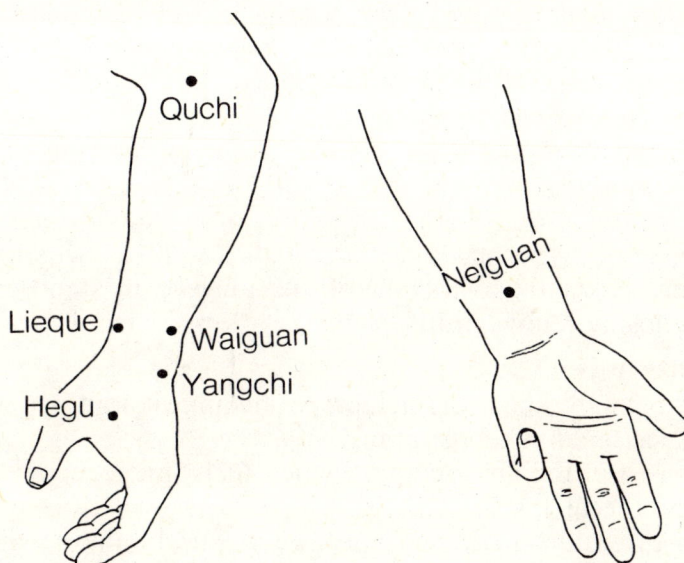

Fig. 62

tissues of the wrist gently. Avoid over pressure, but apply pressure dressing to the wrist to prevent swelling.

b) Start wrist activities the day after the sprain. The massagist gently press-kneads the painful area or the initial and end points of the injured ligament with the thumb.

c) For a case with tumefaction or hydrarthrosis, apply flat-pushing manipulation to remove the swelling by pushing and pressing from the distal to the proximal end with even strength. Use squeeze-pressing manipulation for hydrarthrosis to help with fluid absorption.

3. Chronic wrist strain:

a) Massage extensor and flexor muscle groups of forearm to relieve tension. The massagist holds and tracts the wrist in all directions. In cases with motor impairment, exert stronger force to widen the range of movements such as dorsiflexion and palmar flexion.

b) Stimulate the painful area by nipping; for cords and masses, use flick-poking manipulation to soften and remove them.

c) For chronic sprain of wrist, use wrist pad or adhesive plaster tape for protection in physical training; and enhance strength exercises of wrist to prevent recurrence of sprain.

14. Traumatic Tenovaginitis of Hand

Of all cases of traumatic tenovaginitis of hand, tenovaginitis of flexor tendon of finger is more common, while that of common extensor tendon of finger is rare.

Injury Mechanism

There is a shallow bone groove at the palmar aspect of metacarpal cervix and metacarpophalangeal joint. Together with the sheath-shaped ligament of finger, it forms an "osseofibrous canal" through which pass the deep and superficial flexor of finger and long flexor of thumb.

Long-term continuous forceful flexion and extension of fingers, repeated friction between the muscular tendon and sheath and long-term lifting of heavy objects, such as bar-bells, may cause pressure and stimulation that may cause hyperaemia, edema and hyperplasia of tendon sheath, all of which impair tendon movement. If fibrosis occurs to the sheath, it can lead to stenosed canal cavity, hence causing stenosing tenovaginitis.

Symptoms and Diagnosis

1. Pain in the palmar aspect of metacarpophalangeal joint or interphalangeal joint, which is exacerbated when gripping.

2. Local tenderness at the diseased part which feels thickened with small masses that turn out to be thecal cysts.

3. Flexion and extension of fingers are limited; there may be snapping sounds when flexing and extending them. That is why this disease is also called snapping

finger and trigger finger. The other hand may be needed to help straighten the fingers, possibly followed by repeated locking.

Treatment

1. The massagist grips the patient's wrist with one hand and pulls at the affected finger gently with the other 5-50 times.

2. To remove stasis, the massagist push-presses the medial and lateral aspects as well as the palmar and dorsal aspects of the affected finger with thumb and index finger from finger tip to wrist 5-10 times.

3. Perform stronger scraping and pinch-nipping manipulations at the painful area of snapping area to stimulate the stenosed tendon sheath. In cases of masses, perform heavy pushing manipulation to remove them. There may appear slight swelling and pain in the finger, which is a normal reaction after treatment. If this happens, suspend treatment for two days. Local scraping and nipping are the main methods for curing this disease.

15. Disturbance of Small Wrist Joints

This disease has rarely been reported in the literature. A frequently occurring trauma, though not serious and only temporary, it affects the athletes' participation in competitions. It is liable to be mis-diagnosed and improperly handled.

Injury Mechanism

The wrist area comprises of the radius, ulna, two rows of carpal bones (scaphoid, lunate, triangular, pisiform, trapezium, lesser trapezium, capitate and hamate bones) and five metacarpal bones. Together, they form a number of small joints which are complicated structures, well coordinated with each other and playing specific roles to ensure that the wrist and hand perform their complicated duties well. When the wrist is suddenly pulled, turned, over-extended or over-flexed, the relations among these small joints are disturbed. Also, if some articular synovium is incarcerated into a joint, or the ligaments among joints are twisted, or articular capsules are squeezed, pathological symptoms may also appear at the wrist region.

Symptoms and Diagnosis

1. A sensation of being stuck at the wrist in physical training and competition, with slight pain.

2. Weakness in the wrist, worsening pain when moving, slight limitation of joint activity.

3. No special manifestations on examination.

Treatment

1. The massagist holds the patient's wrist, pulls and rotates in all directions, squeezes the affected wrist with two palms facing each other. The symptoms can vanish when a sound is heard. The patient may then actively practise over-flexion, over-extension and rotation of the wrist.

2. Perform digit-pressing or press-kneading manipulations at the tender area to reposition articular synovium, ligaments and muscular tendons.

3. Perform massage along the forearm and wrist to regulate the hand and restore the soft tissues. The author has given treatment on the spot to many athletes with satisfactory results.

4. Patients with frequently recurring disturbance of small wrist joints should do more wrist strength exercises to increase its stability, and also strap the wrist with wrist pads or adhesive plaster during training.

Chapter 5
INJURY OF HEAD AND NECK

1. Fracture of Nasal Bone

Injury Mechanism

The fracture is caused by direct external impact on the nasal bone.

Symptoms and Diagnosis

1. Apparent history of trauma; pain and tumefaction in the nose.

2. Nasal bleeding, abnormal appearance of nose with one or both sides looking hollow in the shape of a saddle.

3. Tenderness on pressure and a sensation of bone friction; hand can feel that the nose caves in.

4. Front-view and side-view X-ray photos help confirm fracture of the nasal bone.

Treatment

1. For cases with nasal bleeding, apply cold compress or pack the nasal cavity with cotton. If the bleeding persists, pack the nasal cavity with a strip of Vaseline gauze.

2. Manual reduction of fracture: Insert a pair of long tweezers wrapped with sterilized cotton into the nasal cavity to prop up the sunken nasal bone. After completion of fracture reduction on one side, compare with the nasal bone on the opposite side to check for accuracy. If the nasal bone on both sides is fractured, prop up the sunken nasal bone in both nasal cavities and ask the patient to examine the nasal appearance in a mirror after reduction to see if it is normal. If not satisfactory, prop up the nasal bone again.

3. With the reduction completed, the massagist applies gentle kneading from the nose bridge downward to regulate and restore the soft tissues and remove swelling.

4. Reducing nasal fracture with tweezers may stimulate nasal mucosa, causing tears and conjunctival congestion for several hours. The author has performed manual reduction of nasal bone fracture for three athletes, two basketball players and one sprinter, and nasal appearance of all of whom became normal after only one reduction.

5. Swelling in the nose after reduction is caused by fracture bleeding and contusion of nasal soft tissues. Cold compress at the bridge of the nose may help relieve it. The patient is advised not to blow or press the nose within one week after the operation.

2. Dislocation and Subluxation of Mandibular Articulation

Injury Mechanism

The mandibular articulation is composed of the small head of the mandible and the mandibular fossa of the temporal bone. In the articulation is the discoid cartilage. The front wall of the articular capsule is fairly thin, its upper part is connected with the articular prominence and the mandibular fossa of temporal bone, and its lower part adheres to the neck of the mandible. The chewing muscle consists of the masseter muscle, temporal muscle and lateral pterygoid muscle. The mandibular articulation performs four functions, namely, opening the mouth, shutting the mouth, moving back and forth, and moving laterally. When the mouth is open to the upmost, as the front part of articular capsule is thin and weak, the articular disc and the small head of the mandible dislocates from the articular fossa, causing forward dislocation of mandibular articulation, of which most cases are dislocation of both sides, while a small number involves dislocation just on one side. In partial dislocation of the articulation, there is pain and dysfunction in biting, and we call it subluxation. Repeated subluxation is also called dysfunction of biting, while repeated dislocation is called habitual dislocation of mandibular articulation.

Dislocation of mandibular articulation may be caused by direct hit in the face. Even such factors as yawning, opening the mouth wide when bursting into laughter, or chewing hard food, may cause dislocation of mandibular articulation. These affected by mandibular arthritis and local articular flaccidity are apt to suffer from subluxation and dislocation.

Symptoms and Diagnosis

1. The chief complaint of patients affected by subluxation of mandibular articulation is pain at the joint, and weakness and difficulty in chewing although they can open and shut their mouths.

2. The symptoms of total dislocation of mandibular articulation are half-open mouth, inability to close the mouth, speak fluently and swallow of saliva, and slobbering.

3. The mandible protrudes to the front and downward; one-side dislocation shows the mandible deviates to the healthy side and prolapses.

4. For subluxation of articulation, there are no particular clinical manifestations, while for dislocation the small head of the mandible displaces forward with local protrusion and its posterior side shows evident hollowness. There is no difficulty to diagnose this disease.

Treatment

1. Press acupoints Jiache (ST 6), Xiaguan (ST 7) and Hegu (LI 4) for 30-60 seconds on each side with fairly strong force to ease pain and relax the masseter.

(See Fig. 63)

2. Extra-oral-cavity reduction: This method is suitable for old and weak patients, and those suffering from subluxation or habitual dislocation of the mandibular articulation. The massagist holds the mandible at the cheeks and tracts downward and, while the mandible moves, lifts and pushes it back. A sliding sound indicates completion of the reduction. Ask the patient to open and close the mouth. If the bite is still abnormal, push and adjust the mandible for thorough reduction.

3. Inner-oral-cavity reduction: Suitable for patients suffering from total dislocation of the mandibular articulation and cases that cannot be reduced by the extra-oral-cavity method.

a) Wrap the massagist thumbs with gauze, insert them into the patient's mouth and press on the last molar bilaterally with the other four fingers holding the mandible.

b) Press the mandible downward with gradually increased strength with both thumbs to displace it downward, then lift and push it back. A sliding sound indicates completion of the reduction. The massagist must withdraw his thumbs swiftly to prevent them from being bitten by the patient's sudden mouth shutting.

c) Treatment for one-side dislocation of mandibular articulation is the same as above. The force exerted is not by the thumb on the healthy side but by pressing downward on the affected side. This is followed by lifting and pushing back the mandible with both hands. Finally, the massagist pushes the mandible left and right to achieve total reduction.

d) Post-treatment: Massage the cheeks, perform flick-poking manipulation to regulate and restore the masseter, disperse swelling and remove blood stasis to resuscitate the soft tissues. Check to see if the bite of upper and lower teeth is

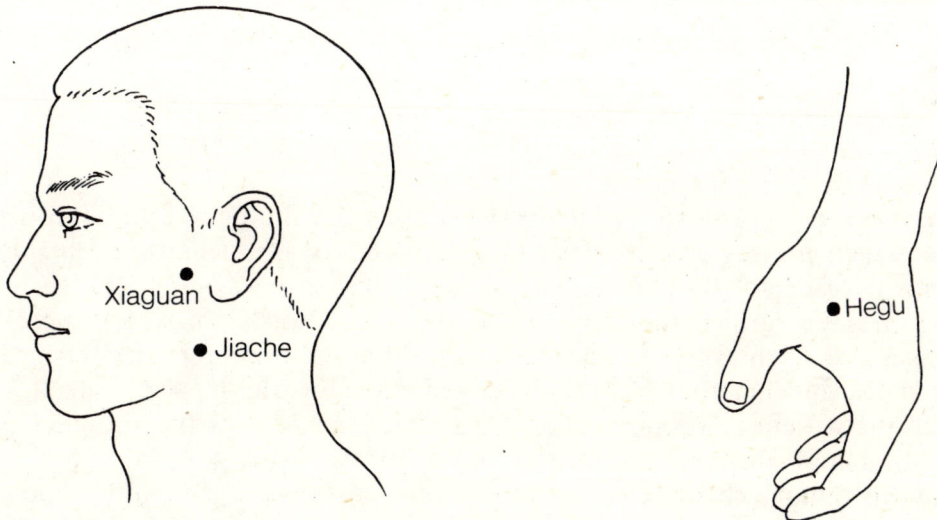

Fig. 63

correct. An uneven bite may suggest subluxation of articulation and require further reduction. Advise the patient to eat soft food and not to open the mouth wide for a week.

3. Acute Cervical Sprain

Acute cervical sprain includes injury of cervical muscles, malposition of small cervical joints and synovial incarceration.

Injury Mechanism
1. Direct external force acting on the head and neck may cause contusion at the neck region, such as contusion of the trapezius, sternocleidomastoid and splenius muscle of head. Violent external force may cause malposition of cervical joints, and even synovial incarceration and injury of ligaments.

2. Indirect cervical sprain may be caused by sudden and violent turning of head and neck, such as rolling movements during falling, head-swing in football games and over lifting of the hand in throwing events.

Symptoms and Diagnosis
1. History of trauma, with possible sound in the sprained neck.

2. Limitation of neck motion, either in one direction or all directions, manifested as leaning of the head to one side and cervical malformation. Cervical motion in any direction can only be accomplished passively, with the patient feeling pain and stiffness in the neck.

3. Neck muscles are strained; cords or scleromata are palpable, usually occurring at the interspinal region or on both sides of the spinous process.

4. X-ray examination reveals changes in physiological curvature in the cervical region but no change in bone structure.

Treatment
1. Acupoint pressing: With patient in sitting position, the massagist stands behind and presses acupoints Dazhui (DU 14), Fengchi (GB 20), Tianzong (SI 11) and Tianzhu (BL 10). (See Fig. 64)

2. The massagist grasps and pinches the muscles of the neck up and down for 3-5 rounds, then presses on the initial muscle points of the neck on both sides of the tuberosity of occipital bone.

3. The massagist grasps the trapezius at the upper border of which there may be tenderness, so the massagist may press with thumb at the intermuscular groove, which is at the upper border of and at the same level as the trapezius itself.

4. With the patient in prone position, the massagist presses the shoulder blade region with major thenar eminence of both hands. Flick-poke any cords and scleromata to remove them. This manipulation may relax the shoulder and neck muscles.

5. Feel out the tender spot and nodes at the interspinal region and at both sides

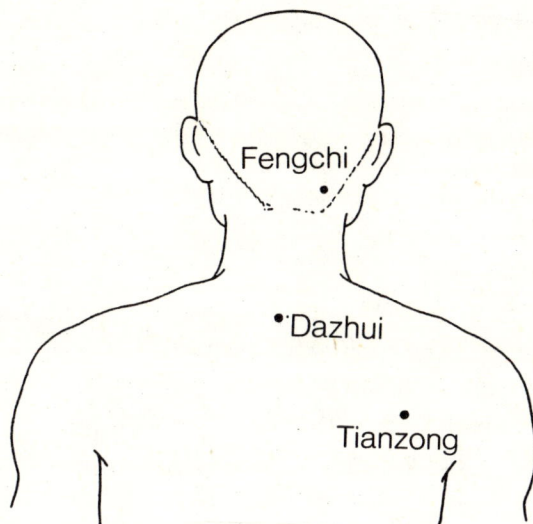

Fig. 64

of the spinous processes, deeply push and press them up and down with the thumb to repair soft tissues.

6. Tract and rotate the head: With the patient in supine position, the head resting at the bed edge, the massagist supports the mandible with one hand and the occiput with the other to tract the head slowly and rotate it by 45 degrees to each side. A snap indicates that the malpositioned small cervical joints have been reduced. Avoid abrupt rotation of the head and too forceful manipulation may exacerbate the cervical injury and even cause such harmful reactions as dizziness.

7. Finally press-knead along the neck, shoulder and back for 3-5 rounds to loosen the muscles, relax the muscles and tendons and activate the flow of qi and blood in the meridians and collaterals.

4. Stiff Neck

Injury Mechanism
1. Stiff neck caused in sleeping: Due to improper height of pillow, the muscles of neck, trapezius and sternocleidomastoid are in abnormal posture, causing myospasm or fracture. Long-term improper posture of the neck may pull the cutaneous nerve of the neck, causing local pain and pain that radiates toward distant sites accompanied by an allergic zone in the skin.

2. Stiff neck caused by spasm of blood vessels: Blood vessels which serve to supply nutrition to the cervical nerves may become spasmodic due to pathogenic wind and cold, inducing ischemia and edema in the tissues of cervical nerves and thus giving rise to symptoms in the cervical region. The patient often has a history of attack by pathogenic wind and cold at night. Hot compress or massage may

111

generate heat locally and produce a satisfactory curative effect.

Symptoms and Diagnosis

1. The patient must have a history of attack by pathogenic wind and cold at night or a history of having had the head and neck in an improper posture.

2. Sudden onset of pain and rigidity at the neck after sleep with the head leaning to one side and difficulty to move the head.

3. In serious cases there may be dizziness, strained back and back pain that might refer to the upper limbs.

4. Medical examination reveals that the trapezius and sternocleidomastoid are strained, with tenderness, cords and masses present.

Treatment

1. With the patient taking a seat, the massagist stands behind and performs press-kneading on acupoints Fengchi (BG 20) and Dazhui (DU 14) bilaterally with the thumb and index finger, and the force applied should be light at the first and gradually grows stronger until the patient feels warmth. Then, the massagist applies pinch-grasping manipulation along the muscles of the neck up and down for 5-10 times followed by pressing and flick-poking manipulation on the tender spot or masses to disperse them.

2. Perform press-kneading manipulation on the upper end of trapezius of both shoulders, i.e., the upper border of shoulder, 5-10 times with the force applied increasing gradually. Then tract and rotate the head slowly.

3. Massage may be applied at the scapula region where the trapezius lies and the first and second thoracic nerves are distributed. This can also relax the muscles and nerves.

4. Perform scrubbing manipulation at the neck, shoulder and back until the skin turns red so as to dispel pathogenic wind and cold.

5. Cervical Spondylopathy

Cervical spondylopathy is a syndrome with hyperosteogeny at the cervical spine as the main symptom and complicated by pathological changes in the peripheral soft tissues of neck, nerves and blood vessels. The incidence of this disease increases with advancing age after thirty.

Injury Mechanism

1. All types of acute injury and chronic strain of the cervical region may lead to injury of the cervical intervertebral disc, ligaments, articular capsule and peripheral soft tissues, reduce the stability of the cervical vertebrae themselves and cause compensatory hyperplasia of bony substance at the cervical vertebrae. This hyperplastic substance may directly or indirectly constrict the nerves and blood vessels, resulting in a series of symptoms. As indicated by domestic records, out of 1,000 patients suffering from cervical spondylopathy 60 percent have a history of

trauma ranging from three to fourteen years.

2. Retrograde degeneration of tissues. Degeneration of cervical intervertebral disk appears after the age of thirty and becomes more apparent after fifty in such forms as ossification of bone plate, dehydration of pulpiform nucleus, rupture of fibrous ring due to loss of elasticity, narrowing of cervical intervertebral disc and cervical intervertebral space, reduction of stability of cervical vertebrae, hyperplasia of cervical vertebral joints and hamate vertebral articulation due to friction, hypertrophy or calcification of articular capsule and ligaments, edema of soft tissues. All these changes may constrict nerves and blood vessels and cause various clinical symptoms, the types of which differ depending on the varied positions and degree of constriction.

3. If it is rare that the nerves and blood vessels are constricted directly; in most cases they are constricted indirectly. Symptoms caused by indirect constriction refer to such ones resulting from hyperplasia of cervical vertebrae as disturbance of intervertebral facet joints, inflammatory edema at ligaments, and poor blood supply and myospasm at local areas caused by attack of pathogenic wind and cold in the neck, i.e., manifestations caused by stagnation of qi and blood vessels. This can explain why some patients who are affected by serious hyperplasia do not show obvious clinical manifestations, while others who have no evident hyperplasia do have apparent clinical manifestations. Surgery is generally required to relieve compression in cases when the nerves and blood vessels are constricted directly, while manual treatment is sufficient to relax symptoms in cases with the nerves and blood vessels compressed indirectly. Manual treatment is mainly to achieve the curative effects of promoting blood circulation by removing blood stasis, expelling pathogenic wind and cold, relieving rigidity of muscles and activating collaterals while restoring and treating the injured soft tissues.

Symptoms and Diagnosis

1. Cervical spondylopathy of the nerve root type — the most common type:

a) The patient has pain in the neck and nuchal regions and radiating pain in the shoulder and upper limbs, accompanied by numbness; the skin in the diseased region is slow in sensation; the upper limbs and hands are asthenic; pain and numbness become more serious when the diseased limb is compressed during sleep. The manifestations differ for pathological changes in different cervical intervertebral spaces — pathological changes above the fourth cervical intervertebral space are manifested as pain or numbness at the neck and occiput; pathological changes between the fourth and fifth cervical intervertebrae are manifested as pain from the neck and shoulder to the anterolateral aspect of the upper arm and the lateral aspect of the forearm to the wrist; pathological changes between the fifth and sixth cervical intervertebrae are manifested as pain and numbness at the neck and back, from the lateral aspect of upper arm and forearm to the thumb, and weakening of biceps muscle strength; pathological changes between the sixth and seventh cervical intervertebrae are manifested as pain and numbness from the neck, back and the posterior aspect of the upper arm and forearm to the index and middle fingers, and decrease of the brachial triceps muscle strength; and pathological changes between the seventh cervical intervertebra and the first thoracic vertebra are manifested as pain and numbness in the medial aspects of the upper arm and forearm, ring and little fingers and the medial border of scapula.

b) Tender points: There are tender points at the injured nerve, at the zone controlled by the nerve, beside the cervical spinous processes, at the lateral aspect of arm and in the region between the scapulae. Scleromata and cords may be palpated at the neck, back and shoulder regions.

c) Traction and pulling test of brachial plexus: The massagist presses the patient's head with one hand so that it leans to the healthy side, holds the patient's wrist on the diseased side and tracts the upper limb with the other. The result will be positive for those patients with pain and numbness in the neck and upper limbs.

d) Vertex-percussion test: With the patient in sitting position, the massagist rests one hand on his head and percusses the back of the hand with the other hand. Those who feel radiating pain in the neck and upper limbs are positive.

e) Cervical intervertebral foramen-squeezing test: With the patient in sitting position with the head falling slightly back and leaning to the diseased side, the massagist presses the vertex downward. Patients feeling radiating pain in the neck and upper limbs are positive.

f) Other conditions to be ruled out: Neck sprain, stiff neck, neck and shoulder fascitis, periarthritis of shoulder, tuberculosis of cervical vertebrae, dislocated fracture of cervical spine and tumour of cervical vertebrae.

g) X-ray photograph: Front-view X-ray photo of the cervical vertebrae shows hyperosteogeny at the hamate cervical articulations; side-way photo shows hyperosteogeny at the front and rear borders of the vertebral body and calcification shadow at the nuchal ligament; while left and right photos show intrusion of spurs into the intervertebral foramen and the change of the intervertebral foramen contour. The degree of cervical hyperosteogeny may not be in direct ratio to that of clinical manifestations.

2. Cervical spondylopathy of the vertebral artery type: Aside from the symptoms apparent in cases of the nerve root type, there are also the symptoms seen in poor blood supply to the vertebral artery, such as dizziness, vomiting, vertigo, tinnitus, deafness and blurred vision. These symptoms may be induced by sudden turning of head and so must be differentiated from Meunière's syndrome, which is related to over-fatigue, inadequate sleep and poor state of mind and is not induced by cervical movement.

3. Cervical spondylopathy of the sympathetic nerve type: The following clinical symptoms may appear due to reflex stimulation of the sympathetic nerves caused by pathological changes in such tissues as dura mater of neck of spinal cord, facet joints, ligaments, nerve root and vertebral artery.

a) Eye and ear region: Blurred vision and swollen eyes, and sometimes deafness and tinnitus.

b) Head region: Headache, dizziness and pain in the nape.

c) Heart: Heart beat quickens and slows down; there is an unwell feeling at the pericardium and chest distress.

d) Four limbs: Feeling of cold, heat, numbness and hyperalgia in the four limbs, hyperidrosis or hypohydrosis in certain parts of the body.

e) Other diseases to be ruled out: Neurovascular migraine, coronary heart disease, neurosis, vegetative nerve functional disturbance and menopausal syndrome.

4. Cervical spondylopathy of the spinal cord type: Symptoms of this disorder are caused by direct constriction of spinal cord due to retrograde cervical intervertebral disc, spurs at the rear aspect of vertebral bodies, hyperosteogeny of facet joints, and thickening and calcification of yellow ligament. This is a serious type of cervical spondylopathy.

a) Light case: Pain in the neck and shoulder, headache and dizziness, aching and distending pain, trembling and asthenia in limbs.

b) Serious case: Asthenia of both upper and lower limbs, inability to hold objects, difficulty in walking, even paralysis of all limbs, difficulty in urination and defection. This must be differentiated from dislocated fracture of the cervical bone, tuberculosis and tumour in cervical vertebra.

Treatment

1. Points for attention:

a) Diagnosis should be definite and correct. Manual treatment cannot be performed for such diseases as dislocated fracture of cervical spine, tuberculosis, tumours and serious hyperosteogeny.

b) If it is not advisable to give manual treatment to patients suffering from hypertension, serious coronary heart disease, poor blood supply to the brain and serious cervical spondylopathy of the spinal cord type, and to the aged and weak patients.

c) The manipulations should be gentle. Avoid forceful rotation manipulation on the head so as to prevent cerebrovascular and cardiovascular accidents as well as spinal cord injury.

2. Functions of manual treatment:

a) Acupoint pressing may relieve pain and numbness as well as dredge the meridians and collaterals.

b) Traction performed through the head may widen intervertebral foramen, intervertebral space and reposition the disordered face joints to reduce constriction on nerves and blood vessels.

c) Relax and ease muscular tension and spasm of the neck and limbs.

d) Improve blood circulation of the head and neck and stimulate adjacent nerves to recover normal body functions.

3. Manual treatment:

a) Press and select proper acupoints from the following according to disease: Dazhui (DU 14), Fengfu (DU 16), Fengchi (GB 20), Tianding (LI 17), Quepen (ST 12), Jiquan (HT 1), Tianzong (SI 11), Quchi (LI 11), Hegu (LI 4), Yangxi (LI 5) and Yanggu (SI 5). (See Fig. 65)

b) With the patient in supine or sitting position, the massagist performs pull-grasping manipulation on neck muscles from the occiput downward 5-10 times; performs pressing on the upper part of both shoulders and back, as well as rolling manipulation to relax muscles of the shoulders, back and neck.

c) The massagist performs push-pressing manipulation with thumbs from the second cervical vertebra along the spinous processes and on both sides of the spinous processes; use heavier pressing manipulation at the tender points and at the hypertrophy or masses along the spinous processes to disperse them. This is an important method for curing the disease, so the location of pathological changes should be carefully palpated.

d) With the patient in supine position, the massagist stands at the head of the bed with one hand holding the patient's mandible and the other the occiput, tracts the head slowly with force for 3-5 minutes while turning the head left and right to a 45-degree angle. A "crack" may be heard. This method is safer and more reliable than that of lateral sudden pulling of the head with the patient in a sitting position and is thus more suitable for the aged and those with serious symptoms.

e) With the patient in sitting position, the massagist presses one hand on one shoulder and holds the head with the other, then with both hands exerts force toward the opposite directions to tract the neck, i.e., the brachial plexus. Apply this same manipulation on the other side.

f) For patients with pain and numbness in various regions of the limbs, perform

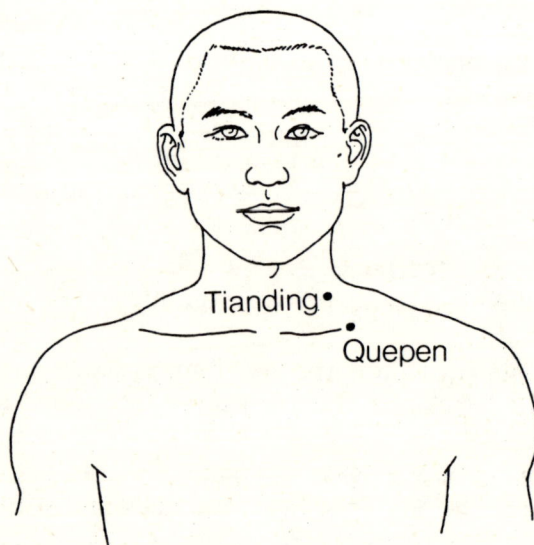

Fig. 65

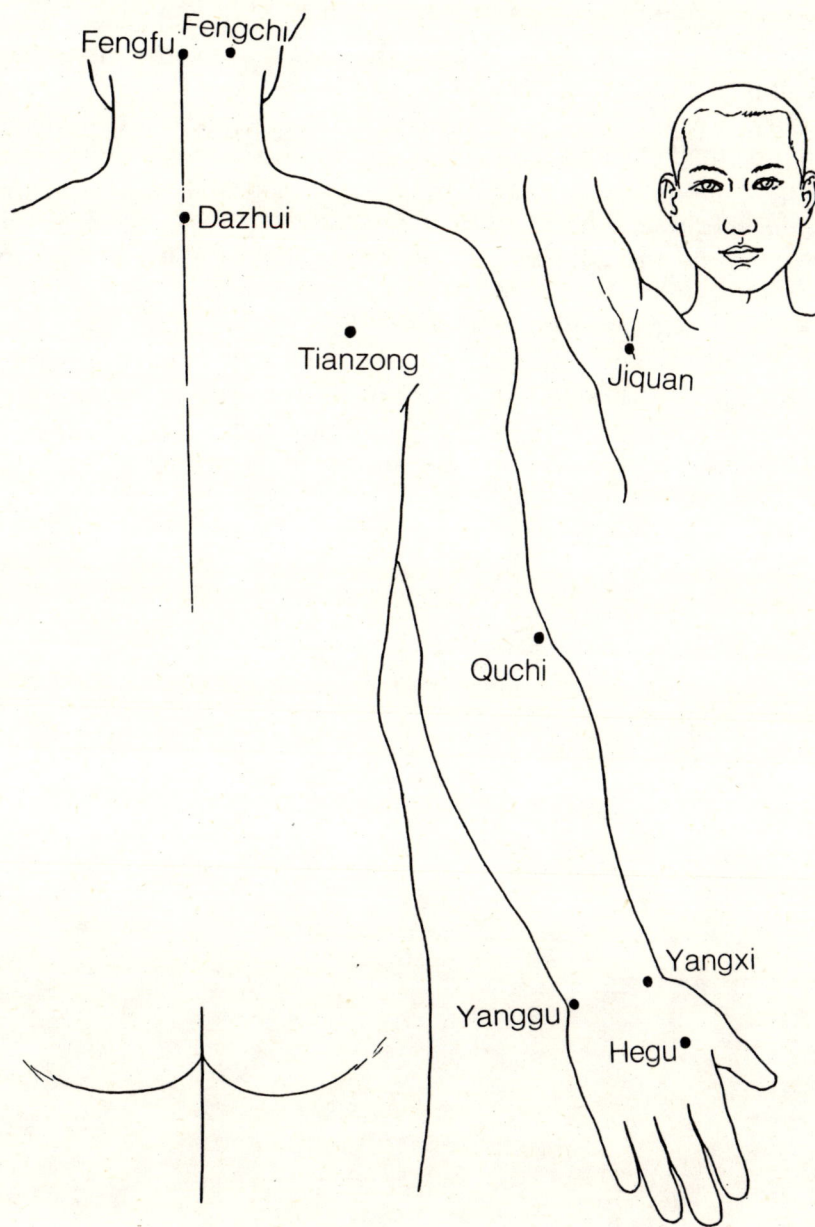

Fengfu

Fengchi

Dazhui

Tianzong

Jiquan

Quchi

Yangxi

Yanggu

Hegu

Fig. 65

117

digit-pressing manipulation accompanied by press-kneading on soft tissues to relieve myospasm and improve nerve and blood vessel functions. Pressing the acupoints Tianding (LI 17), Quepen (ST 12) and Zhongfu (LU 1) may stimulate and excite the brachial plexus. Pressing acupoints Jiquan (HT 1) and Quchi (LI 11) may temporarily block blood supply to the axillary and brachial arteries. Then suddenly releasing the pressing causes the blood flow to impact on the blood vessels, promptly improving blood supply.

g) The patient who has the symptoms of headache, dizziness, blurred vision and deafness can be made to take a sitting position with the massagist standing behind and pressing acupoint Fengfu (DU 16) on both sides. The patient may feel heat generated at the head and neck. Then the massagist presses or kneads both temples for one minute and digitally presses acupoint Baihui (DU 20) and push-presses acupoint Yintang (EX HN 3) with both index and middle fingers toward both sides of the forehead to the temples 5-10 times. Scrapes with the ten finger tips from the front hair line, passing the vertex to the back hair line as in combing the hair until the scalp feels warm and slightly painful; performs scraping with the middle section of the index fingers from both temples backward 10 times; and finally performs gentle push-pressing along the supercilliary arch and the zygomatic bone horizontally, i.e., push-presses the regions above and under the eyes 5-10 times.

Chapter 6
INJURY OF THORACO-ABDOMINAL REGION

1. Disturbance of Posterior Thoracic Vertebral Joint

The posterior thoracic vertebrae include the upper and lower small zygapophyseal joints, costovertebral joints and costotransverse joints.

Injury Mechanism

Forceful simultaneous turning of the upper limbs and the thoracodorsal region, such as in the movement of throwing, may cause malposition of various small thoracic vertebral joints, especially the small joints between the fifth and sixth, and between the 10th and 11th thoracic vertebrae. Such malposition is often accompanied by injury to the articular synovium and may be acute injury or chronic strain.

Symptoms and Diagnosis

1. Back pain: In acute injury the pain is prominent while in chronic strain the back feels stiff. The pain may radiate to the shoulder and neck or to the front thoracic region along the intercostal nerves.

2. Examination may reveal limited tenderness beside the thoracic vertebrae as well as tenderness at the spinous processes and the interspinal regions; the back muscles feel tense, and there are possibly scleromata and cords.

Treatment

1. Press acupoints Tianzong (SI 11), Jianjing (GB 21) and Fengmen (BL 12). (See Fig. 66)

2. The massagist presses the back muscles on both sides with overlapping palms and grasps these muscles during rolling manipulation to relax them.

3. Sudden and forceful pressing on the back may evoke a sound at the joints, indicating the reduction of the small joints, and then most patients will feel the back pain eased. For patients with well-developed muscles, press the back with both fists. The strength should be deep but bounding and it should never be rude. Otherwise, it will cause rib fracture.

4. Place the palm or palm end of one hand on the thumb of the other and press downward hard along both sides of the spinous processes to regulate and restore the posterior small thoracic vertebral joints and ligaments; then perform transverse plucking with the thumb on the spinous processes to regulate and restore the

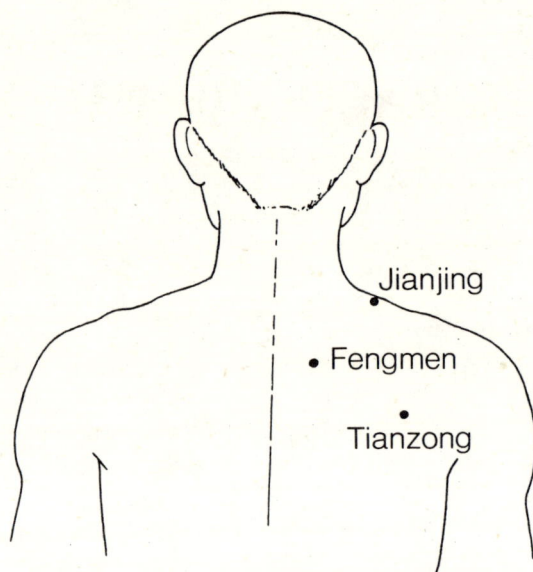

Fig. 66

supraspinal and interspinal ligaments; and finally beat the back fast and gently with both fists or palms to relax the muscles and tendons and promote blood circulation. Do sufficient warm-up exercises before physical training and competition.

2. Rib Fracture and Dislocation

Rib fracture, whether of one or more ribs, is a serious injury. There may also be fracture and dislocation of costal cartilages.

Injury Mechanism

1. Causes of rib fracture and dislocation:

a) Direct external force: Any external force may directly cause this injury. For instance, collision in basketball games may cause the elbow to hit the thoracic region, or the thoracic region may bump on the apparatus in the gymnasium. The fracture occurs at the site of the injury.

b) Indirect external force: When the external force acts on the front and back aspects of the thoracic region, bilateral rib fracture is likely to occur, such as in crush injuries in the thoracic region and in motorcycle accidents.

c) Sudden and forceful muscle contraction: Sudden and violent turning of the body and fierce contraction of the intercostal muscle may also cause rib fracture and dislocation.

2. Site of rib fracture and dislocation:

a) Rib fracture: The first, second and third ribs are not easily fractured as they are protected by the clavicle and scapula; the costal cartilages under the seventh rib also are not easily fractured as they are not linked to the sternum but above the costal cartilage and have good elasticity; and fracture of the 11th and 12th ribs is even rare as they are floating ribs. Those ribs most commonly seen fractured are the fourth, fifth and sixth.

b) Fracture and dislocation of costal cartilage include dislocation of sternocostal joint, fracture of costal cartilage, dislocation of costochondral joints and separation of neighbouring costal cartilages.

3. Complications of rib fracture: The fractured rib may pierce the pleura, lung tissues and blood vessels, causing such serious complications as injury to the lungs, pneumothorax, haemothorax and shock.

Symptoms and Diagnosis

1. Chest pain, which becomes more serious during deep breathing, coughing and chest-expanding movements.

2. Local tumefaction and ecchymoma, distinct tenderness and bone crepitation. Tenderness at the fractured region is felt when squeezing from any direction. This is the key point for diagnosis.

3. Local protrusion or hollowness.

4. The patient may find it difficult to breath when there is pneumothorax or haemothorax. Haemorrhage in the thoracic cavity may cause symptoms of shock and require emergency treatment.

5. X-ray examination may confirm rib fracture but not fracture or dislocation of costal cartilage. So there may be mis-diagnosed for the latter, for which the diagnosis should be based on clinical manifestations.

Treatment

1. Press acupoints Zhangmen (LR 13), Qimen (LR 14) and Danzhong (RN 17). (See Fig. 67)

2. Making the patient to sit down with both arms up behind the head, the massagist slowly press-squeeze on the protrusion of fracture of dislocation to diminish it and achieve reduction.

3. Apply pressing and restoring manipulation on the chest wall from the back to the front along the ribs to better reduce the fracture, regulate the muscles and tissues and dredge the meridians and collaterals to remove blood stasis and promote blood circulation.

4. Adhesive plaster strapping: With the patient taking in a deep breath, the massagist apply the strapping by winding several pieces of 7-cm wide adhesive plaster starting from the upper chest, passing around the back to the front of the chest again. The tapes should overlap, the range of strapping in line with the number of fractured ribs. Each tape should exceed half the circumference of the thorax in length. Strap for three weeks, and after removal of the strapping, practise deep breathing and chest expansion with the doctor applying gentle massage on the chest wall.

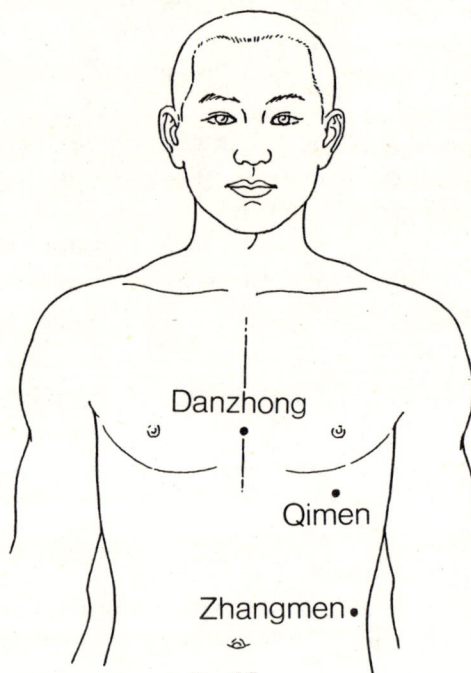

Danzhong

Qimen

Zhangmen

Fig. 67

3. Contusion of Chest Wall

A common injury, the contusion of chest wall includes contusion of chest wall muscles, subluxation of costovertebral joint and synovial incarceration (i.e., *cha qi* or chest pain on breathing).

Injury Mechanism

1. Direct trauma: Impact of dull force on the chest may cause injury of chest wall soft tissues, causing pain, swelling and blood stasis. This may occur in mutual collision in basketball, from a boxing blow in the chest, bumping of gymnasts against the apparatus during failure in athletic performance, and a direct hit in the chest by a football.

2. Improper exertion of force in the chest and upper limbs, such as over-extension and sudden body turning, may lead to spasm of chest muscles, subluxation of costovertebral joint and synovial incarceration. The contusion can also be caused by sudden sneezing, jumping, weight lifting, throwing and carrying heavy load. Over-strain of muscles can cause spasm and stimulate the intercostal nerve, thus causing pain that radiates along the intercostal nerve.

Symptoms and Diagnosis

1. Most patients have a history of trauma and pain in the chest that becomes serious during coughing or breathing deeply. The pain may refer to the chest or

the back. Because some thoracic muscles are linked with the upper arm, there is pain in the chest when the upper limbs are lifted.

2. Tenderness occurs at or around the injured area. When there is myospasm, subluxation of small joints or synovial incarceration, the chest pain becomes reflex in the intercostal nerve, so normally it is hard to find a distinct tender spot.

3. Tumefaction: Local swelling and ecchymoma may be found in serious contusion of soft tissues, and masses may be felt.

4. X-ray examination do not find abnormal symptoms except for cases of rib fracture.

Treatment

1. With the patient in supine position, the massagist performs palm-rubbing on the chest area along with digit-pressing on the acupoints Zhangmen (LR 13) and Danzhong (RN 17).

2. Push-kneading manipulation: The massagist push-kneads along the ribs downward with both palms or palm ends 5-10 times, then do the same on the back. The force used should be even and deep-reaching. Use flat-pushing to disperse any masses or blood stasis.

3. The massagist presses the patient's back until a "crack" being heard, indicating completion of reduction of the subluxation of small joints. The patient will feel an immediate relaxation of the pain at the chest and back.

4. Injury of Abdominal Muscles

The abdominal muscles include the external oblique, the internal oblique, the straight and the transverse muscles of the abdomen.

Injury Mechanism

1. Direct external force: Such as hitting the abdomen by a football, blow at the abdomen in boxing and bumping against the apparatus during failure in athletic performance.

2. Pulling of abdominal muscles: Sudden throwing out and contraction of abdomen in long jump may pull the abdominal muscles, so do in pole vault and back-style high jump. The most common is the pulling of the abdominal straight muscle, followed by the pulling of the external and internal oblique muscles. The abdominal muscles are more likely to be pulled in cold weather when there is not enough warming-up or there is fatigue.

3. Spasm of abdominal muscles may also cause the pulling. Excessive physical exercises can lead to spasm of abdominal muscles as well as spasm of gastrocnemius. In addition, myospasm can also be caused by water-electrolyte imbalance due to rapid loss of body weight.

Symptoms and Diagnosis

1. Only abdominal pain occurs in light cases of direct abdominal trauma, while

in serious cases there is severe abdominal pain, tension of abdominal muscles and tenderness. Direct impact of a heavy force on the abdomen can bring a strong stimulation to the solar plexus in the abdominal cavity, probably resulting in the patient's collapse or coma. When the abdomen bumps against something hard, there may be slight trauma to the skin and subcutaneous bleeding. As violent external force can also cause injury to organs in the abdominal cavity and to such parenchymatous organs as the liver, spleen, kidney, stomach and intestines, serious injury to the abdominal muscles must be differentiated from injury to these organs. In serious injury to the abdominal wall, injury to the organs should not be ruled out light-heartedly and the condition must be observed closely to prevent mistaken diagnosis.

2. Pulled abdominal muscles cause pain, the area of which is extensive and there is no distinct tender point, with tenderness in the center of the abdomen being more serious. In a light case of abdominal muscle pulling pain is felt when throwing out and contracting the abdomen, while in a serious case the patient cannot straighten the back, the body tends to bend forward and there is muscular tension.

3. Abdominal myospasm does not necessarily come with trauma and pulling. It gives rise to severe pain in the abdominal wall, for which the patient has to bend the body and cannot straighten the back; the abdominal muscles feel definitely tense and scleromata may be felt. These symptoms may disappear spontaneously after a while though mild pain in the abdomen may persist.

Treatment

1. Timely surgical operation should be given to injury of abdominal muscle complicated by injury of internal organs.

2. Spasm of abdominal muscles: Digit-press the acupoint Zusanli (ST 36) on both sides with strong force. Perform rub-stroking manipulation on the surface of the abdomen, with the force applied developing from light to heavy. The result should prompt relaxation of symptoms. To avoid recurrence, the amount of physical training should be cut and water-electrolyte replenished to correct the water-electrolyte imbalance.

3. Pulling of abdominal muscles: Press acupoint Zusanli (ST 36) on both sides, and press and stroke the abdomen with a force mild enough not to increase the pain. Press, stroke and scrub the abdomen the next day to promote blood circulation. Starting from the third day, these manipulations should be added with plucking and pushing to disperse any cords and scleromata. Finally, relax the muscles with gentle press-kneading. In order to prevent re-pulling of the muscles, the patient should gradually increase strength exercises of the abdomen.

4. Trauma of abdominal muscles: All the manipulations discussed in the previous paragraph can be applied in cases of slight trauma of the abdominal muscles, while for serious cases, local cold compress or external application of traditional Chinese medicine is needed for pain control, detumescence and removal of blood stasis. Starting from the next day of injury, rub-stroking and press-

kneading manipulations can be applied on the abdomen; and from the third day pushing and plucking manipulations are used to remove blood stasis and disperse scleromata, and pull-grasping manipulation is applied 5-10 times to relieve swelling of subcutaneous tissues. The patient can gradually start contraction of abdominal muscles after a week but is not advised to resume physical training too soon when the muscles are not fully healed. Unhealed trauma might leave scars and weaken the strength of the abdominal muscles.

Chapter 7
INJURY OF LUMBAR REGION

1. Acute Lumbar Sprain

Acute lumbar sprain, the most frequent among lumbar injuries, is one cause of lumbago and backache.

Injury Mechanism

1. Bending the waist to lift heavy objects: Over-extension in weight-lifting may cause strain due to unbalanced exertion of the two sides of the body. Over-extension of such muscles as the sacrospinal muscles, the quadrate muscles of loins, the greater psoas muscles and certain deeply located small muscles may also cause injury to lumbar ligaments (the anterior longitudinal, posterior longitudinal, interspinal and supraspinal ligaments as well as the yellow ligaments). Lifting over-heavy objects causes contraction of the back and buttock muscles, and if the load cannot be lifted, the strong force transmits to the lumbar region and causes sprain. Lifting heavy objects in a squatting position may avoid lumbar sprain.

2. Improper position of rotation of the lumbar region may cause sprain of the muscles and dislocation of the small vertebral joints, such as in discus and hammer throwing incoordinate movements in swift rotation of the body can cause sprain in the lumbar region.

3. Direct impact of external force on lumbar region: External force from sudden mutual collision in football and ice-hockey games may cause sprain of the back muscles and ligaments and may even cause laceration of ligaments and fracture.

4. Over-flexion and over-extension of spine may lead to lumbar strain. A gymnast not fully warmed up for doing somersaults is subject to lumbar sprain.

5. Lumbar sprain can also be caused by incorrect standing position, sudden turning of the lumbar region and even by coughing or sneezing.

If spinal movements exceed the normal range due to external force, temporary over-pulling and turning may occur, causing extension and laceration of muscles, ligaments and articular capsules as well as swelling, hyperaemia and bleeding in soft tissues. Rupture of articular capsules is accompanied by haemarthrosis. Organization of haemarthrosis causes adhesion in the joints. Organization of muscular and ligamental tissues may induce fibroid adhesion. Over-pulling of ligaments may cause avulsion fracture of vertebral column. In some cases lumbar sprain is complicated by injury of superior clunial nerves, piriformis and lumbo-dorsal fascia.

Symptoms and Diagnosis

1. Lumbago and backache: The pain is distinct and confined to a certain area which the patient can locate precisely and is important in diagnosis. Some patients hear a snap and feel laceration in the affected part followed by constant pain. Light-case patients can walk with some effort, while those seriously affected cannot. The pain becomes more serious when coughing, yawning, defecating or urinating. All movements are possible only in fixed position; the patient has difficulty standing up or sitting down.

2. Tender area: As a chief complaint, local tenderness is often found at the initial stage. In order to palpate the tender area, inspection at various areas of the lumbar region is necessary. Different from other types of lumbago, the tender area of lumbar sprain usually occurs at the sacrospinal muscle and at both sides of the lumbosacral joints, a difference that helps the diagnosis.

3. Myospasm of lumbodorsal muscles: Most such patients suffer from muscular tone of lumbodorsal muscles of one or both sides, and cords or scleromata are palpable. The pain and muscular tone gets worse in waist-bending or standing positions and is somewhat relieved with rest. The muscles are again strained on pressure; movement of lumbar region in all directions is limited. When only one side is affected, spasm is apparent when bending at the waist toward the opposite side.

4. Lateral curvature of spine: No signs of swelling are seen in the lumbar region, though lateral curvature of spine is apparent in some patients in standing position; in others lateral curvature is apparent in forward-bending position, while in some other cases it disappears in forward-bending position. The direction of lateral curvature is referable to the area of injury to muscles and ligaments.

5. Radiative and referrable neuralgia: About half of the patients suffering acute lumbar sprain suffer from radiative and referrable neuralgia mainly in the buttocks (superior clunial nerves and piriformis), lateral aspect of thigh (distributive area of cutaneous nerve at the lateral aspect of thigh), posterior aspect of thigh (distributive area of sciatic nerve), and the anteromedial aspect of thigh. The patient may feel radiative pain in defecation and urination and referrable pain when lifting the lower limbs.

Treatment

Early and effective treatment is necessary for relieving pain and preventing sequelae. The treatment should be given to both the principal and secondary aspects as well as the symptoms and causes of the disease simultaneously.

1. Digitally press acupoints Shenshu (BL 23), Huantiao (GB 30), Weizhong (BL 40), Chengshan (BL 57), Taixi (KI 3) and Yaoyan (Extra) to relax spasm of lumbar muscles and relieve pain. This is to make preparation for the ensuing manual treatment. In particular, press and knead the acupoints Taixi (KI 3) and Kunlun (BL 60), i.e., the Achilles tendon bilaterally for 3-5 minutes with the thumbs and fingers to relieve lumbago and improve the mobility of the lumbar area. (See Fig. 68)

2. Manual relaxation of muscles and tendons with the patient in standing

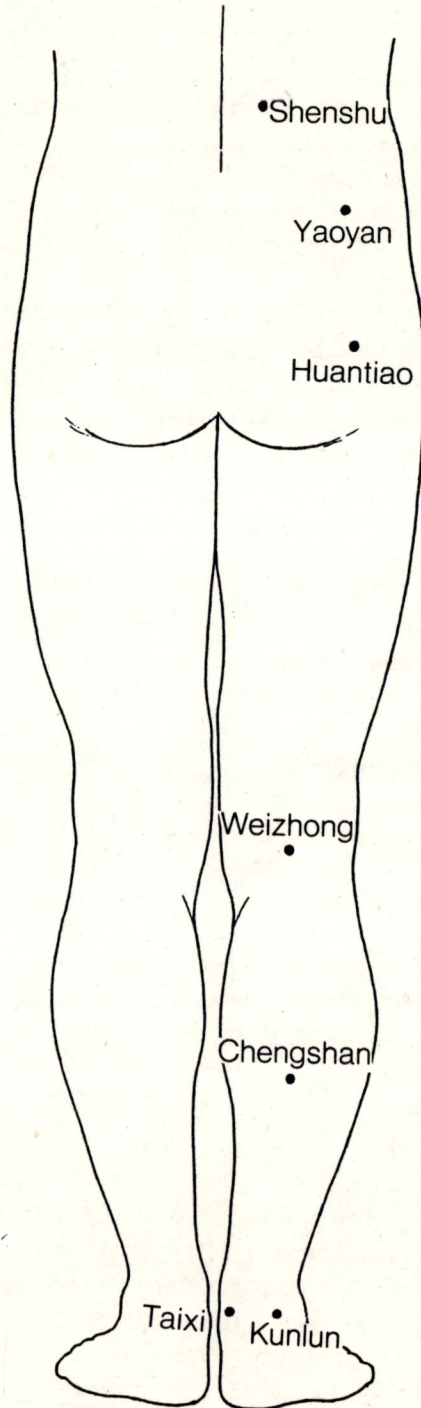

•Shenshu

•Yaoyan

•Huantiao

Weizhong
•

Chengshan
•

Taixi• •Kunlun

Fig. 68

position: (See Fig. 69)

a) With the patient in standing position, an assistant supports the elbow of the affected side and asks the patient to raise both hands and head, relaxing back muscles. The massagist pushes and presses the lumbar and back muscles from the back downward. This treatment may also be applied with the patient leaning his body against a wall and raising both hands.

b) The massagist stands beside the patient with one hand pressing the abdomen, the other pressing the painful site, and push-pressing hard. A snap may be heard. The patient is advised to turn, flex and extend the waist. (See Fig. 70)

c) Pat the back up and down with fist and palm, especially the injured parts.

d) Holding the back of the patient whose pain is aggravated when extending the waist. The massagist and the patient stand back to back with the massagist holding both the patient's arms and bending over to hold the patient on his back with both the latter's feet off the floor, and rocks right and left. Upon hearing a click, the massagist places the patient down gently for bed rest. (See Fig. 71)

3. Manual relaxation of muscles and tendons with the patient in prone position:

a) With the patient in prone position, the massagist kneads and presses with both palms from back to waist for spasmolysis and to promote the flow of qi and blood.

b) The massagist presses both sides of the spinous process with the thumb of one hand and places the palm of the other hand atop the thumb to increase the pressing force. This manipulation can help restore the soft tissues along the spinous process, relax the sacrospinal muscles and restore the malpositioned small joints.

c) Grasp the sacrospinal muscles of both sides to extend them passively, and scrape the existing cords and scleromata with thumbs repeatedly to dispel them.

d) Inverse pulling method: If the right side is affected, the massagist stands to the left, presses the painful area hard with the palm of the left hand, flexes the elbow of his right arm to bring the patient's right leg backward so that the right side of the pelvis is off the bed. Then press the waist downward with sudden and strong force to ensure an over-extension movement of the lumbar and hip region. A click indicates completion of the treatment. This method can also be applied to both lower limbs. (See Fig. 72)

e) While asking an assistant to pull the patient's lower limb downward to widen the articular space and stretch the lumbar muscles, the massagist presses the affected area hard. A click may be heard. Then, making the patient in supine position, the massagist holds the leg, flexes the knee and hip to effect flexion and traction of the waist. This is to be repeated 5-10 times. (See Fig. 73)

f) Lateral pulling method: Making the patient lying on the side with the leg on the bed stretching straight and that on top flexing, the massagist stands behind the patient and presses the anterior part of the shoulder and buttock with both elbows respectively and pushes and pulls hard in opposite directions to turn the waist

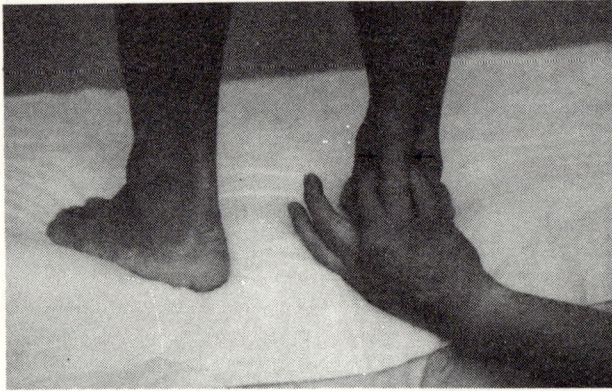

Fig. 69

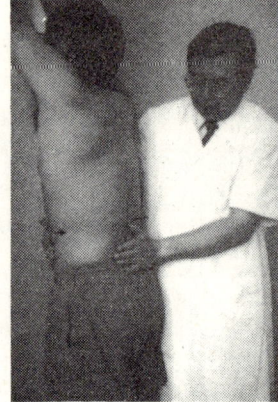

Fig. 70

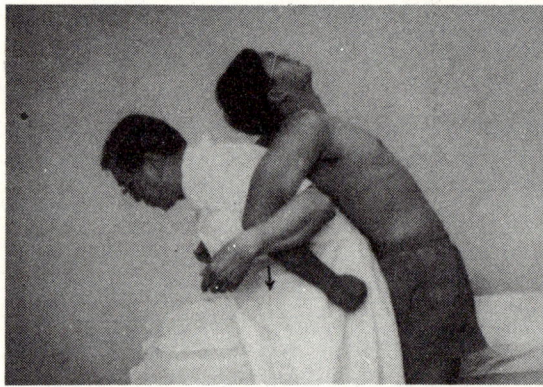

Fig. 71

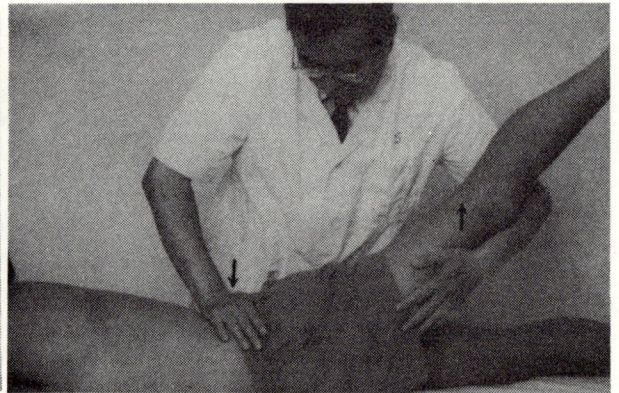

Fig. 72

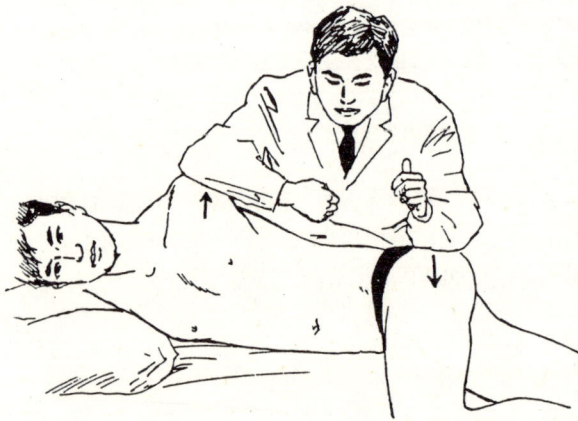

Fig. 73

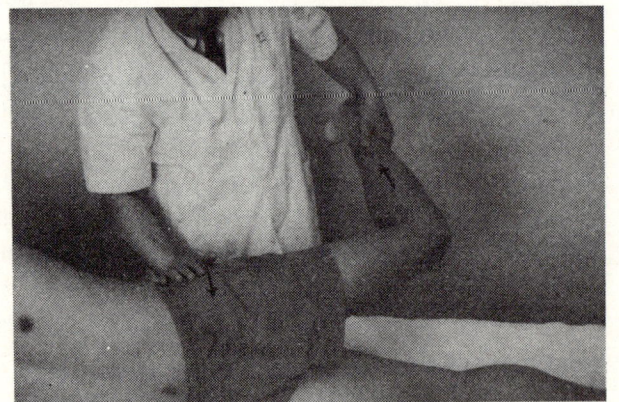

Fig. 74

passively. A click indicates completion of the treatment. Or, push the affected area with one hand and tract the lower limb backward with the other. (See Fig. 74)

4. Suspension traction method: Making the patient hold a high horizontal or transverse bar with both hands, the feet off the floor to ensure traction by the body weight for 1-2 minutes, while the massagist pushes the injured part and shakes the waist when a click is heard. Then make the patient lie flat while the muscles are relaxed by pressing and kneading.

After treatment of lumbar sprain by various manipulating methods, the patient should be advised to do a few flexion and extension exercises, but no rotation. He should also be advised to take bed for 2-3 days, keep the lumbar area warm so as to promote the rehabilitation of the injured muscles and ligaments and the relieve of edema and haematoma.

Example: Mr. Ma is a shot putter. His back was injured in May 1988 when receiving training in the United States. He even could not bend over to tie his shoelaces. Because of his well-developed muscles and body weight, pulling was not suitable in this case, so the author strapped his hands onto a horizontal bar with a cloth belt, held him by the waist and pulled downward, then pushed and shook his waist. The pain was eased immediately after treatment. He resumed normal training after a rest of two days.

2. Lumbar Strain

Lumbar strain refers to chronic injuries of lumbar and back muscles, fasciae, ligaments, articular capsules and bony tissues. This injury is a main cause of lumbago and backache.

Injury Mechanism

1. In normal conditions, the intervertebral discs, small joints and ligaments are well coordinated and they facilitate and support each other automatically. This kind of coordination is usually referred to as internal balance and is not subject to control by subjective will. Long-time activity exceeding certain limits, incorrect movements or improper exertion of strength can all cause chronic injuries. Lumbar muscles are well coordinated in action. We call this external balance, or active coordination subject to control by the subjective will. However, injury may also occur when muscular movements exceed certain limits or the muscles are in a state of prolonged tension.

2. Inadequate treatment and recuperation of acute lumbar injury may result in such sequelae as repeated lumbar injury, local bleeding and exudation, tissue fibrosis and abrading of bone joints.

3. Lumbar strain can also be caused by long-time incorrect position of lumbo-dorsal region in sports activities, excessive training and frequent repetition of a single movement.

4. Fatigue and long-term exposure to exogenous cold, wind and dampness may

lead to dysfunction of nerves and blood vessels as well as qi stagnation and blood stasis.

Symptoms and Diagnosis

1. Some patients may have a medical history of acute or repeated lumbar strain, while others, though without an obvious history of traumatic injury, must have had prolonged training with excessive burden on the lumbar region, causing a course of disease ranging from several months to several years.

2. Lumbago and backache: In most cases the pain is dull; there is heaviness and tension in the lumbar and back region, repeated recurrence of symptoms may become more serious when tired and be relieved after resting. The athlete can manage to go on with training but feels feeble in the lumbar region. Lumbago may occur in rainy or overcast weather.

3. Tender area: The patients feels painful over a large area in the lumbodorsal region; a tender area may be palpated though its location is not fixed, examination revealing the tender area changing from time to time. Cords and scleromata may be palpated in the lumbar region, but seldom myospasm. Movements of lumbar region is slightly impeded. In some cases the lumbar region becomes flat and straight with the physiological curvature diminishing.

Treatment

1. Press acupoints Mingmen (Du 4), Shenshu (BL 23), Yaoyan (Extra), Dachangshu (BL 25), Huantiao (GB 30) and Weizhong (BL 40). (See Fig. 75)

2. Apply heavy grasping and strong press-kneading for five minutes each to the back muscles on both sides, combined with forearm-rolling at the lumbar and back regions to stimulate the muscles and promote blood circulation, until a sensation of heat is felt in the affected part.

3. For athletes with well-developed muscles and heavy body weight, press the lumbodorsal muscles with both fists and perform strong elbow-tip pressing at the local focus to ensure that the force reaches deep to the muscles. (See Fig. 76)

4. The massagist presses the acupoint Dachangshu (BL 25) with fingers or elbow-tip, often finding the tender area. The patient feels eased and comfortable after strong stimulation at this point, which is located about 5 cm. from the spinous process of the fourth lumbar vertebra.

5. Points for attention after manual treatment:

a) Sufficient rest and sleep are conductive to rehabilitation of chronic lumbar injuries. The central nervous system provides good coordination between the internal and external balance in the lumbar region, so sufficient rest may fully relax the muscles.

b) Strengthen lumbodorsal and abdominal muscles by various exercises such as dumb-bell sit-ups, body turning, lifting head and feet in prone position, and stationary exercises. Increasing muscular strength is an effective measure for preventing and curing lumbar injury. Unobstructed blood circulation may help remove local blood stasis, spasm and ankylosis. With the protection of strong

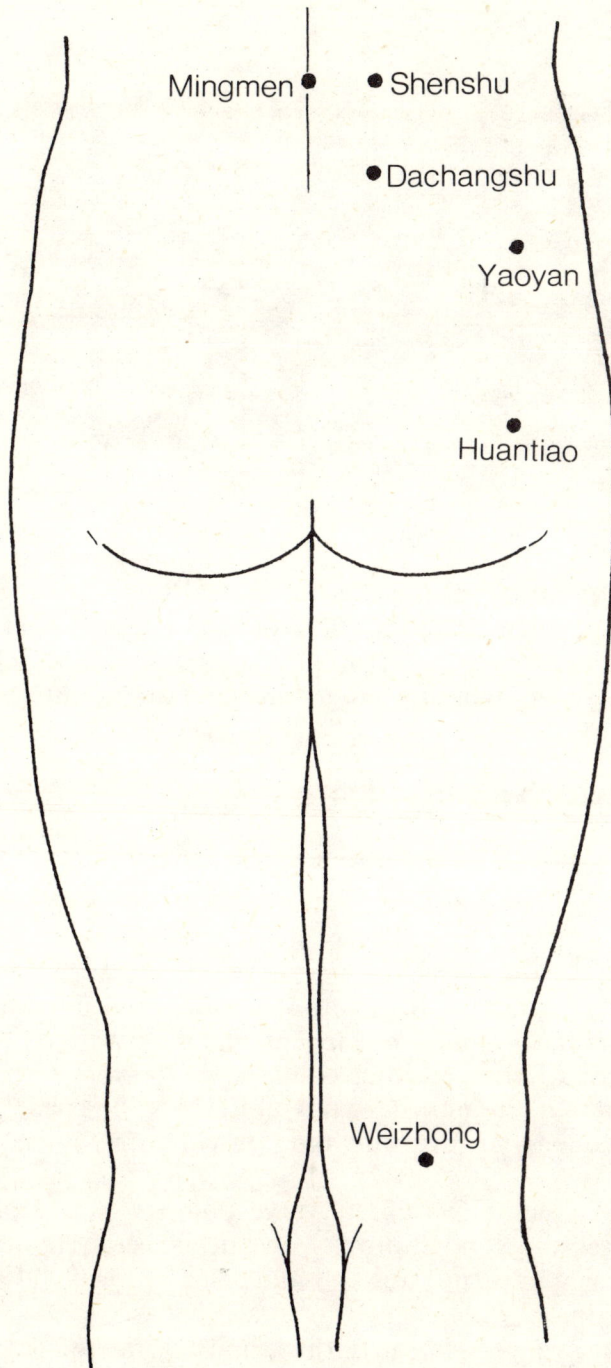

Mingmen ● ● Shenshu

● Dachangshu

● Yaoyan

● Huantiao

Weizhong ●

Fig. 75

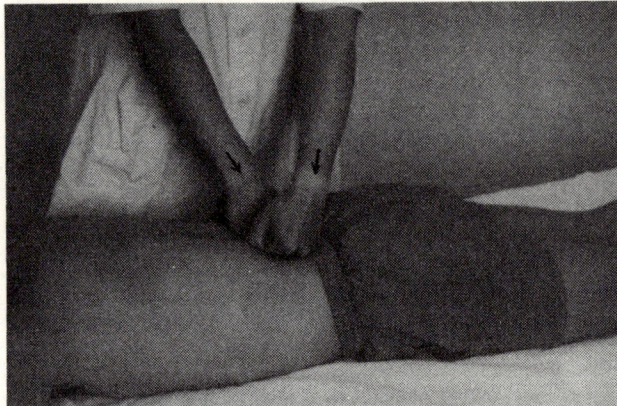

Fig. 76

muscles, a light lumbar injury is not likely to develop into a serious one.

c) Use a waist guard during training to avoid lumbar strain. However, not use it for any length of time to prevent atrophy of lumbodorsal muscles.

d) Keep the waist warm, avoiding exogenous cold and dampness, especially on summer nights.

3. Lumbar Articular Synovial Incarceration

Lumbar articular synovial incarceration presents obvious lumbago while the function of the lumbar region is totally lost, with bending at the waist impossible. Timely treatment, however, yields satisfactory curative effects.

Injury Mechanism

1. Lumbar articular synovial incarceration usually occurs at the posterior lumbar vertebral joint. When doing the movements of forward over-flexion, lateral over-flexion or rotation of the vertebral column, the posterior space of posterior lumbar vertebral joint is open and the synovium enters the space; if the vertebral column straightens suddenly at this time, the synovium may be incarcerated in the joint.

2. The articular synovium is rich in verve endings producing pain, so the squeezing of the nerves and synovium may produce severe pain and reflex spasm of the muscles, the spasm in turn fixing the squeezing on the synovium in the joint and continuing the pain.

3. Lumbar articular synovia are fairly thick and the range of movement of the lumbar region is wide; small joints are pulled widely apart, increasing the occurrence of incarceration in the lumbar region over that in the thoracic vertebral

134

region. Synovial hyperaemia and edema appear after incarceration. Synovial incarceration may be removed by prompt manual treatment, though 1-2 weeks are needed for lesions at the synovia to be cured.

Symptoms and Diagnosis

1. In most cases there is evident flexion, lateral and turning at the waist. Sudden, severe lumbago is the main manifestation of this condition.

2. Lumbar movement is limited and the pain becomes more serious when moving the waist; increased abdominal pressure in coughing, defecating or urinating will aggravate the pain, which may only be somewhat eased when the patient lies on the side.

3. Tender area: Apparent tender area is often found at small lumbar vertebral joint. Thickening is felt at the site of the synovial incarceration, and this is the main symptom to be treated by manual manipulation.

4. Board-like waist: The waist becomes stiff and straight or bends backward. Due to the protective spasm of muscles, the lumbar muscles are tense and feel like a wooden board.

Treatment

1. Press acupoints Mingmen (DU 4), Shenshu (BL 23), Huantiao (GB 30) and Weizhong (BL 40).

2. With the patient in prone position, the massagist applies press-kneading manipulation from the back to the waist to remove myospasm and relax squeezing on the synovium.

3. Traction: With the patient grasping the bed frame with both hands, two assistants tract both of the patient's lower limbs simultaneously for 2-5 minutes, while the massagist scrapes or push-presses the tender area with thumbs to relieve the synovial incarceration.

4. Suspending traction: The patient hangs suspended from a horizontal bar or parallel bars for 3-5 minutes or longer to widen the articular space, while the massagist supports the abdominal region with one hand and performs pushing, scraping and pressing manipulations over the tender area with the thumb of the other to force the incarcerated synovium out of the joint. This done, the pain can be remarkably eased and the lumbar movement improved.

5. The patient should be advised to rest in bed for one or two days after treatment and to cut activity for one week, especially waist-bending movement. Resume lumbar muscles exercises to increase elasticity of synovium and avoid recurrence of synovial incarceration.

4. Posterior Articular Disturbance of Lumbar Vertebrae

Also called disturbance of vertebral facet joint and malposition of lumbar vertebrae, posterior articular disturbance of lumbar vertebrae is a common cause

135

of lumbago.

Posterior articulation of lumbar vertebrae is composed of articular processes of two adjacent lumbar vertebrae, i.e., the two inferior articular processes of a superior lumbar vertebrae and the two superior articular processes of an inferior lumbar vertebra, which are encircled by thin and tight articular capsules. Their main function is to stabilize the vertebral column. When the range of movement of posterior articulation of lumbar vertebrae is large, they also participate in partial lumbar movement.

Injury Mechanism

1. Subluxation of posterior articulation of lumbar vertebra: This injury may be induced by such causes as the lumbar region not being adequately warmed up before vigorous activity, being tired after physical training so that the muscles lose the ability of control, i.e., the external balance is lost; sudden flexion, extension or rotation movement.

2. Chronic strain: This is the main cause of posterior articular disturbance of lumbar vertebrae. Long-term over-vigorous movement of the lumbar region results in retrograde changes intervertebral disc and stenosis of interspace of lumbar vertebrae. Correspondingly, the interspace of posterior articulation of lumbar vertebrae is also stenosed. Long-term friction of articulation leads to hyperosteogeny, thickening of synovium and osteoarthropathy of posterior articulation of lumbar vertebrae.

3. If acute subluxation of posterior articulation or synovial incarceration is not reduced promptly, inflammation and thickening of synovium may result. Friction of bony tissues in abnormal position may cause lumbago.

Symptoms and Diagnosis

1. Pure subluxation of posterior articulations of lumbar vertebrae is often associated with incoordination of lumbar movement. The patient may hear a "click" accompanied by pain in the lumbar region. However, the symptoms are not as serious as those in synovial incarceration; the painful area is wide so that the patient can scarcely point out the tender spot but feels deep pain and limitation of lumbar movement. Medical examination reveals definite pain deep down along both sides of the spinous processes.

2. Chronic strain: Onset is gradual; there is a history of lumbago, and the pain comes and goes intermittently, assuming an aching and distending pain seldom radiating on one or both sides. The pain becomes more serious after physical training, with unclear tender spot; tender spots are found along both sides of the spinous processes.

Treatment

1. Press acupoints Dachangshu (BL 25), Huantiao (GB 30), Weizhong (BL 40) and Chengshan (BL 57).

2. The massagist applies both palms to press down the back to the buttocks to

relax the muscles.

3. Oblique pulling manipulation: Making the patient in a lateral recumbent position with the lower leg stretching straight and the high bent, the massagist presses the anterior shoulder and buttock with the two elbows respectively and pulls in opposite directions. After a "click," in most cases the pain is relieved, indicating reduction of the articular dislocation and completion of treatment. The massagist may also apply inverse pulling or suspending traction.

4. Apply heavy pressing on both sides of the spinous processes with either palm end or thumb, five times each side, to regulate and restore posterior articulation of lumbar vertebrate and adjacent soft tissues.

5. For strain-type posterior articular disturbance of lumbar vertebrae, either the above manipulations or methods for treatment of lumbar strain are applied.

5. Periostitis of Spinous Process

A frequent occurring disease, periostitis of the spinous process occurs most often in the lumbar area and next in the lumbosacral area while it is seldom seen in the thoracic area.

Injury Mechanism

1. Excess dorsiflexion exercises of the vertebral column causes mutual squeezing and collision between spinous processes, causing injury of supraspinal and interspinal ligaments. In chronic cases there may be hyperosteogeny of the spinous process and calcification of ligament.

2. Excess over-flexion exercises of vertebral column causes the supraspinal and interspinal ligaments to pull hard on the spinous process, resulting in pathological changes in the terminal of the spinous processes.

3. Delay in treatment of supraspinal and interspinal ligaments; frequent recurrence of pulling.

4. Lack of physical training results in poor lumbodorsal muscle strength, so in order to sustain forward flexion and backward extension of the vertebral column, the burden on the supraspinal and interspinal ligaments is increased, pulling on spinous processes is aggravated and chronic strain results.

Symptoms and Diagnosis

1. Aching and heaviness in the lumbodorsal region; limited pain in the center of vertebral column, which becomes worse with fatigue after physical training and relieved after rest.

2. Tender spot: There is evident superficial tenderness on pressure at one or two spinous processes, interspinal areas and along both sides of spinous processes. This is the key in diagnosing this disease.

3. The spinous process feels thickened, the supraspinal ligament slides sideways on the spinous process, a snap may be heard. This is also called stripping of supraspinal ligament.

4. X-ray examination at the early stage may not show any changes while a more recent one may show osteosclerosis, hyperosteogeny and ligament calcification shadow of spinous processes.

Treatment

1. Perform pressing manipulation from the back to the waist along both sides of the spinous process for 5-10 minutes to relax the sacrospinal muscles.

2. Pluck at the spinous process to relax the ligament, then push-press along the vertebral column to restore and treat the injured soft tissues around the spinous process and activate the meridians and collaterals.

3. Press or scrape on the tender spot with heavy thumb force to remove blood stasis and promote blood circulation so as to help repair the soft tissues. This is the major method for treating periostitis of spinous process.

4. Acupuncture and moxibustion: Insert the needle through the tender spot onto the spinous process, burn a Chinese mugwort roll to heat the needle tail until the patient feels the warm in the lumbodorsal region and the skin around the needle turns pink. A course of treatment takes 20-30 minutes once a day for six days, and one course should relieve the symptoms. (See Fig. 77)

6. Syndrome of the Third Lumbar Vertebral Transverse Process

Injury Mechanism

1. This is also a frequent occurring disease. The third lumbar vertebra is the center of lumbar motion, the sacrospinal muscle, the quadrate muscle of loins, the

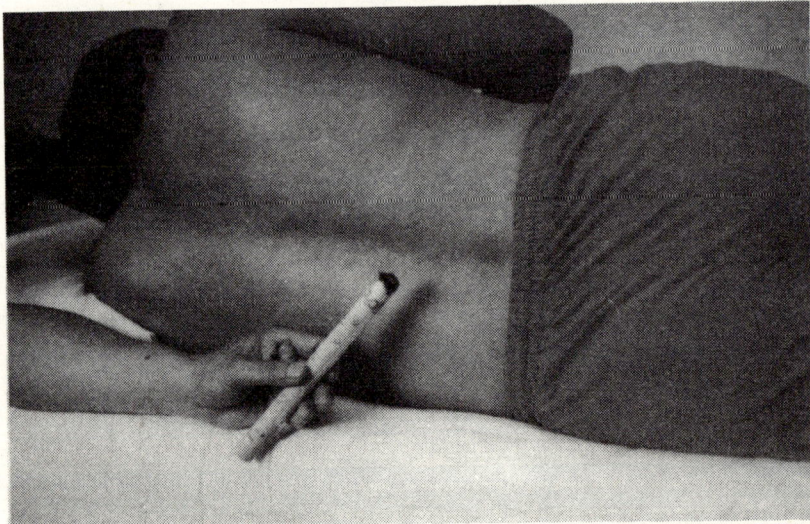

Fig. 77

138

greater psoas muscle and the iliopsoas muscle all adhering to it. The longest of all, the third lumbar vertebral transverse process bears the greatest pulling force. Both repeated violent motion of the lumbar region and repeated minor injuries to the ends of tendons may cause local enthesiopathy.

2. Trauma in the lumbar region, tension or violent contraction of lumbodorsal muscles on one side may pull and injure the muscles adhered to the third transverse process. In light cases there may be local haematoma, while in serious ones there may be avulsion at the transverse process, causing fracture.

3. Since the third lumbar vertebral transverse process is long and links closely with the depths of lumbodorsal fascia, any over-motion of muscular fascia may stimulate the apex of the transverse process and cause local synovitis, local tumefaction and pain, and synovial bursa.

Symptoms and Diagnosis

1. In the acute period of injury, there is backache, evident tenderness on pressure at the apex of the third transverse process and tension in the lumbar vertebrae.

2. Chronic strain causes a feeling of weakness in the lumbar area; pain deep down in the lumbar area which radiates to the buttocks and the posterior aspect of thigh; and apparent tenderness on pressure at the third lumbar vertebral transverse process, which may become very sharp when pressing the apex of the transverse process obliquely; and masses, i.e., the transverse process and the synovial bursa formed therein may be palpated in the depth of the lumbar area. Tenderness on pressure at the apex of the third lumbar vertebral transverse process is the main manifestation for diagnosis of this disease.

3. X-ray examination: The third lumbar vertebral transverse process is remarkably larger than the others.

Treatment

1. Press acupoints Dachangshu (BL 25), Huantiao (GB 30) and Weizhong (BL 40).

2. The massagist presses the lumbodorsal region with both palms, pulls and grasps the lumbar muscles heavily or performs rolling manipulation in the lumbar area with forearm to fully relax the muscles.

3. The massagist push-presses together with scraping and plucking on the apex of the third transverse process obliquely with both thumbs and the force applied should grow from light to heavy to give local stimulation for absorption of inflammation. This is an important method for treating this disease. If the patient has well developed muscles and the force applied by the thumbs cannot go deep, the massagist may press obliquely with the elbow tip. This is done when the patient takes a kneeling position with his lumbar area being flexed to the utmost, as in this way the third transverse process may be felt easily. Keep the lumbar area warm after treatment.

7. Subluxation of Sacro-iliac Joint

One cause of lumbago, subluxation of sacro-iliac joint is an obvious clinical manifestation caused by slight dislocation of joints due to pulling of ligaments and turning of the body.

Injury Mechanism

1. Anatomical characteristics: The sacro-iliac joint is an amphiarthrosis composed of the auricular surfaces of ilium and sacrum. The two surfaces, uneven by well coinciding, are enveloped by tight articular capsules. The anterior and posterior aspects of the joint are protected by various ligaments, such as the sacrotuberous, the sacrospinal, the anterior sacro-iliac, the posterior sacro-iliac and the interosseous sacro-iliac ligaments. These ligaments constitute an important structure for linkage with the sacro-iliac joint to strengthen joint stability. Due to the above characteristics of joint surface, any slight malposition of joint surface may cause total malposition of the entire uneven joint structure, producing severe pain.

2. The posture of the back appears deformed and trunk of the body looks a bit twisted. Sudden turning of the lumbar region causes imbalance due to muscular construction, and thus leading to disturbance of the internal balance of the ligaments. Also due to the leverage function, the malposition, which occurs at the ilium and sacrum, may cause arrangement disturbance at the uneven joint surfaces, loss of normal interposing relations as well as partial incarceration of synovia in the joint.

3. When the back suffers from fatigue and exogenous cold, the protection for the ligaments becomes poor. So any slight turning of the waist can cause malposition of the sacro-iliac joint.

Symptoms and Diagnosis

1. There is pain in the lumbosacral region and the buttock of the affected side. The patient cannot stand straight and bend at the waist, and the pain becomes worse when standing on the foot of the affected side. When sitting, the body weight falls on the buttock of the healthy side. In a serious case the patient cannot even turn his body in bed and the pain refers to the lower limb.

2. Tender area: Pain is felt on pressing the sacro-iliac joint and the upper back iliac spine and gets worse when tapping the diseased part. There is no skin-deep pain on pressure but lumbar muscular tension.

3. Figure "4" test is positive, so are pelvis-separation and pelvis-squeezing tests.

4. No abnormality is shown by both front or oblique X-ray examination.

Treatment

1. Press acupoints Mingmen (DU 4), Shenshu (BL 23), Yaoyan (Extra), Weizhong (BL 40), Kunlun (BL 60) and Taixi (KI 3). (See Fig. 78)

2. Kneads and presses the lumbodorsal region with both palms to relax the muscles.

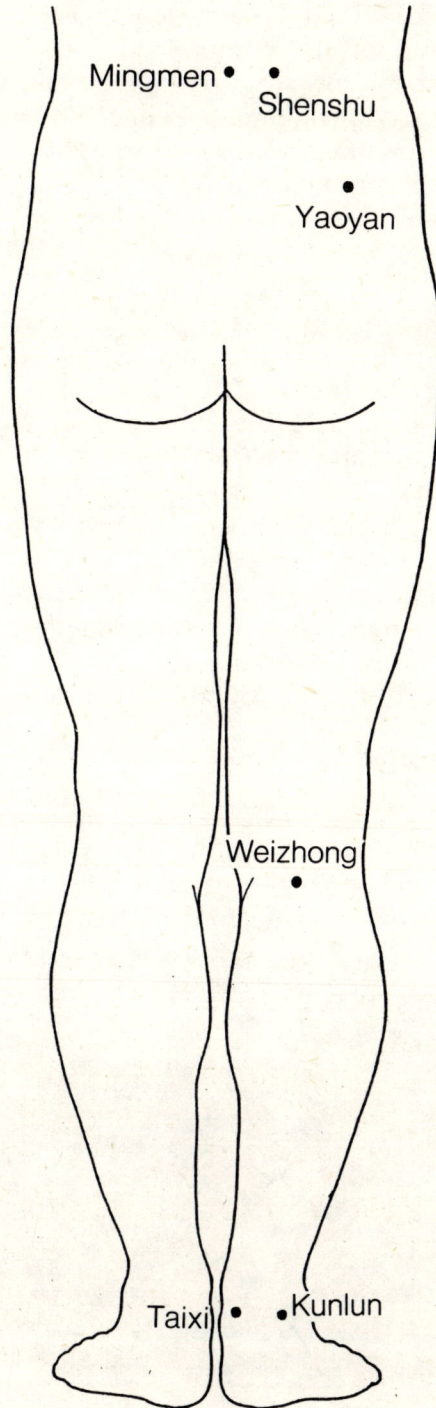

Fig. 78

3. Lateral pulling therapy: With the patient in supine position, the massagist holds the patient's lower limb and stretches it backward with one hand, in the meantime applying sudden backward pressing on the sacro-iliac joint with the other. A snap may be felt, showing success in the treatment. The pain becomes more serious during the treatment, but is substantially eased after the treatment. The treatment should be performed gently.

4. Knee-carrying therapy: The patient holds the knee on the affected side with both hands, while the massagist pushes his shoulder, back and buttock hard to open the sacro-iliac joint so as to reduce it and pull out the incarcerated synovium. (See Fig. 79)

5. In case the above two therapies fail or when the patient is overweight, ask an assistant to tract and stretch the leg backward while the massagist presses the sacro-iliac joint region, a snap indicating reduction of the malposition. Suspension method can be applied to ensure traction of the waist by body weight, with the massagist pushing and pressing the sacro-iliac joint.

Example: Miss Hou, a discus thrower, suffered from pain in the lumbar and right buttock region due to attack by exogenous cold after training. She could not straighten the back or stand on the right leg alone. Tenderness was felt on pressure on the right sacro-iliac region. The case was diagnosed as subluxation of right sacro-iliac joint. The pain was relieved after just one treatment and the patient resumed normal training after three rounds of treatment.

8. Lumbodorsal Fascitis

A main cause of lumbodorsal disorders, this disease is also called myofascial

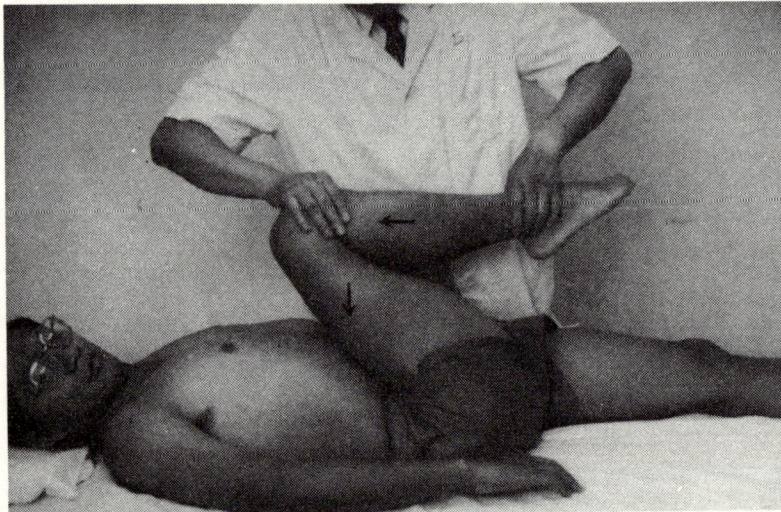

Fig. 79

fibrositis, myofascitis, rheumatism, myofascial pain syndrome and myofibrositis.

Injury Mechanism

1. Injury: Lumbodorsal fasciae cover the trapezius, the broadest muscle of the back and the sacrospinal muscle. Violent movement in the lumbodorsal area may cause acute injury to the fasciae and muscles; fibrosis of injured tissues results in focus of pain. When the lumbodorsal fasciae rupture, the adipose tissues under them protrude from the split, forming adipocele, incarceration of which in the fasciae causes pain. Small foci may also result from repeated minor injuries to the lumbodorsal fasciae due to lumbar strain.

2. Cold and dampness: The patient has a history of attack by exogenous cold and dampness before the onset of the disease. This may occur in taking a cold bath right after training, exposure to cold at night, especially when the lumbar area is exposed to direct blowing by electric fan for a long time. Prolonged exposure to cold and dampness may also cause this disease, which is more serious in bad weather.

3. Infection: With common cold or tonsillitis the patient may also suffer from lumbago and stiffness in the lumbodorsal region which will ease when the infection is controlled. This disease may also caused by such factors as fatigue, prolonged anxiety, weakening of neuro-regulation function and the body's protective ability against exogenous wind, cold and dampness.

Symptoms and Diagnosis

1. Pain and tingling and distending sensation in the waist and back, weakness in the waist accompanied by radiating pain to the buttock and legs, which become worse when sitting or standing for a long time, tiredness, and when the weather is cold, rainy or overcast. Proper activity may, however, ease the pain somewhat.

2. Tender spot: Tender spots are found most often in the scapular region, both sides of the vertebral column, the lumbar vertebral transverse processes and areas around the ilium and the sacro-iliac articulation. There is reflex pain on pressing a tender spot.

3. Muscular tension: When the pain in the waist and back is severe, there will evident muscular tension; when the pain abates, cords may still be felt, caused possibly by fascial adhesion. These cords are painful on pressing. Also be palpated are nodes of varying sizes, from that of soybeans to that of rice grains. Most are around the sacro-iliac articulation and the wing of the ilium. These nodes are adipocele formed by protrusion of fat from ruptured fasciae, which is a manifestation of stagnation of qi and blood stasis.

Treatment

1. Press acupoints Huantiao (GB 30), Fengshi (GB 31), Weizhong (BL 40), Dachangshu (BL 25) and Baliao (literally "eight holes," a collective term for the eight-liao points). (See Fig. 80)

2. Perform press-kneading manipulation on the back, waist and the sacral region

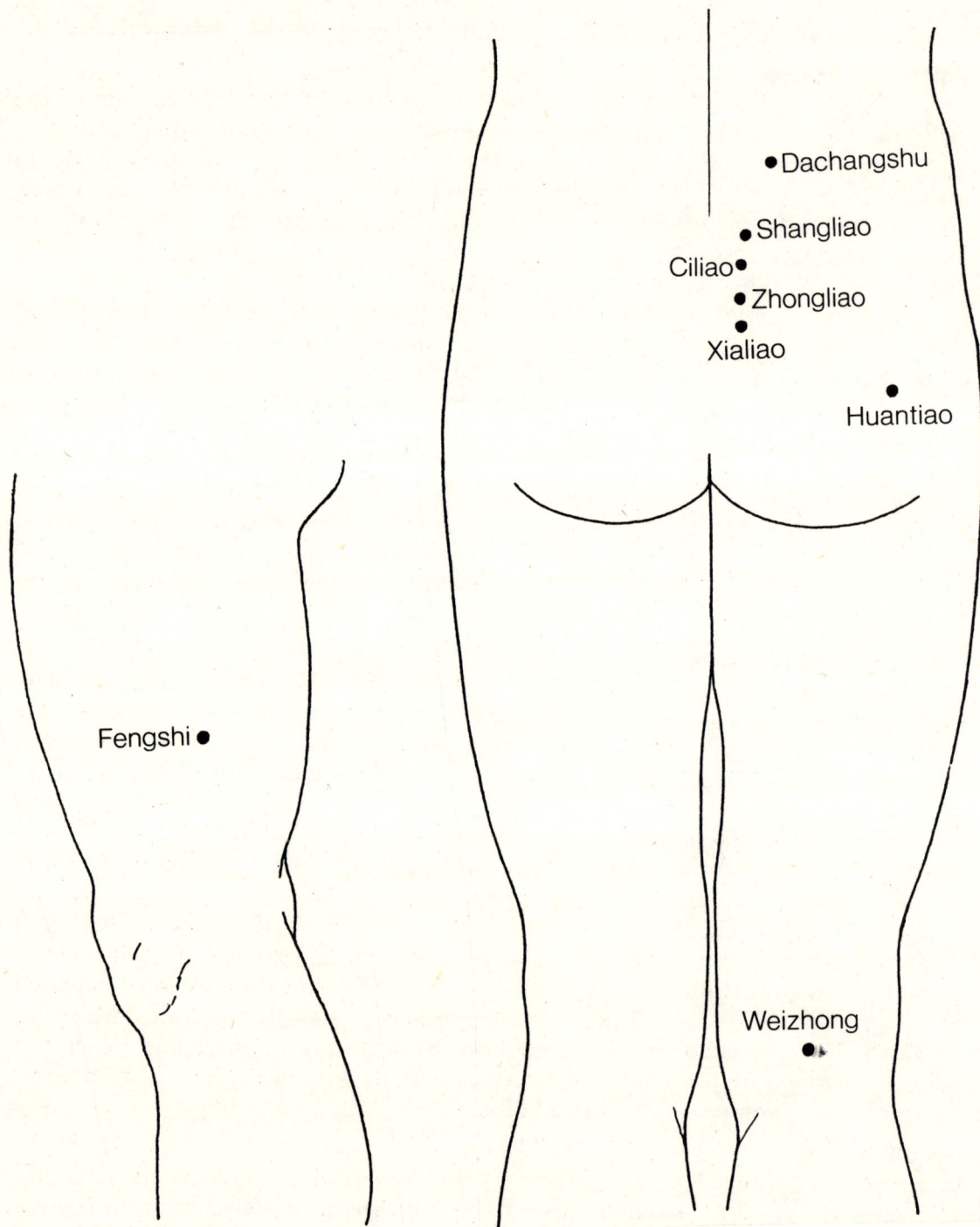

• Dachangshu

• Shangliao

Ciliao •

• Zhongliao

Xialiao •

• Huantiao

Fengshi •

Weizhong

•

Fig. 80

144

with both hands, with emphasis on the painful areas, supplemented by rolling, patting and scraping to relax the tissues and make the skin warm.

3. Stimulate the tender spot with strong manipulations such as digit-pressing, elbow-pressing, pinching and scraping to relieve pain by causing pain and remove the foci.

4. Pluck the cords with force together with heavy push-pressing and kneading to separate any adhesion; then press-knead along the longitudinal axis of cord to relax the muscles and tendons and activate the flow of qi and blood in the meridians and collaterals.

5. Dispersing masses: First palpate the location of the masses and relax the adjacent tissues with gentle manipulation, then apply heavy pushing, pressing, scraping and pinch-nipping to reduce or remove the masses. The force should not be too violent lest it causes local tumefaction and hyperaemia and increases the pain.

6. Beat the waist, back, sacral region and buttocks with fist or palm until the skin turns pink to relax the muscles and tendons, promote blood circulation as well as expel exogenous cold and remove blood stasis. Keep the waist warm after treatment and avoid attack by pathogenic wind and cold. In serious cases the amount of physical training must be reduced. During the treatment the patient can do exercises to strengthen the strength of the lumbodorsal muscles. But he or she should be advised to avoid monotonous movement for the lumbar region.

9. Protrusion of Intervertebral Disc

Protrusion of intervertebral disc is a common sports injury. Although it can be treated by surgery, it is liable to recur.

Injury Mechanism

1. Anatomical characteristics: There is an intervertebral disc for each vertebral body from the second cervical vertebra to the first sacral vertebra, 23 in all and accounting for one-fourth of the total length of the vertebral column. Of all these intervertebral discs those at the lumbar region are the largest and are wedge-like, wide in front and thin in back. Each of the disc is composed of three parts: the upper and lower parts are two discoid cartilages that link closely with the surface of the upper and lower vertebral bodies and with the peripheral fibrae. Their function is to prevent the pulpiform muscles from protruding upward and downward. The middle part is a fibrous ring, which is a fibrocartilaginous tissue rich with ligaments and links with the periphery of the discoid cartilages to ensure firm contact between the two discoid cartilages so as to prevent the pulpiform nucleus from protruding in any direction. The pulpiform nucleus is residue of notochord and is a glue-like elastic substance of greyish white colour that contains 88 percent water. Encircled by the fibrous ring and the discoid cartilages it has no special form, which varies according to vertebral activity. It performs a spring function

145

to lessen vibration of the vertebral column. Since the intervertebral discs have no blood circulation themselves, their generative ability is very poor once ruptured.

2. The intervertebral discs have the characteristic of denaturation. After the age of 20, their elasticity gradually weakens and there appears a split in the fibrous ring due to denaturation, allowing the pulpiform nucleus to protrude. This change constitutes the endopathic cause of intervertebral disc protrusion. The region of the fourth and fifth intervertebral discs is the area most often injured because the waist bears most of the torso's movement and weight. The fibrous ring is often ruptured by trauma, and the types of trauma vary, such acute lumbar sprain and lumbar strain. Most such patients have a medical history of some trauma in the lumbar region.

3. Attack by pathogenic wind, cold and dampness in the lumbar region. Some patients have no evident medical history of trauma. Yet, they do have a history of attack by pathogenic wind and cold.

4. The main physiological change in cases of intervertebral disc protrusion is rupture of the fibrous ring accompanied by backward protrusion of the pulpiform nucleus into the vertebral canal to constrict the nerve roots. The size of the protruded substance varies though it is usually the size of a soybean. The protrusion squeezes, constricts or pushes up the nerve roots or adheres to them. Another type of intervertebral disc protrusion is the central type, such as that constricting the cauda equina nerve and bilateral nerve roots, thus giving rise to symptoms of constriction on the cauda equina nerve.

Symptoms and Diagnosis

1. Lumbago: The onset of lumbago can either sudden or gradual. About half of the patients may have a medical history of trauma. The lumbago can be either dull pain and angina, or sharp pain, even difficulty in walking, inability to turn over in bed and take care of daily needs. It can be eased or cured after a bed rest of several days or several weeks due to absorption of local edema and hyperaemia. Yet, it will recur.

2. Radiating pain in the legs: In most cases lumbago is accompanied by radiating pain in the legs while in some cases there is radiating pain without lumbago, showing that there is no natural connection between the two. Severe lumbago may not be accompanied by evident pain in the legs. Inversely, severe pain in the legs may not be accompanied by marked lumbago. The pain often manifests as "numb pain," or electric shock, tingling or twitching pain. It refers from the buttock downward to the posterior aspect of the thigh, popliteal fossa, the posterior or lateral aspect of the leg, and further to the lateral aspect of the instep or even the heel and toes, i.e., the area through which the sciatic nerve passes. In some cases the pain refers to the medial aspect of the thigh. The pain becomes worse when walking and standing up, or when increasing the abdominal pressure as in deep breathing, coughing, sneezing, defecating and urinating. The pain may occur at one leg or both legs, or at each leg alternately, depending on the location of the

rupture on the fibrous ring.

3. Subjective sensation of numbness: Patients with a long history of this disease often experience a subjective sensation of numbness at the posterolateral aspect of the leg, instep, heel or sole. Examination may reveal dysesthesia at the lateral aspect of the thigh, and the posterolateral aspect of the leg and instep.

4. Lumbar activity is limited: Seventy percent of patients suffer from dyskinesia, particularly backward extension of lumbar region in all directions. Because backward extension of the lumbar region stenoses the vertebral spaces and more intervertebral disks are squeezed, constriction of nerve roots results. In cases where the fibrous ring is totally ruptured, backward extension will no longer affect the form of the protruded substance; on the contrary it helps relax the nerve roots. In such cases the range of backward extension of vertebral column is large, while the forward flexion is limited.

5. Posture of waist: Some 80-90 percent of patients have functional scoliosis, varying from very serious to very slight. Three-finger palpation may reveal slight scoliosis. In most cases, the scoliosis is to one direction, usually toward the normal side and widening the vertebral spaces of the affected side so as to reduce constriction on the nerve roots by protruded intervertebral discs. This is a sort of compensatory manifestation. In some cases the scoliosis is not limited to one side, physiological curvature of lordosis reduces or diminishes, and there may appear kyphosis to relax the constriction on the nerve roots.

6. Tender spot: Where there is distinct radiating pain in the legs, a tender spot may be found at or around the prolapsed intervertebral discs. The radiating pain will become worse by heavy pressure on the tender spot. When manifestations of neuralgia appears less serious or the period of constriction on the nerve roots by the prolapsed intervertebral discs has been there for a long time, the tender spot may be located only after a series of examinations or on examination after the patient has made to do physical exercises. Tender spots are highly significant in diagnosing and locating the protrusion of intervertebral discs. The method of examination is as follows: Making the patient in a standing position with the lumbar region extended slightly backward and muscles completely relaxed, the massagist presses the pubic symphysis with one hand and palpates the tender spot around the lumbar region with the other. Tender spots may also be found on the buttocks, posterolateral aspects of the thigh, popliteal fossa and lateral aspect of the leg and sole.

7. Straight-leg-raising test: The result of the test is positive for most patients. Yet, it is necessary to consider the circumstances. It may be negative when the pain is eased and change to positive when the conditions become worse. In some cases, the test is positive only for one leg, while in others it is positive for both legs or is positive alternately for the two legs. Because for athletes and people who regularly do physical exercises the range of hip joint movement is large, the positive reaction in their straight-leg-raising test is not distinct as compared with

that for the usual patient. Neck sign and jugular vein compression test made when the symptoms are distinct are all positive, i.e., the lower limbs feel numb and painful when bending the neck or compressing the jugular vein.

8. Tendon reflex: Knee reflex and Achilles tendon reflex show abnormality in 70-80 percent of patients, mainly with the knee reflex remaining normal while the Achilles tendon reflex being weakened or fading. Both reflexes seldom weaken or fade at the same time. Abnormality of knee reflex favours the diagnosis but cannot locate the position of the intervertebral disc protrusion. Knee reflex is controlled by the femoral nerve while the Achilles tendon reflex is controlled by the sciatic nerve.

9. Great-toe-dorsiflexion test: In some patients with intervertebral disc protrusion, the strength for dorsiflexion of the great toe considerably weakens on the affected side, especially in patients whose fourth and fifth intervertebral discs protrude. The test is important in diagnosing and locating the lesion. Method of examination: The massagist presses the dorsal aspect of both great toes of the patient with both thumbs and asks the patient to dorsiflex the great toes to test their dorsiflexion strength.

10. Myotrophy: This develops in patients with a long history of pain in the thigh and leg. It is caused by malnutrition affecting the nerves.

11. X-ray examination: Front, sideways, left oblique and right oblique photos are necessary. X-ray examination seldom reveals obvious pathological changes, but only a narrowness in the interspace of the lumbar vertebrae, scoliosis and unevenness between the left and right or front and rear parts of the interspace of the lumbar vertebrae. X-ray examination may rule out pathological changes in spinal bony substance. Special means, such as CT scanning and nuclear magnetic resonance, may indicate the location and degree of the protrusion of intervertebral discs.

It is not difficult to diagnose protrusion of intervertebral disc with typical symptoms. But attention should be paid to differentiating those without typical symptoms from lumbar strain, piriformis syndrome, injury of superior clunial nerves, hyperosteogeny, sciatica and posterior articular disturbance of lumbar vertebrae.

Treatment

Manual treatment plays three functions: a) To re-situate the prolapsed tissues of intervertebral discs; b) to separate adhesion between the prolapsed substance and nerve roots; and c) to crush the prolapsed pulpiform nucleus so that the prolapsed substance can be absorbed. The basic manipulations are to flex, extend, rotate the vertebral column to achieve re-situation, separating adhesion and crushing the prolapsed intervertebral discs. It should be specially pointed out that the manual treatment must be gentle at the initial stage for patients who have a fairly long course of disease, suffer from severe pain and experience pronounced constriction on the nerves and whose situation is swiftly worsening lest more nerves be injured. Manual treatment is forbidden for patients who show distinct symptoms of constriction on the cauda equina nerve, i.e., sensory disturbance in the perineum, muscle paralysis, foot drop and incontinence of faeces and urine. Emergency surgery is necessary for such patients.

Example: Mr. Zhang, a football coach, had suffered from pain in the lumbar region and both legs for a week. The case is diagnosed as protrusion of intervertebral disc. Massotherapy, physiotherapy and acupuncture all failed and the symptoms had become more serious. Further examination revealed loss of sensation in the perineum, retention of urine, weakness in both legs, inability of dorsiflexing the great toe and constriction of the cauda equina nerve. So, an emergency operation was performed. Half a year later, the defecation and urination returned to normal, though the sequelae of slight paralysis of peroneal nerve in the right leg and foot drop remained.

1. Press acupoints Taixi (KI 3), Chengshan (BL 57), Weizhong (BL 40), Chengfu (BL 36, located at the middle of the plica under the buttock) and Huantiao (GB 30). As these acupoints closely follow the course of the sciatic nerve, manipulations should be gentle when symptoms of sciatica are evident so as to avoid increasing the pain, which may cause reflex spasm. Acupoints to be massaged in the lumbar area include Mingmen (DU 4), Shenshu (BL 23), Yaoyan (Extra) and Dachangshu (BL 25). (See Fig. 81)

2. With the patient in supine position, the massagist gently press-kneads the waist, buttocks and legs to relax the muscles, alleviate pain, relieve nervousness and promote the circulation of qi and blood.

3. Traction: The patient holds the headboard with both hands while the massagist and an assistant hold both ankles of the patient and pull with force to widen the interspace of the lumbar vertebrae and reduce pressure on the interver-

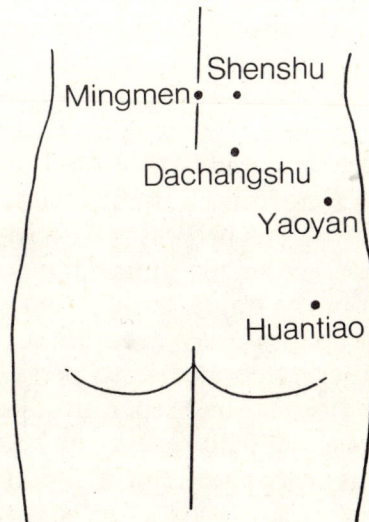

Fig. 81

tebral discs so that the prolapsed substances can be re-situated. The traction lasts 1-2 minutes each time and is repeated 3-4 times. The hip joint ligaments of gymnasts are loose and the force of traction may not reach the lumbar area. The massagist may tract the pelvis with a wide cloth belt or apply mechanical traction instead of manual traction.

4. Local pressing: Find the tender spot, which is often located beside the fourth and fifth lumbar vertebrae where the focus usually lies. Push-press the tender spot with the thumb, first gentle and then with force, until there is a feeling of pins and needles in the lower limbs.

With the patient in prone position, insert a pillow under the chest and ilium region respectively to raise the abdomen slightly. The massagist overlaps both palms and push-presses the waist downward swiftly 10 times as one session. After a rest of five minutes, repeat 4-5 sessions. The pressure should not be abrupt but strong enough to ever-extend the waist. (See Fig. 82)

With the patient in prone position, insert a pillow under the chest. An assistant carries the leg with his shoulder to over-extend the lower lumbar region and suspend the abdomen, while the massagist presses and shakes the lumbodorsal region with both hands. After press-shaking a dozen times, rest for 3-5 minutes, then repeat the whole course 4-5 times. (See Fig. 83)

5. Vertebral column rotation:

a) Oblique pulling: With the patient lying sideways, stretching the leg at the foot and bending it above, the massagist presses the posterior part of the buttock with one hand and presses the shoulder with the other and pulls in opposite directions. A snap may be heard in the vertebral column. This is repeated on the other side.

b) Reduction by rotation: The patient sits on a stool with an assistant standing in front, facing the patient and putting the patient's left thigh between his knees and holding the thigh with both hands to keep the patient sitting upright. The massagist stretches his right hand forward from under the patient's armpit with the palm pressing on the back of the neck. The patient lowers his head slightly while the massagist holds the fourth and fifth spinous processes with his left thumb and uses his right upper limb to turn the patient's trunk backward and inward, and at the same time pushing the spinous processes with his left thumb. The massagist may feel the spinous processes under his thumb moving slightly and hear a snap. Repeat the same procedures in the opposite direction.

Rotation of the vertebral column may generate a torsional force between the lumbar vertebrae and the intervertebral disc to press the intervertebral disc and re-situate it or to rupture the fibrous ring, separate adhesion between the prolapsed substances and the nerve roots, and help relieve the posterior articular disturbance of the lumbar vertebrae. It is thus an effective therapy for treating this disease. The strength used should not be so strong as to aggravate the pain. (See Figs. 84 and 85)

6. Straight-leg raising: Raise the affected leg straight to tract the sciatic nerve and the posterior muscle group of thigh. Be sure to raise the leg gradually, with no sudden movement. When the leg is raised to a certain height, dorsiflex the foot to tract the gastrocnemius and help separate the adhesion.

7. Restore the injured soft tissues: With the patient in prone position, the massagist presses, kneads, grasps, rolls and strikes the back, waist, buttocks, the posterior aspect of both thighs and legs several times to repair the injured soft tissues and promote the circulation of qi and blood. After the treatment, the patient should be advised to lie on his back with both knees bent for half an hour, then start walking.

8. Rehabilitation after treatment: Patients with definite symptoms should rest in bed, while those less affected may receive treatment while continuing physical training with belt protection. Exercises of the lumbar region should be light. Keep

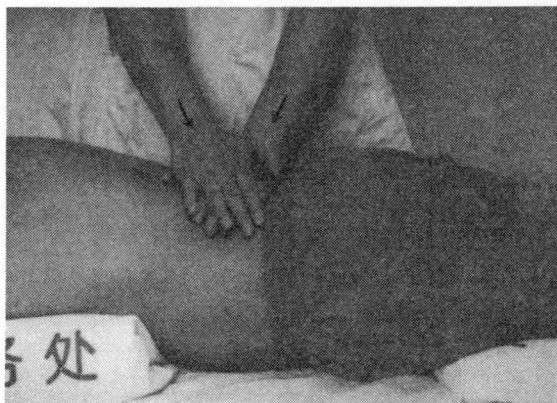

Fig. 82

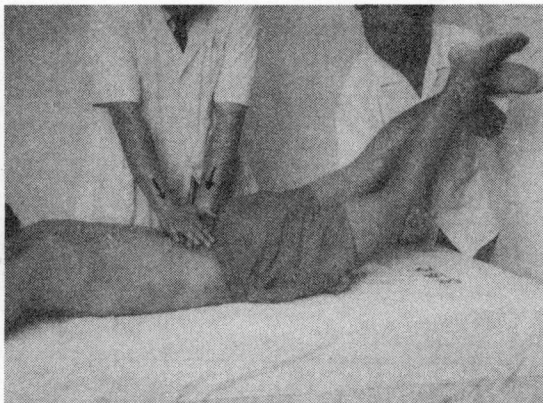

Fig. 83

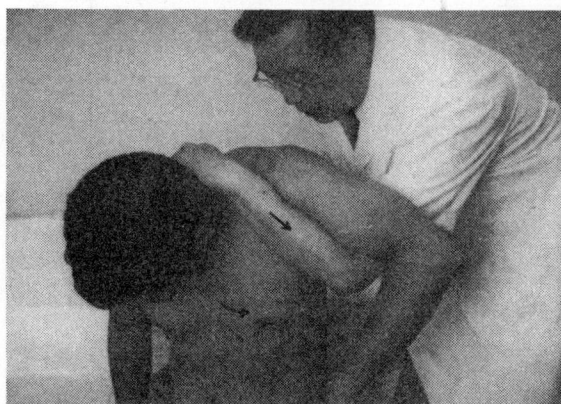

Fig. 84

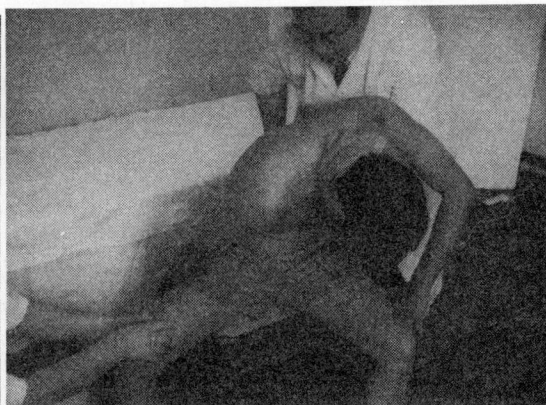

Fig. 85

the lumbar region warm, away from attack by wind and cold.

Example: Mr. Tong, gymnast, suffered from protrusion of intervertebral disc. After training every day, four people performed traction while the massagist pressed the lumbar region and buttocks with the elbow. The patient continued training while receiving treatment, and some time later won a world champion title.

10. Lumbar Isthmic Dehiscence and Spondylolisthesis

The narrow part of the upper and lower spinous processes of lumbar vertebrae is called isthmus. Disunion of isthmus caused by injury or hereditary malformation is called isthmic dehiscence or vertebral disintegration. A third of such patients may suffer from vertebral displacement, called spondylolisthesis.

Injury Mechanism

I. Lumbar Isthmic Dehiscence

1. Acute fracture of lumbar vertebra: Isthmic fracture of lumbar vertebra may be caused by direct impact on the lumbar region due to falling from a great height or by sudden over-extension of the lumbar region, both rare accidents.

2. Hereditary malformation and disunion of isthmus.

3. Chronic injury: Repeated activities of the lumbar region with burden, such as clean and jerk in weightlifting and backward somersault in gymnastics, cause the lower articular process of the upper lumbar vertebra and the upper articular process of the lower lumbar vertebra (or the sacral vertebra) to squeeze and impact the isthmus, resulting in fatigue fracture. To lift heavy object by bending the waist, such as lifting barbells or repeated turning of the waist may generate a shearing force at the isthmus and thus cause fracture. Isthmic dehiscence may occur on one or both sides, mostly at the fifth lumbar vertebra and seldom at the fourth lumbar vertebra. Most cases of isthmic dehiscence involve only one isthmus. Yet, there are a small number of cases that involve two or more isthmuses.

The isthmus, being very narrow, is easily acted on by shearing force, and since its blood circulation is poor, a natural cure is difficult.

II. Spondylolisthesis

Physiologically, there is a forward curvature at the lumbosacral portion with a tendency of forward displacement of the lumbar vertebrae and backward displacement of the sacral vertebrae. In bilateral isthmic dehiscence, due to the effect of the shearing force from the lumbosacral portion, the lumbar vertebra slips forward and the sacral vertebra correspondingly displaces backward. Spondylolisthesis may be accompanied by protrusion of intervertebral disc. In cases of serious displacement, the cauda equina nerve is constricted, giving rise to a series related symptoms.

Symptoms and Diagnosis

1. Pain in the waist and back: The waist is painful and weak with forceful

movements, and the pain at times refers to the sacro-iliac region.

2. In case of spondylolisthesis, the pain refers to the posterior aspect of both thighs and there are typical symptoms of sciatica accompanied by the symptoms of cauda equina nerve constriction such as pain in the lower limbs, incontinence of stools and urine, and change in perineal sensation. This situation is seldom seen.

3. Medical examination reveals tenderness beside the spinous process of the fifth lumbar vertebra with tenderness referring to the lower limbs. There may also be lumbar dyskinesia and muscle tension. In serious cases of spondylolisthesis there is forward hollowness in the lumbosacral region as well as tenderness.

4. X-ray examination: Patients suffering from prolonged lumbago require X-ray photo to provide a basis for diagnosis of this disease. Left and right oblique X-ray photos of the lumbar vertebra will show in oblique projection of a normal vertebral column in the form of "dog head," while in isthmic dehiscence a rupture shows at the "dog neck." In spondylolisthesis, front-view X-ray photo reveals narrowing of the intervertebral space, and side-view ones show forward slipping of the lumbar vertebrae, the slipping displacement falling into grades I, II, III and IV according to the degree of displacement.

Treatment

1. Press acupoints Kunlun (BL 60), Weizhong (BL 40), Huantiao (GB 30) and Dachangshu (BL 25).

2. Press-knead the lumbodorsal portion to relax the muscles; pluck or push-press to remove scleromata; scrape and nip to ease tenderness. Pain may usually be relieved by performing fairly strong stimulations to promote local blood circulation. Patients with pain in a lower limb may raise it high or have strong traction performed at it to separate adhesion of the nerve roots and reduce constriction of the isthmus by posterior small articulations of the vertebral body.

3. For patient of spondylolisthesis without apparent nerve symptoms, make the patient take a supine position while the massagist lifts the sacral region with both hands to minimize the slipping. Do not perform oblique and backward pulling or vertebral column rotation which could aggravate the slipping and injure the nerves.

4. In order to prevent recurrence of lumbago resulting from lumbar isthmic dehiscence, it is necessary to exercise the lumbodorsal muscles. Power lumbodorsal muscles can maintain the stability of the vertebral column and prevent forward displacement of lumbar vertebrae. The patient is advised to protect the waist with a belt during physical training. However, for those with serious lumbago it is necessary to reduce the amount of training and rest in bed. Symptom-free patients can continue normal physical training and competition.

11. Spine Fracture

Spine fracture is a serious injury. It can be divided into stable fracture and unstable fracture. The following is a brief introduction of stable fracture.

153

Injury Mechanism

1. As the central axis of the trunk, the spine is a part of the thoracic cavity, the abdominal cavity and the pelvis. It bears the burden, facilitates movements, cushions vibration and balances the body. As the range of activity of the thoracic and lumbar portion of the spine is the largest, it bears the heaviest burden and serves as the turning point for forward and backward bending of the physiological curvature. Therefore, fracture of the spine often occurs here. Fractures between the 12th thoracic and the second lumbar vertebrae account for 70 percent of all spinal fractures. Deformation displacement may remain after injury. Chronic fracture may cause disuse atrophy of lumbodorsal muscles and local tissue adhesion, resulting in weakening the lumbar functions and chronic lumbago.

2. Spinal fracture is often caused by external force. Landing on the ground on the foot or buttock in a fall from a great height will cause over-flexion of the spine due to external force, causing flexion-type fracture. Direct impact on the lumbar region while in standing position may cause extension-type fracture, a type rarely seen.

3. Spine stability after a stable fracture is fine, without the possibility of displacement, such as in simple compression fracture, simple fracture of spinous and transverse processes. Fracture displacement may occur in the unstable type because the spine is no longer stable, such as in serious compression fracture and dislocation of posterior spinal articulation, which may injure the spinal cord.

Symptoms and Diagnosis

1. Obvious history of trauma: Pain in the lumbodorsal region, dyskinesia, inability to stand up; and exacerbating pain on moving the body. Be sure not to move the patient too much.

2. Spasm of muscle, flat and straight waist; evident tenderness in the diseased area, or local tumefaction or abrasion. Kyphosis malformation may occur and would be a manifestation of fracture displacement.

3. X-ray examination may reveal the type of fracture and degree of injury, providing a basis for manual treatment of spine fracture.

Treatment

1. Manual reduction: The principles for treatment of the stable compression fracture of the thoracic lumbar vertebra are to reduce fracture, correct malformation, and restore normal physiological curvature of the spine so as to lessen the sequelae of lumbago. For young patients, reduction may be achieved by over-flexion of the lumbodorsal portion. This is performed with the posterior spinal articulation acting as the fulcrum and by using the pulling force of the anterior longitudinal ligament to achieve reduction. The specific methods are as follows:

a) Pillow-insertion method: With the patient lying supine in a hard bed, insert a 10-cm-wide piece of cloth at the fracture part, the massagist stands on the bed and lifts the cloth to over-flex the patient's spine to achieve reduction. An assistant then inserts a thick pillow under the suspended lumbar region to maintain the over-flexed position of the spine. The patient lies supine in bed for 2-3 days before the pillow is lowered. A gentle manipulation with little disturbance of the spine and with little side effect, this is the method of first choice.

b) Suspension-extension method: First, apply local anaesthesia by injecting 40-60 ml. of 0.5-1 percent procaine into the injured area on both sides of the spinous process. The patient lies prone in bed with both ankles in traction to raise both feet gradually until the body forms a 45-degree or larger angle with the bed surface. The massagist then presses the diseased area with the palm to reduce the fracture.

c) Back-holding method: With the patient lying on the side, the massagist stands behind the patient back to back and holds the patient's arms tightly. Then with the help of an assistant, the patient is lifted gradually; the massagist supports the fracture area with his lumbodorsal portion while the assistant performs downward traction on both legs of the patient. The massagist bends his waist gradually, within the patient's tolerance, to 90 degrees and at the same time rocks the pelvis. This may achieve reduction in 2-5 minutes. Then, ask the patient to lie supine in bed with a cushion under the fracture area.

2. Treating the soft tissues and removing blood stasis: Massage treatment on the lumbodorsal region may be started the day after reduction. With the patient on the side or in prone position, the massagist performs gentle kneading or scraping on the lumbodorsal region to clear the meridians and relax the muscles, and plucks to remove scleromata. Pressing is forbidden on the lumbar region, but press-kneading and pulling-grasping along both lower limbs can promote blood circulation to prevent myotrophy. After treatment, the patient should rest in bed in a supine position.

3. Lumbodorsal muscle exercises: Lumbago is eased a week after the treatment. Then, lumbodorsal muscle exercises should start, using various methods. One easy and simple exercise is to lie in prone position with the spine dorsiflexed and the chest raised. Ten such dorsiflexion movements per session are done, 2-3 times a day. Sit-ups for muscle exercise are forbidden.

4. After bed rest for four weeks, the patient may try walking with the help of a spine support or wide waist belt. When X-ray photo shows union of the fracture, the support is removed, the range of waist activity gradually enlarged and the exercise intensified.

12. Fracture of Coccyx

Fracture of coccyx is not often seen, but if not given timely manual treatment, local pain may remain.

Injury Mechanism

Slipping or falling from a height with buttocks hitting the ground may cause fracture or dislocation of the coccyx. This is more common in females. Direct impact on the coccyx could also cause fracture.

Symptoms and Diagnosis

1. Apparent trauma: There is pain in the sacrococcygeal region, which becomes worse in sitting position. So the patient prefers sitting on one buttock. Pain may also be felt on defecation.

2. Tumefaction, blood stasis, tenderness and the sensation of friction of bone may be found in the sacrococcygeal region.

3. A side-view X-ray photo of the sacrococcyx reveals fracture or dislocation of the coccyx. However, dislocation of coccyx should be differentiated from unciform coccyx which produces no pain.

Treatment

1. Gentle pushing manipulation: For cases of coccyx fracture without displacement, perform gentle pushing manipulation on the sacrococcygeal region for subsidence of tumefaction, removal of blood stasis and alleviation of pain, but do not press the painful area.

2. Anus manual reduction: The massagist puts a finger cap on the index finger of the right hand, inserts the index finger into the anus to push-press the distal end of the coccyx toward the dorsum of the patient, and presses the proximal end of the coccyx from skin surface of the sacrococcygeal region with the left hand. A snap or a sensation of moving at the fracture area indicates completion of reduction. Due to pulling by muscles around the anus, recurrence of dislocation is possible. So, an X-ray examination should be taken 2-3 days after the treatment. If there is dislocation, repeat the treatment again.

3. Within two weeks after treatment, the patient may walk but not sit. Take sitz bath 1-2 times a day to promote subsidence of tumefaction, improve blood circulation and accelerate union of fracture.

Chapter 8
INJURY OF BUTTOCKS AND THIGH

1. Injury of Superior Clunial Nerve of Buttock

The superior clunial nerve of buttock refers to the cutaneous branches of the lumbar nerves 1, 2 and 3. It starts from the intervertebral foramen, passing through the sacrospinal muscles and the lumbodorsal fascia to subcutaneous fat, then goes over the ilium and ends at the buttock skin. The injury of superior clunial nerve of buttock is a common disease that manual treatment can satisfactorily treat.

Injury Mechanism
1. The injury of the superior clunial nerve of buttock is directly related to injury of lumbodorsal muscles. The posterior branch of lumbar nerves pierces the lumbar muscles which may become, in certain conditions, spasmodic to stimulate the nerve and aggravate the pain in waist and back, leading to radiating numbness, delayed sensation or allergy.
2. Anatomic variation and improper position: Pulling or friction due to eversion of the ilium and constant lateral rotation of the spine thickens the superior clunial nerve of buttock.
3. Acute injury: Violent and sudden movement of the lumbar region changes the relations between the superior clunial nerve of the buttock and its adjacent tissues, causing it to change position and giving rise to definite symptoms.

Symptoms and Diagnosis
1. One side of the waist and buttock has pain radiating to the lower limb on the same side, which, however, does not go beyond the knee.
2. Lumbar movement is limited; the patient cannot stand up quickly from a bending position and needs the hand to support the buttock to straighten up.
3. Examination of buttock: In the soft tissues at a point 3-4 cm. directly under the mid-point of the iliac crest, cords may be felt, which move about by pushing and cause soreness, numbness distention and aching in the local area. This provides an important basis for diagnosis of this disease.

Treatment
1. Press acupoints Yaoyan (Extra), Huantiao (GB 30) and Weizhong (BL 40).
2. Press the lumbar area and buttocks to relax the buttock muscles.
3. Palpate the cords along the mid-point of the iliac crest, push and pluck the cords with the thumb left and right like plucking strings of a muscle instrument.

Push-pluck from top to bottom 5-10 times, then press along the direction of the cords 5-10 times for re-situate and restore the peripheral soft tissues. After treatment, the patient will immediately feel relaxed and comfortable in the buttock area. For a case of acute injury, the patient should be advised not to bend and rotate the waist after manual treatment. The injured area should be kept warm.

2. Piriformis Syndrome

Deep in the buttock, the piriformis is closely related to the sciatic nerve. It starts from the anterior border of the sacral vertebrae, emerges from the smaller pelvic cavity through the lower border of the greater sciatic notch and gradually becomes tendons and terminates at the posterosuperior part of the hip joint capsule and the trochanter of femur. Its function is to help abduction and outward rotation of the hip joint. The sciatic nerve normally emerges from the pelvis through the lower border of the piriformis.

Injury Mechanism

1. Acute injury and chronic sprain: Contusion or sprain in the piriformis may be caused by direct impact or kicking at the buttock, sudden outward rotation of legs and quick standing up from a squat position, giving rise to tension, swelling, hyperaemia and spasm of the muscles. In such situation, the sciatic nerve under the piriformis can also be affected, hence pain in the buttock and the posterior aspect of thigh. Repeated squatting and standing up, such as in lifting barbells, cause chronic sprain, muscular hyperaemia and edema, even hypertrophy, stiffness and adhesion in the piriformis, and stimulate the adjacent nerves and blood vessels and result in chronic pain in the buttocks and legs.

2. Anatomical variation: Normally, the sciatic nerve emerges from under the piriformis. One type of change shows that the sciatic nerve falls into the tibial nerve and the common peroneal nerve into the piriformis, with the tibial nerve emerging from under the piriformis and the common peroneal nerve from the belly of piriformis. Sudden abduction and outward rotation of the thigh or attack by exogenous cold in the buttocks narrows the muscular space and constricts the nerve, causing constricting symptoms on the common peroneal nerve.

Symptoms and Diagnosis

1. Most patients have a history of trauma and attack by exogenous cold. There is dull pain, soreness and heaviness in the buttocks. The pain may refer downward to the legs, causing hipgout, and the pain becomes worse by coughing and defecation when abdominal pressure is increased.

2. Transverse cords or raised scleromata may be felt in the depth of buttocks and there are apparent local tenderness and radiating pain in the lower limbs. In chronic cases, the pathological changes are manifested in amyotrophy and flaccidity of buttock muscles.

3. Adduction and inward rotation of hip joint is restricted, which increases the

·pain. Straight leg raising test is positive. There is no lumbago, which helps differentiate this disease with protrusion of intervertebral disc.

Treatment

1. Press acupoints Huantiao (GB 30), Weizhong (BL 40) and Kunlun (BL 60).

2. With the patient in prone position, the massagist presses or rolls with forearm the buttock to relax the greatest gluteal muscle and stretch the leg backward passively. This represents a preparatory step for manual treatment of the deeply located piriformis.

3. When the greatest gluteal muscle is relaxed, the piriformis can be felt clearly. The massagist should press the piriformis outward from the center and pluck the muscles slowly and deeply. If the gluteal muscle is well-developed, press and pluck it with the tip of elbow. But be sure the force applied is not too heavy. This is a key method for treating this disease. The pressing and plucking should be repeated 5-10 times.

4. Restore the muscles and tendons: Push and press along the direction of the muscles to restore the soft tissues, supplemented by large-range backward extension and abduction of the leg. Most patients feel the heaviness in the buttocks eased after the treatment. Keep the lumbar and buttock regions warm and avoid attack by exogenous cold.

3. Bursitis of Hip Joint

There is bursa wherever there is frequent friction and heavy pressure, such as between the bony processes, muscles, tendons and skin, between different muscles and between muscles and tendons. There is usually only a small amount of synovial fluid to reduce the friction and pressure. Of the few bursae around the hip joint, three are clinically important and they are:

a) The iliopectineal bursa, which is located between the iliopsoas muscle and pelvis and is linked with the hip joint capsule.

b) The greater trochanteric bursa, which is located between the attaching point of the greatest gluteal muscle and the greater femoral trochanter.

c) The sciatic bursa, which is located at the ischial tuberosity and deeply inside the greatest gluteal muscle.

Injury Mechanism

1. Chronic injury: This type is the most common. Long term repeated friction or constriction on the bursae may cause bursitis. For example, repeated hip extension and leg swing of gymnasts, pulling and friction of bursae by the posterior leg in hurdling may cause iliopectineal bursitis; repeated friction or direct impact on the lateral aspect of hip as when a goal keeper dives with the ball while playing soccer, may cause greater femoral trochanteric bursitis; sprinters may suffer injury to the posterior femoral muscle group, which is often complicated by sciatic bursitis; and hitting the pit with buttocks in long jump may repeatedly produce

impact on the sciatic tuberosity, giving rise to sciatic bursitis.

2. The injury mechanism for acute injury is the same as for chronic injury, the only difference being that the trauma is more obvious. Acute injury often happens in the situation of chronic injury. The symptoms of bursitis are more obvious and is often marked by exudation and bleeding, such as in acute bursitis caused by impact on the greater femoral trochanter in soccer games.

Symptoms and Diagnosis

1. Iliopectineal bursitis: At the acute stage there is pain in the anterior part of hip joint and the hip appears at semi-flexed; there are tumefaction and tenderness at the outer aspect of groin. The pain becomes worse when the hip joint is being flexed or extended; when the femoral nerve is constricted, the pain radiates along the anterior aspect of high to the medial aspect of leg. At the chronic state the hip feels painful and weak, there is tenderness at the depth of the affected area while the tender area cannot be defined. A snap may be felt in the hip, with pain felt on passive overextension of the hip joint. A definite diagnosis is difficult in this situation because the pathological changes are deep down.

2. Greater femoral trochanteric bursitis: Pain is felt at the greater femoral trochanter when running or jumping. In serious cases the patient cannot lie on his side, tenderness is felt at the lateral side of the greater femoral trochanter, and the pain is worse when flexing and extending the hip joint. In a chronic case there is local swelling and hypertrophy. If complicated by contracture of iliotibial tract, a snap may be heard at the greater trochanter when flexing or extending the hip, this is also called "snap hip." In such cases, cords or moving cystic mass may be palpated. As the pathological changes are superficial, a definite diagnosis is easy to make.

3. Sciatic bursitis: For sprinters pain in the posterior femoral muscle group is always accompanied by pain at the ischial tuberosity, which is more obvious on pressing, and hypertrophy of the bursa can be felt. It is necessary to compare the diseased side with the healthy side for accurate diagnosis. The pain is worse in sitting position and also felt when contracting the buttocks. Attention should be paid to differentiating this disease from injury of piriformis. Tenderness at the ischial tuberosity is the main basis for its diagnosis.

Treatment

1. Iliopectineal bursitis: The deep location of pathological changes require deep and heavy manipulations in treatment. With the patient lying on the side with the knee and hip slight bent, the massagist presses the acupoint Chongmen (SP 12), which is at the inferolateral aspect of the mid-point of the inguinal ligament, over-flexes the hip joint to bring the bursa close the body surface, then presses the tender spot with fingers and pluck-poke the thickened tissues. Since the skin at the groin is thin, be careful not to injure it while directing the manual force to the deep part. Then, roll, pull-grasp and press-knead the anterior aspect of thigh to relax the muscles and relieve detumescence. The treatment is given once a day. (See

Fig. 86)

2. Greater femoral trochanteric bursitis: With the patient lying on the healthy side with the hip and knee slightly bent, the massagist digit-presses the superior aspect of the greater femoral trochanter, followed by pressing from the wing of ilium downward to the lateral aspect of knee. Gentle manipulations are used to relax the greatest gluteal muscle, the middle gluteal muscle and the tensor muscle of fascia lata. Then, digit-press the tender area around the greater femoral trochanter and scrape it with relatively strong force 5-10 times to stimulate the inflamed bursa and promote the circulation of blood and the absorption of the inflammation. The treatment for "snap hip" is to heavily scrape or pluck the iliotibial tract, particularly the snapping area. This method can relax the contracture of the iliotibial tract and cure bursitis under it. Most snap-hip cases are curable.

3. Sciatic bursitis: With the patient in prone position, the massagist presses acupoints Huantiao (GB 30) and Chengfu (BL 36), and press-kneads from the buttocks downward to the popliteal fossa to relax the greatest gluteal muscle, the piriformis and the posterior femoral muscle group so as to ease the pulling at the ischial tuberosity. Grasping manipulation can also be applied, i.e., strongly pressing, scraping, nipping and plucking the ischial tuberosity with both thumbs. If the buttock muscles are well developed, press the ischial tuberosity with the elbow tip to stimulate the diseased bursa. The patient then lies on his back, carries the thigh with his own hands and bends the hip hard to bring the ischial tuberosity closer to the skin surface, while massagist push-presses the ischial tuberosity with his thumb and thumps it briskly to stimulate the diseased area. This method is quite effective in treating this disease.

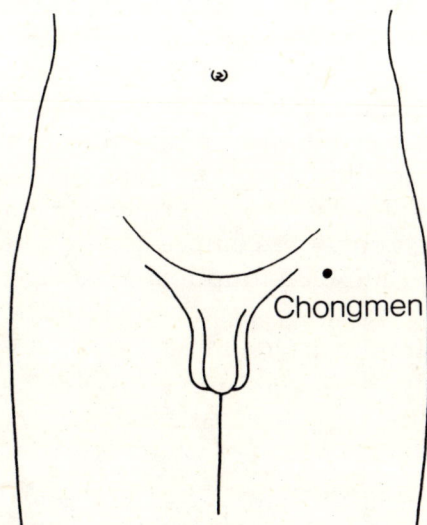

Fig. 86

4. Injury of Posterior Femoral Muscle Group

The posterior femoral muscle group includes:

a) The biceps muscle of thigh: Located at the posterolateral aspect of thigh, it has two heads, one long and one short, with the long head starting from the ischial tuberosity and the short head from the thick line of femur; these heads meet at the posteroinferior one third of thigh, with the muscular tendon terminating at the head of fibula. The functions of the biceps muscle of thigh are to extend the hip, flex the knee and slightly rotate the knee outward.

b) The semi-tendinous muscle: It starts from the ischial tuberosity and ends at the medial aspect of the superior part of tibia, with the functions of hip extension, knee flexion and inward rotation of the knee.

c) The semi-membranous muscle: It starts from the ischial tuberosity and ends at the posterior part of the medial condyle of tibia, with the same functions as the semi-tendinous muscle.

Injury Mechanism

1. Acute injury: Accelerated running as in the final dash of 100-meter race may cause injury to muscles. The athletes' hard drive and overextension of knee joints may pull the belly of the muscle. In hitting the ground with the toes during take-off, run-up and jumping, the gravity moves backward and the posterior femoral muscle produces an active force for contraction, causing injury to the superior part of the posterior femoral muscle group or to the ischial tuberosity. Pulling of the muscle group may also be caused by accelerated running from a state of jogging or running with the knee raised high. Passive pulling of the posterior femoral muscle group is often seen in leg-pressing or leg-swinging in gymnastics and wushu exercises. Top athletes with strength and good elasticity in the thigh are not apt to suffer passive pulling while those with poor training and muscular elasticity are.

2. Chronic injury: It is the result of accumulated minor and small injuries. Chronic injury is often seen at the muscle attachment area of ischial tuberosity, which is a type of enthesiopathy. The symptoms may occur repeatedly if acute pulling of muscles of an athlete is not given prompt treatment and patient undertakes much physical training or competition.

3. The posterior femoral muscle group may also be injured if an athlete only pays attention to strength exercises of the quadriceps muscle of thigh while neglecting those of the posterior femoral muscle group due to incoordinate training and unbalanced muscles of the anterior and posterior muscle groups of thigh.

Symptoms and Diagnosis

1. Acute injury:

a) The patient must has a medical history of injury. When the muscle is pulled, a snap may be heard or a sensation of laceration may be felt at the posterior aspect of thigh, suggesting laceration of some of the muscles. Pain, lameness and limitation of activity of the diseased limb will be evident soon after the injury, and physical training must be stopped.

b) Tenderness: There may be tenderness at the belly of muscles or at the ischial tuberosity. Because the posterior femoral muscle group is well developed and the tissues are deep inside the muscles, tumefaction is not apparent; bleeding and edema may follow laceration of muscles, and tumefaction may manifest at the posterior aspect of thigh. In muscle rupture, transverse groove and tenderness can be found.

c) Resistive check of the posterior femoral muscle group is positive, i.e., performing resistive test during hip and knee flexion will cause pain in the injured area; there is also pain during over-dorsiflexion and forceful resistive test of thigh.

2. Chronic strain: There is definite pain during intensive physical training, which however is eased after rest. Inspection finds the posterior femoral muscles stiff; pressing on the muscles may cause pain and palpation reveals cords or scleromata.

Treatment

1. Digitally press acupoints Huantiao (GB 30), Chengfu (BL 36), Yinmen (BL 37) and Weizhong (BL 40). (See Fig. 87)

2. In the acute stage of injury, briskly but gently press-knead from the posterior aspect of thigh down to the posterior aspect of the leg to alleviate pain, relax muscles, promote blood circulation and disperse blood stasis. In serious pulling of muscles, apply pressure dressing and raise the affected limb and start manual treatment the day after injury.

3. Apply pressing, nipping and grasping manipulations to a week-long or chronic injury with the painful spot as the center. To reach the depth of the muscle, press with both fists. For cords or scleromata, apply heavy plucking or pushing to remove them. The manual treatment should continue for 10-20 minutes. Less than that will not produce satisfactory results.

4. Treatment of enthesiopathy of the ischial tuberosity: Apply nipping, pressing and plucking manipulations. For patients with well-developed muscles, press hard with the elbow tip to stimulated the affected area, i.e., to cure pain by generating pain, and to repair the tissues. Ask the patient to flex the hip and carry the knee to keep the posterior femoral muscle group tight and the ischial tuberosity protruded for manual treatment. After the manual treatment, the posterior muscles of thigh must be relaxed.

Prevention

1. It is necessary to do strength exercises for the posterior femoral muscles in a planned way to have them well balanced with the quadriceps muscle of thigh.

2. Note any pain or sense of tightness in the posterior femoral muscle group, which may mean a pulling injury. Now massage the thigh to relax the muscles or stamp on both legs with the feet, the force varying with different patients.

3. Before physical training, sufficiently warm up the muscles of thigh and make

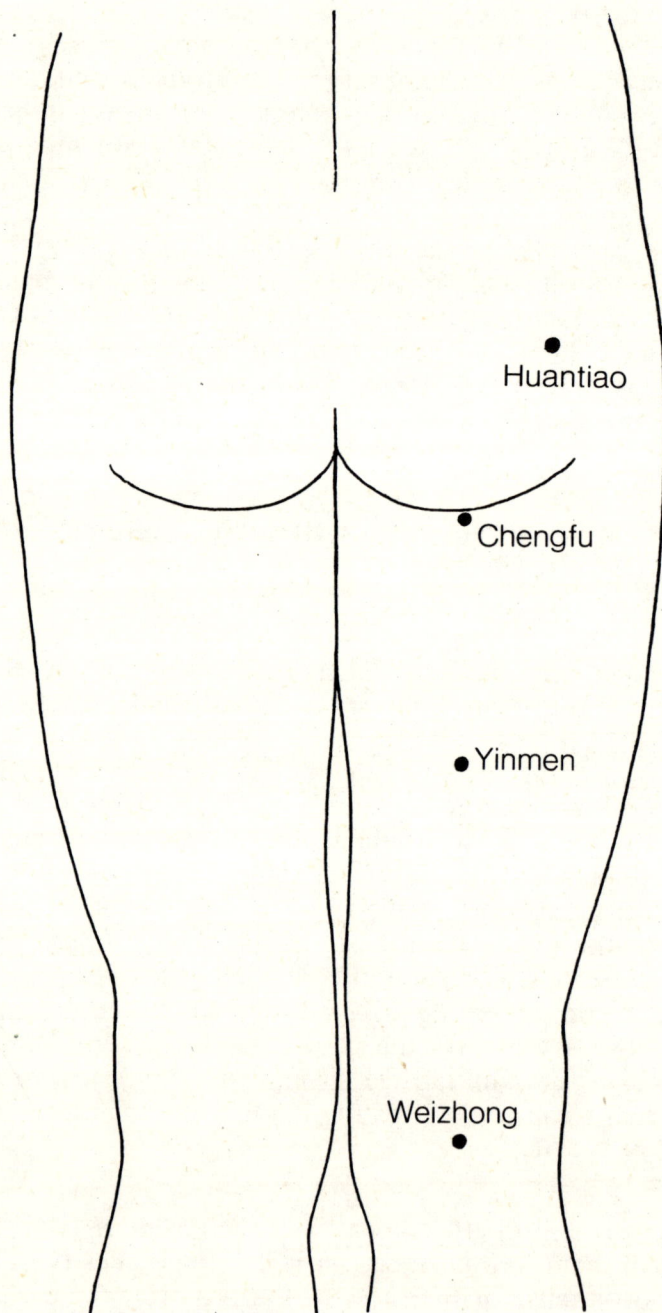

Huantiao

Chengfu

Yinmen

Weizhong

Fig. 87

the body warm in cold weather to strengthen elasticity of the muscles.

5. Injury of Adductor of Thigh

The adductor muscle group of thigh includes the gracilis muscle, the pectineal muscle, the long adductor muscle, the short adductor muscle and the great adductor muscle. Starting from the upper branch of the pubis and the pubic tubercle and terminating at the medial aspect of femur, the long adductor muscle has the functions of adducting, outwardly rotating and flexing the thigh and is most likely to be pulled. Next comes the pulling of the great adductor muscle. As injury of the adductor muscle group of thigh is common in horse riding, it is also called "rider's sprain."

Injury Mechanism

1. Passive pulling of the adductor of thigh due to sudden and strenuous adduction of the thigh, such as in strenuous adduction of both legs to press the belly of the horse during riding. When the horse veers left and right, the rider abducts the thigh suddenly, pulling the adductor. Also, side sliding or striding steps in table tennis and badminton games may cause pulling of the muscle, passive pulling and rupture of muscle fibre or pulling of the point of muscle attachment. Clinical manifestations include local edema and exudation, even haematoma in muscles in serious cases, followed by adhesion and organization of haematoma and even myositis ossificans.

2. Strain of the adductor of thigh due to long-term strenuous adduction of thigh, such as splitting movements in horse riding and gymnastics, and kicking a ball with the medial aspect of the instep as in a football game. The muscles may become spasmodic give stimulation to the obturator nerve, giving rise to more serious symptoms.

Symptoms and Diagnosis

1. Pain at the medial aspect of thigh. In acute injury the pain is more serious and accompanied by tumefaction of ecchymoma.

2. Tenderness: The tenderness is found at the pulled muscle; if the belly of muscle is ruptured, the tenderness is at the mid-thigh, and hollowness of rupture may be felt. In an old injury, cords and scleromata are palpable at the medial aspect of thigh, a condition known as myositis ossificans.

3. The medial aspect of thigh feels painful when abducting the thigh, even cause limitations to the lateral striding of the leg. Resistive test of the adductor muscle proves positive: The patient makes strenuous adduction of both thighs while the massagist holds back the adductor at the medial aspect of thighs with both hands, at which time pain is felt in the affected area at the medial aspect of thigh. Any movement of pulling the adductor muscle at the acute stage of injury should be avoided and resistive test of the adductor muscles not be done frequently lest bleeding and edema occur.

165

Treatment

1. Digitally press acupoints Fengshi (GB 31) and Chongmen (SP 12). (See Fig. 88)

2. The patient lies on the healthy side with the body in semi-bending position. The massagist presses with both palms from the pubic symphysis downward, passing the medial aspect of thigh to the medial aspect of the leg. 5-10 times, using force from superficial to deep. In acute cases the manipulating force should be gentle while in chronic ones the force should be heavy. This may achieve spasmolysis, detumescence and pain relief. For a patient with well-developed muscles, apply grasping or stamping but not by the heel so as not to aggravate pain.

3. Remove cords and repair tissues. The massagist plucks and push-presses along the cords with both thumbs 5-10 times. The action should go deep to lessen the adherent tissues. Yet, it is necessary to avoid violent push-pressing to prevent further injury to the tissues. If there are masses, thumb push-press to disperse them. If the tender spot is deep, test the lower limb for adduction resistance to precisely locate it. Manual treatment should concentrate on the tender spot.

4. With the patient in prone position, the massagist presses the ischial tuberosity and the posteromedial aspect of the thigh and adducts and abducts the leg to increase elasticity of the adductor muscle group of thigh. In acute injury, physical exercises of the lower limbs must be suspended for 1-2 weeks. For chronic injury the patient may receive treatment while continuing physical training, but protect the muscles with shinguards and thigh protectors against pulling in strong movements.

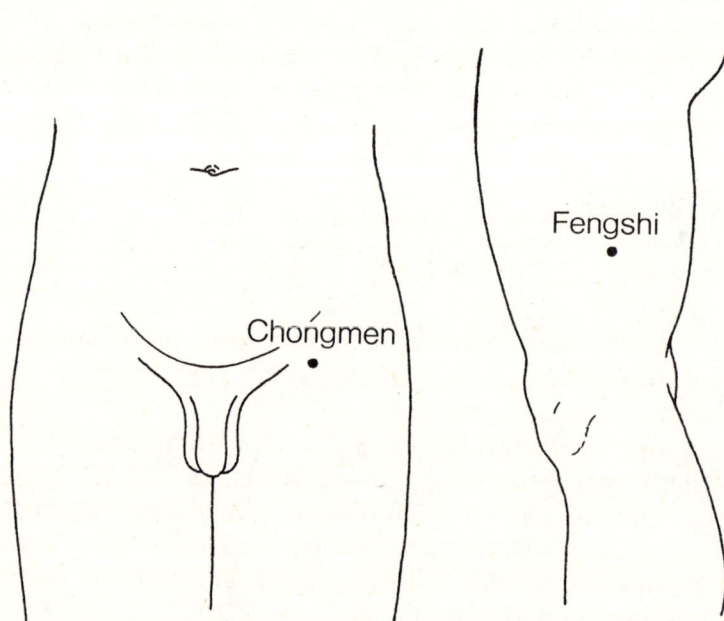

Fig. 88

6. Injury of Quadriceps Muscle of Thigh

A strong knee-extension muscle group, the quadriceps muscle of thigh are composed of the straight head, the musculus vastus lateralis, the musculus vastus medialis and the musculus vastus intermedius. The four muscles constitute a common muscular tendon encircling the patella from the anterior aspect and both sides. They then form the patella tendon and terminate at the tuberosity of the tibia. The quadriceps muscle of thigh performs the function of pulling the patella upwards and stretching the knee joint. Completion of various movements of the lower limbs depends entirely on the coordination and contraction of the quadriceps muscle of thigh.

Injury of quadriceps muscle of thigh includes pulling, contusion, laceration and rupture of the muscles as well as myositis ossificans and subcutaneous haematoma of quadriceps muscle of thigh. This is a common sports injury.

Injury Mechanism

1. Indirect external force: When the knee joint is semi-flexed, sudden contraction or over-pulling of the muscles may cause injury. In light cases muscles may be pulled, while in serious ones the muscles may be torn or ruptured.

2. Direct external force: The quadriceps muscle of thigh is located at the anterior aspect of thigh, so direct face-to-face collision may injure this muscle, and in serious cases cause bleeding and haematoma.

3. Fatigue injury: Continuous running and bouncing with excessive burden may lead to fatigue in the quadriceps muscle of thigh, with reduction of excitation in this local area. In this situation, even slight external force or muscular contraction may cause injury. Retrogressive changes may be seen in the muscles and tendons with a chronic injury in quadriceps muscle of thigh, so even slight external force may cause spontaneous rupture of muscles, a condition rarely seen.

4. Disuse amyotrophy: Injury of the lower limbs, especially the knee joints, leads to reduction of activity of the joint and to secondary amyotrophy of the quadriceps muscle of thigh, which is more evident at the musculus vastus medialis and weakens the strength of the quadriceps muscle of thigh. This muscle may be pulled soon after physical training is resumed.

Symptoms and Diagnosis

1. Pain: After the contusion of the thigh quadriceps muscle the transient numbness at the injured area soon turns to pain, which occurs in the thigh when the muscles are pulled.

2. Tumefaction: In a light case of muscular contusion the tumefaction is not marked, while in a serious one there may be ecchymoma and tumefaction, which is especially serious when the muscle is ruptured. Tendon rupture may be accompanied by swelling at the knee joint and hydrarthrosis. Subcutaneous haematoma of quadriceps muscle of thigh is caused mainly by rupture of large blood vessels, giving rise to tumefaction that increases fast.

167

3. Tenderness: Tenderness of varying degrees may be found at the injured area; scleromata may be palpated due to disturbance of muscle fibre or haematoma. In muscle rupture, hollowness may be found at the ruptured ends and, at the late stage, hard scleromata or cords may be felt, which could be myositis ossificans. When there is myositis ossificans, X-ray examination would reveal a calcification shadow.

4. Function impairment: The quadriceps muscle of thigh feels week or painful when the knee is extended, while knee-extension resistive test shows positive. Yet, the test may lead to mis-diagnosis because, although the straight head is injured, the musculus vastus medialis and the musculus vastus lateralis are still complete and the knee extension function remains. It is therefore important to feel out the tender spot for a reliable diagnosis.

Treatment

1. In acute rupture of the quadriceps muscle of thigh and serious haematoma, timely surgery is necessary to cure the ruptured muscles, or possibly to puncture to withdraw extravasated blood. In serious cases, pressure dressing and cold compress should be applied to the thigh, and the legs raised to reduce exudation.

2. Manual treatment: The following manipulations are suitable for light injury, while fairly serious injuries and old injuries of the quadriceps muscle of thigh require pressure-dressing for one day.

a) Press acupoints Chongmen (SP 12) and Futu (ST 32). (See Fig. 89)

b) Initial stage of trauma: With the patient lying on his back, the massagist press-kneads the anterior aspect of thigh gently with both palms to soften the muscles, and remove cords and scleromata by push-pressing or plucking. This is followed by swift and light patting on the anterior aspect of the thigh with the minor thenar eminence to promote blood circulation and absorption and to relieve muscular fatigue.

c) Old injuries: Heavily press-knead the thigh in combination with large area of pull-grasping or pinching. For patients with well-developed muscles, use the foot-stamping method to relax the muscles and promote tissue metabolism. Painful areas, scleromata and cords are the foci for the manipulations, so heavy pressing, nipping, pinching or plucking are normally applied to resolve masses and remove blood stasis. However, if the cords or masses are not dispersed and, on the contrary, become even harder after a certain period of treatment. In such a situation, X-ray examination is necessary. If any signs of myositis ossificans appear, stop the manual treatment so as not to accentuate these signs. When the myositis ossificans is stabilized, surgical excision may be considered.

3. Actively exercise the thigh quadriceps muscle to prevent amyotrophy and adhesion. Isotonic exercises are preferable, i.e., stretch the knee joint and contract the muscles to that the patella moves up and down. Also perform flexion and extension exercises of knee joint. Try jogging as pain in the thigh is relieved and increase training gradually. Protect the thigh quadriceps muscle with elastic

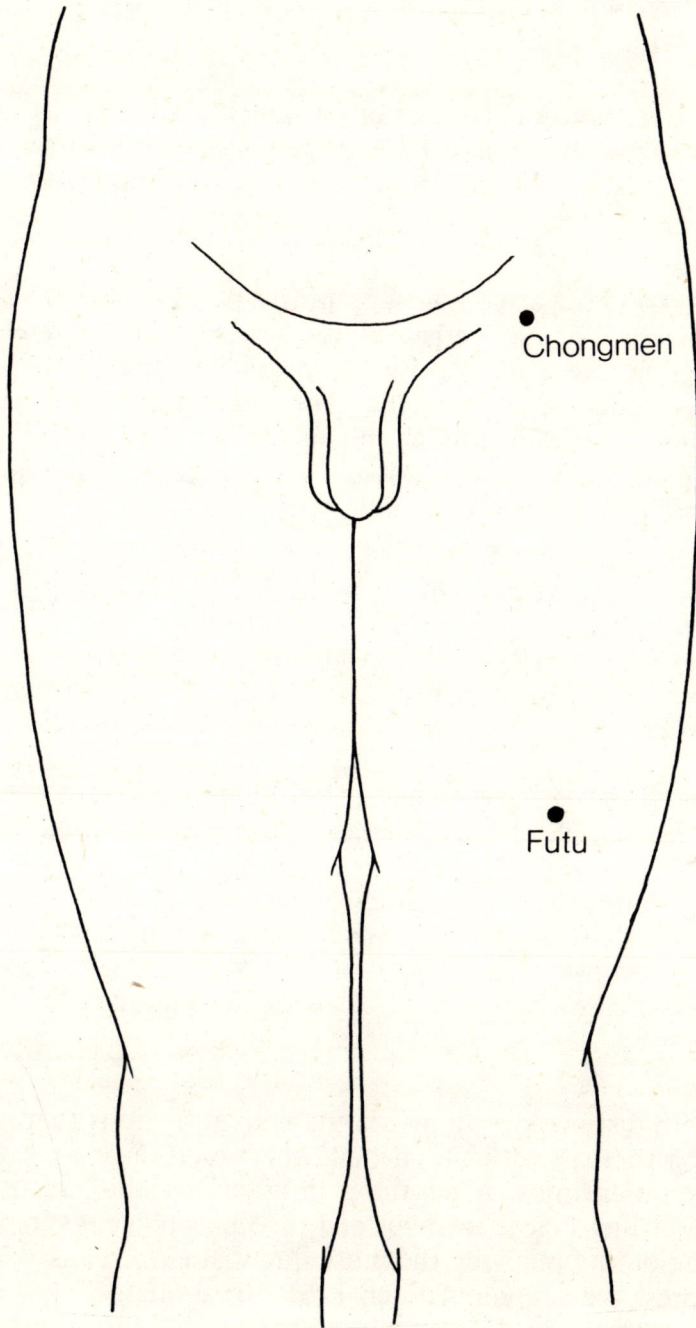

● Chongmen

● Futu

Fig. 89

shinguard and tight protector during training.

7. Pubic Osteitis

Pubic osteitis frequently occurs among footballers as well as athletes in such events as hurdling, tennis and fencing. It can also occur during the period of gestation and labour in women as well as after operation around the pubic symphysis.

Injury Mechanism

Pubic osteitis is an idiopathic non-suppurative pathological change occurring at the pubic symphysis. When a football player performs knee-stretching abduction, the pubis suffers repeated pulling by the pectineal muscle, the great adductor muscle, the long adductor muscle, the short adductor muscle and the gracilis muscle. This causes enthesiopathy at the end of tendon, leading to pathological changes in the bone and cartilage. Pubic osteitis is referable to prolonged strain though it may occur following an action.

Symptoms and Diagnosis

1. Pain: There is pain at the pubic symphysis and pubic branch which spreads along the adductor muscle group on both sides. Pain may also be felt when kicking football with the medial side of foot. Adduction resistive test of the lower limb may aggravate the pain. But there is no swelling and fever. In some cases, the pain may affect walking. Though this condition persists for many years, a natural cure is possible.

2. Tenderness: Tenderness is found at the pubic symphysis and at the end of the thigh adductor muscle. Pelvis separation test shows muscular tension at the adductor muscle.

3. Early X-ray examination reveals no changes while that at the late stage shows such changes as decalcification, widening of space and uneven border of the pubic symphysis, which shows a saw-tooth or cup-like damage. It is necessary to differentiate this disease from separation of pubic symphysis and pubic tuberculosis.

Treatment

1. Patients with distinct symptoms should stop all actions that may cause pain, such as kicking a football with the medial aspect of foot or repeatedly abducting and rotating the lower limbs. When the pain is serious, the patient must take bed rest with the lower limbs close together and the hips and knees in bending posture to reduce pulling on the pubis by the musculus vastus medialis.

2. Digitally press the acupoints Xuehai (SP 10), Jimen (SP 11) and Chongmen (SP 12). (See Fig. 90)

3. Perform press-kneading and grasping manipulations with both palms from the pubic symphysis to the superomedial aspect of knee along the medial aspect of

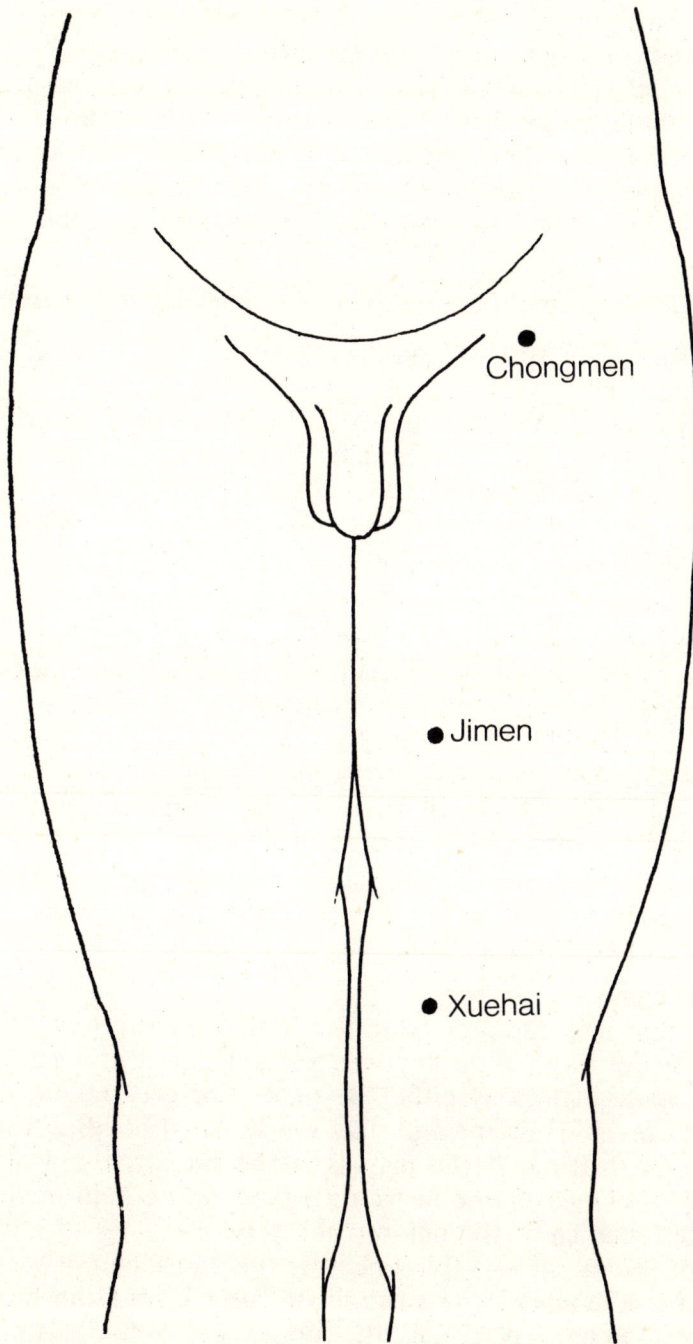

Chongmen

Jimen

Xuehai

Fig. 90

thigh 5-10 times. In case there are cords, use plucking manipulation to soften them. Abduct and outwardly rotate the lower limbs to tract the muscles together with press-kneading and plucking on stiff and painful muscles.

4. Find the tender spot and heavily scrape or push-press the area around it to improve blood supply to the attachment point of the muscles and the cartilages and promote tissue repair. The manipulation should not be too strong when the symptoms are present. Yet, the force applied can be gradually increased each day. Manual treatment has proved to be satisfactory in treating pubic osteitis.

8. Sciatica

A common disease, sciatica is a syndrome rather than a single disease. It may be caused by a number of factors. The sciatic is the largest nerve system of the human body. It passes through the greater sciatic foramen, runs downward under the piriformis, passes between the greater tuberosity of femur and the ischial tuberosity, then proceeds downward along the posterior aspect of thigh to the popliteal fossa where it is divided into the tibia nerve at the medial aspect and the common peroneal nerve at the lateral aspect.

Pathogenic Mechanism

1. Peripheral neuritis: This is often seen as sciatica on one side. Exogenous cold and dampness are the direct causes. Traditional Chinese medicine holds that when there is deficiency of qi and blood and insufficiency of yang in the human body, exogenous cold, wind and dampness are likely to invade the human body, blocking the medians and collaterals and stagnating blood flow.

2. Reflex sciatica: disturbance of small lumbar vertebral joint, subluxation of sacro-iliac joint and coxitis may all cause sciatica.

3. Constriction of sciatic nerve: The sciatic nerve can be constricted by prolapse of lumbar intervertebral disc, injury of piriformis, hypertrophic spondylitis and lumbar spondylolisthesis, thus causing sciatica.

Symptoms and Diagnosis

1. Pain: The pain may radiates from the lumbosacral portion to the buttocks, the posterior aspect of thigh and the posterolateral aspect of leg and further to the sole. The onset of the pain may either be sudden or gradual; it in time becomes either continuous or intermittent and may worse when bending the waist, coughing, defecating or urinating. If the pain is at the proximal end of the nerve, the condition is called sciatica of the nerve-root type, while pain at the distal end of the nerve is called sciatica of the nerve-trunk type.

2. Tender spot: Tenderness is felt wherever the sciatic nerve passes and spreads to the lower limbs. The tender spots usually occur 1-2 cm from the midline of the fourth and fifth lumbar vertebrae, the upper sacro-iliac articulation, or the buttocks, the popliteal fossa, the bottom of the small head of fibula, or the center of sole. Pain also occurs when the gastrocnemius muscle is constricted. In sciatica

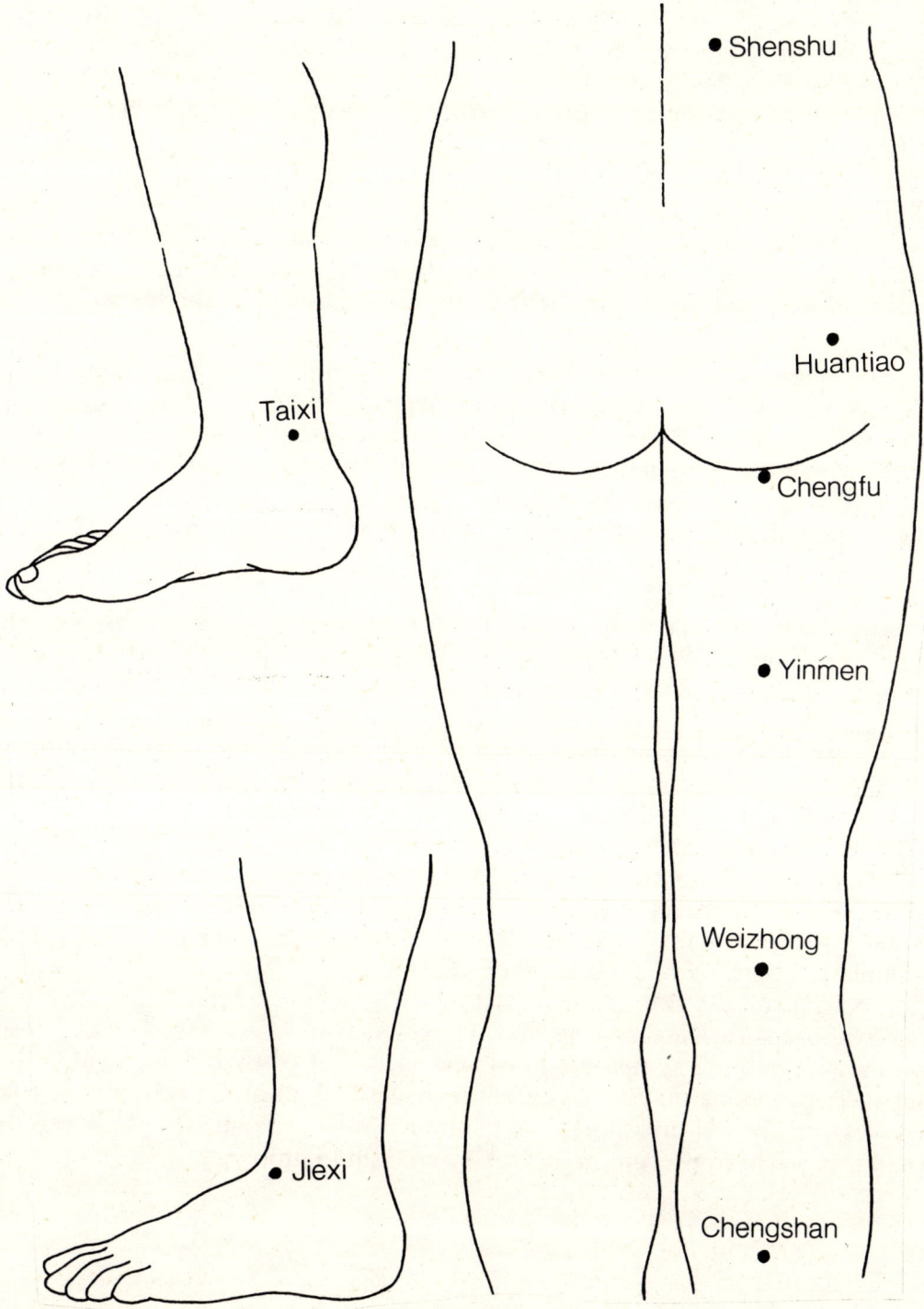

Shenshu

Huantiao

Taixi

Chengfu

Yinmen

Weizhong

Jiexi

Chengshan

Fig. 91

of the nerve-root type, tenderness is mainly at the waist though it may also be felt in other areas. In sciatica of the nerve-trunk type, tenderness often starts at the buttocks and spreads downward.

3. The straight leg raising test is positive. However, athletes have ample pliability in the hip joint, so the angle of straight leg raising is larger than that ordinarily seen, a factor to be considered.

4. Impaired sensation due to muscular atrophy: In a chronic case of sciatica, there is slight muscular atrophy or a certain degree of flaccidity on pressure at the buttock, thigh and leg, making the corresponding portion of the sciatic nerve feel numb or be slow in sensation, especially at the lateral aspect of the leg and instep.

Treatment

1. Digitally press acupoints Shenshu (BL 23), Huantiao (GB 30), Chengfu (BL 36), Yinmen (BL 37), Weizhong (BL 40), Chengshan (BL 57), Taixi (KI 3) and Jiexi (ST 41). Acupoints where there is pain or radiating pain on pressure are the key points for finger pressing. At Huantiao (GB 30) and Chengfu (BL 36) press with the elbow tip to increase the pressure. (See Fig. 91)

2. With the patient in prone position, the massagist presses both sides of the spinous processes of lumbar vertebrae with the thumbs, and scrapes the painful point and presses the buttock with both palms or both fists. The pressing may also be performed with the elbow tip. Perform hard plucking if there are cords at the piriformis, press and pull-grasp on the posterior femoral muscle and the triceps muscle of the leg to relax the muscles and ease pain.

3. Tapping the sciatic nerve: Perform swift fist-tapping or palm-tapping at the waist, buttocks, the posterior aspect of thigh and the posterior aspect of leg and sole to alleviate pain, promote blood circulation and improve nerve function. Heavy tapping is not advised if the symptoms are pronounced.

4. Moving the joints and pulling the nerves: Pull at the ankle of the affected limb 4-5 times for 1-2 minutes each time, followed by passive knee and hip flexion 5-10 times. Raise the affected limb with the leg straight 5-10 times to tract the nerves and ease nerve pain, avoiding forced raising of the lower leg, which could over-stimulate the sciatic nerve and increase pain.

5. Scrape and rub the skin from waist to foot to produce heat that expels wind and cold pathogens, relaxes muscles and relieves spasm.

Patients with definite symptoms must rest in bed after treatment, while those without such symptoms may receive treatment while continuing training, supplemented by swinging and pressing down of the leg with it being straight. Keep the waist and legs warm to prevent affliction by cold and dampness.

Chapter 9
INJURY OF KNEE AND LEG

1. Injury of Medial and
Lateral Accessory Ligaments of Knee

Knee joint ligaments include the medial accessory, the lateral accessory, the anterior cruciate, the posterior cruciate and the patellar ligaments. The superficial layer of the medial accessory ligament is triangular in shape while the deep layer is the thickened part of the joint capsule. This ligament, linking the medial meniscus, originates from the adduction tuberosity of femur and ends at the medial aspect of tibia. The lateral accessory ligament, weak and not linked with the lateral meniscus, originates from the external epicondyle of humer and ends at the small head of fibula. Injury of knee joint ligament is a common sports injury, with the injury of the medial accessory ligament accounting for a considerable percentage.

Injury Mechanism

1. Injury of medial accessory ligament of knee: The knee joint stability is poor when it is slight turned (at an angle of about 30°). In sudden eversion of the knee at this juncture the medial accessory ligament will be pulled, causing partial or complete rupture of the ligament. A strong external force acting on the lateral side of the knee can cause an obvious eversion of the knee joint, possibly causing simultaneous injury to the knee medial accessory ligament, the medial meniscus and the anterior cruciate ligament. Yet, the injury of the medial meniscus and the anterior cruciate ligament are liable to be misdiagnosed clinically.

2. Injury of lateral accessory ligament of knee: Due to protection by the other knee, external force seldom acts on the medial aspect of a knee, so over-inversion of knee seldom occurs. Injury of the lateral accessory ligament is therefore rare.

Symptoms and Diagnosis

1. At an obvious history of trauma; pain at both the medial and lateral aspects of a knee; tenderness, tumefaction and ecchymoma are found at the diseased area.

2. Knee joint movement is impaired, pain appears when the knee flexes and extends with complication by injury of the medial meniscus as well as symptoms of hydrarthrosis. Test of lateral stability is conducted in the following steps: Stretch the knee joint straight or flex it to an angle of 30° and abduct the leg. Increased pain indicates partial rupture of the medial accessory ligament; widening of the medial articular space with a sensation of "opening" indicates complete

rupture of the ligament. Some athletes' joints are loose, however, so the articular space may be widened on pulling the leg sideways. This alone cannot be taken as the base for the diagnosis. A comparison should be made with the other knee joint to decide whether the ligament is injured.

3. X-ray photos can show passive eversion of both knees, while the front-view photos of both knees showing the medial articular space of the affected knee widened. This indicates rupture of the medial accessory ligament.

Treatment

Manual treatment can only be applied to incomplete knee accessory ligament injury and chronic injuries, while complete rupture of the ligament requires surgical repair.

1. Acute injury: If pain after injury is not prominent, apply a supportive belt at the medial or lateral aspect of knee for protection so that the patient may continue physical training. If the pain is severe, activity must stop. Elastic pressure dressing is applied for 24 hours to avoid hyperaemia and edema, and manual treatment is given the next day. For this, the patient is in supine position, stretches the affected leg straight and turns the foot outward while the massagist gently press-kneads the medial aspect of the knee joint to clear the meridians and collaterals to promote blood circulation and remove blood stasis, followed by light plucking on the medial accessory ligament and push-pressing along the ligament to restore the disturbed ligament and promote the healing of the tissue. Finally, scrape the medial aspect of the knee until the skin produces a hot feeling. The patient may resume physical training after 1-3 weeks.

2. Old rupture and injury of the medial accessory ligament: Apply press-kneading from the medial aspect of the thigh, passing the knee, to the medial aspect of the leg to clear the meridians and collaterals; perform forceful plucking and push-pressing on the injured area to promote healing, supplemented by active exercises of the thigh quadriceps muscle to improve stability of the knee joint. Treatment for 3-6 months plus exercise should achieve the desired improvement. No surgery is needed. The above steps of manual treatment also apply to injury of the lateral accessory ligament.

2. Peritendinitis of Patellar Tendon

Peritendinitis often occurs at the apex of the patella, so it is also called enthesiopathy of patellar apex and pain of patellar apex.

Patella, important in the knee extension mechanism, has attached to it the quadriceps muscle of thigh; at its superolateral corner is attached the tendon of musculus vastus lateralis; at its superomedial part is attached the tendon of musculus vastus medialis; at its superior central right is attached the tendons of straight head and musculus vastus intermedius; at its medial aspect is attached the medial patella retinaculum; and at the lower border and apex of patella is attached

176

the patellar ligament.

Injury Mechanism

1. Injury of patella: Repeated contraction of the thigh quadriceps muscle with overload gives repeated over-pulling at the joint of attachment of tendons, which may lead to inflammation around the patella, i.e., enthesiopathy. The thigh quadriceps muscle is a tissue with fine elasticity that can produce a cushioning effect against the pulling force at the attachment point of patella. When the muscle is overwhelmed by fatigue because of overload, muscular tension, stiffness and spasm occur, damaging the muscle's elasticity and making it lose its cushioning effect. Forceful pulling at the attachment point of patella can cause injury. The occurrence of peritendinitis is therefore definitely related to fatigue of the thigh quadriceps muscle.

2. Traumatic injury: Direct impact on patella and sudden local pulling can also cause peritendinitis of the patellar tendon.

Symptoms and Diagnosis

1. Painful knee: Pain is felt when half squatting and starting to run. In serious cases the patients suffer pain during walking and going up and down stairs, and feels sore and weak in the knee joint. Normal training is hampered.

2. Tenderness: There will be obvious tenderness when the massagist pushes the patella downward with the part of the hand between the thumb and the index finger of one hand and presses the lower border of patella or the apex of patella with the thumb of the other hand with the patient stretching the knee joint. Tenderness may also be found at other spots of the patella. This is the key in diagnosing this disease. Uneven border of patella and thickening of soft tissues can also be palpated.

3. Changes in the thigh quadriceps muscle: Stiffness and even scleroma are palpable; there is slight amyotrophy in a long-standing case, especially at the musculus vastus medialis.

4. Single leg standing and squatting test: Pain is felt at the anterior part of the knee when the test is conducted with the affected limb. Resistive knee-extension test: With the affected knee flexed, the massagist holds the ankle and exerts some resistance, then when the affected knee is extended, it feels painful and weak.

5. X-ray examination may show local decalcification or cystic changes in the patella, hyperosteogeny at the border of the patella and at times calcification of ossification in the muscles.

Treatment

1. Digitally press acupoints Dubi (ST 35) and Futu (ST 32). (See Fig. 92)

2. With the patient in supine position, the massagist presses and kneads the thigh muscle evenly with both palms, grasps the front part of the thigh, then pats the muscles quickly with the palms to relax the thigh quadriceps muscle, relieve spasm and increase muscle elasticity.

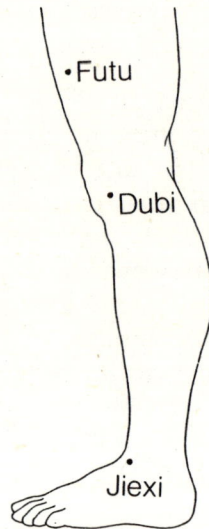

Fig. 92

3. Scraping: Scraping is a very effective manipulation. It is applied with the thumb along the border of the patella, and the strength applied goes from light to strong. The patient may experience severe local pain at first. After several treatments, however, the sensation of pain weakens as the strength becomes stronger and stronger.

4. Nipping: Nip hard around the patella with all five fingers, applying more strength on the painful spots.

The patient is advised to adjust his or her training program for the legs, and not to run, jump or bounce on hard ground. But, he or she should do exercises to build up the strength of the thigh quadriceps muscle, and protect the leg from attack by exogenous cold and dampness.

3. Chondromalacia of Patella

Chondromalacia of patella is a retrogressive disease with such symptoms as chondromalacia, rupture and falling of cartilages.

Injury Mechanism

1. Repeated flexion and extension of the knee joint at halt-squatting position cause malposition, collision or abrasion between the patella, the femoral articular surface and the femoral joint. This occurs when basketball players crouch slide sideways in semi-crouching position for defence and when volleyball players jump and save the ball in semi-crouching position. At such moments, the knee joints bear all the weight and the articular surfaces tilt mutually, causing chondromalacia in the joints. In time this may spread to the entire patellar femoral joint. When the chondromalacia of patella becomes serious, it may spreads to the articular surface

of the condyle of femur and finally to the whole knee joint.

2. Excessive training and hard ground are also main causes of this disease. Falling of the articular cartilage results in free bodies in the joint (also called "articular mouse"), which may lead to locked joint. Moving of the free bodies in the articular spaces in turn cause abrasion against the normal cartilage surface, thus aggravating the pathological changes.

3. Secondary chondromalacia of patella: It is mainly caused by trauma. Direct crush on the patella may cause cartilage fracture. Subluxation or dislocation of patella may also injure the cartilage. Due to eversion of the knee, the patellar is subject to outward displacement and cannot stay stable in the intercondylar trochlear. Repeated compression and friction on the cartilage of patellar femoral joint surface may cause chondromalacia of patella.

Symptoms and Diagnosis

1. Painful and weak knee: Pain occurs at semi-squatting position; it becomes more serious when going up and down stairs, and relaxing in rest. In serious cases any movement of the knee joint may cause pain, which is worse at night and may affect sleep.

2. Tenderness: Pressing the patella with the palm induces pain and friction is felt when pushing the patella. Tenderness at the border of the patella and in the adjacent soft tissues indicates secondary inflammation at the end of the patella, the articular capsule and fat pad.

3. One leg semi-squatting test: When standing on one foot and squatting down gradually weakness and pain in the knee suggest a positive reaction.

4. In the early stage, X-ray examination reveals no special change. In the late stage, however, there may be hyperosteogeny and free bodies in the patella. In making diagnosis, this disease must be differentiated from meniscus injury, chronic synovitis and thickening of knee fat pad.

Treatment

1. Digitally press acupoints Futu (ST 32), Dubi (ST 35) and Zusanli (ST 36).

2. With the patient in supine position, the massagist presses and rubs the middle and lower thigh and relaxes the thigh quadriceps muscle as well as the exterior muscle group of leg by grasping manipulation. The massagist then presses the patellar area with the hypothenars of hand to relax the peripheral tissues, and also presses the lateral aspect of thigh with strong manipulation to help relieve pain in the knee.

3. Scrape with the thumb and index finger along the border of patella to raise the patella border. Push and press the superior border of patella with the thumb and index finger to raise its inferior border. Bend the knee at an 15° angle, push and press the patella apex upward to raise its superior border and scrape it. Then push and press the lateral border to raise it. Repeating the manipulation so that each border of patella is raised and scraped in turn. Stronger manipulation is applied gradually to the painful area within the patient's tolerance. Finally nip

around the patella with all five fingers, with the force penetrating deep beneath the patella, followed by drawing the patella upward and moving it about in all directions. This is a major method in treating this condition. (See Fig. 93)

4. Scrubbing around the knee and the patella until the skin turns red. Keep the knee warm after treatment to ward off exogenous cold and dampness.

5. Strengthen exercises of the thigh quadriceps muscle to prevent recurrence of this disease.

a) Squatting exercise: Flex the knee joint at an angle of 30-50 degrees, i.e., in a semi-squatting position, to straighten the back without forward flexion until the thigh feels sore and aching and trembles slightly. Then rest 2-3 minutes and repeat the exercise 4-5 times in a run.

b) Standing up and squatting with load: Put a barbell on the shoulder, squat and stand up 30-40 times, rest 3-5 minutes and repeat the whole exercise 4-5 times each day.

c) Do exercises to build up the strength of the thigh quadriceps muscle as well as posterior muscle group; avoid excessive training in a single movement with load on the knee joint. Be sure to make timely adjustment in the training program and seek prompt treatment for any injury or symptoms in the knee.

4. Injury of Knee Meniscus

Injury of knee meniscus includes injury of the meniscus caused by crush and rupture of the meniscus. The meniscus of the knee joint on the medial side is large, assuming a C-shape, while that on the lateral side, which is more likely to be injured, takes an O-shape. The function of the meniscus is to increase the depth

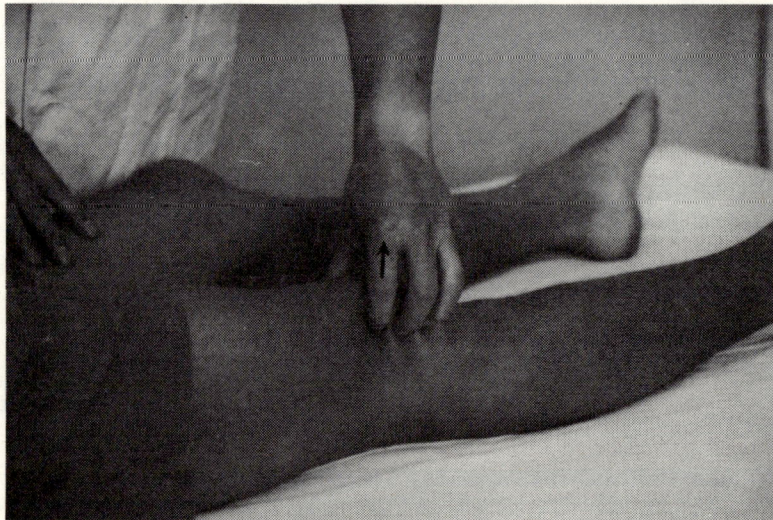

Fig. 93

the condyle of tibia for the condyle of femur to fit in so as to stabilize the joint. When the knee joint flexes, extends and rotates, the meniscus slides harmoniously; it slides forward when the knee extends and slides backward when the knee flexes; and when the knee joint rotates, one meniscus slides forward while the other backward. When the knee joint is semi-flexed and the leg turns inward, the meniscus is crushed and will not be able to move. Healing is possible for injury at the border of the meniscus as there are blood vessels there. But for injury in other parts, because there is no blood supply and their nutrition depends on synovial fluid, natural recovery is impossible.

Injury Mechanism

1. There are four causes of meniscus injury: Crush of the meniscus due to abduction, and adduction and rotation of the knee when the knee joint is semi-flexed. Crushing or even rupturing of the meniscus may result from sudden extension of the knee accompanied by rotation with the knee joint in semi-flexed position and the meniscus sliding backward. Also, when the leg is fixed, sudden rotation or inversion of thigh may cause crush injury to the meniscus by body weight, hence rupture.

2. Rupture of meniscus: Rupture of the meniscus may be caused by mutual pulverizing between the condyle of femur and the surface of tibia. In terms of rupture types, there are longitudinal rupture, laceration at the anterior, middle and posterior portions, laceration of the anterior apex and laminated rupture. The lacerated border may move out of the joint, impeding joint movement and causing locked joint. In such cases immediate manual treatment is necessary to restore knee joint functions.

3. Crush injury of meniscus: Sufficient attention is paid to rupture of meniscus but little is known about crush injury of meniscus. Some patients have typical symptoms after knee injury, the symptoms disappearing after a short course of manual treatment, indicating crushing and no rupture of the meniscus, and contraindicating surgery. In cases with light symptoms and locked joint manual treatment is the prime therapy.

4. Discoid cartilage and meniscus cyst: Congenital discoid cartilage of knee is popularly called discoid meniscus, a malformation that does not occur in a semi-lunar meniscus but is due to maldevelopment during the course of discoid cartilage occur at the lateral aspect located between the condyle of the femur and the tibia. Long-term friction and crushing may cause rupture, especially after heavy exercise. Meniscus cysts, which contain a gluey substance and vary in size, often appear at the lateral meniscus and may show symptoms in the knee.

Symptoms and Diagnosis

1. Most patients clearly have a history of trauma, very few without a knee injury. There are pain, hydrarthrosis and tumefaction at the knee joint, which cannot fully extend voluntarily. Old meniscus injury shows signs of weakness in the knee joint, with both legs feeling weak, especially when going up and down

stairs. In the course of time amyotrophy may appear at the quadriceps, muscle of the thigh, more obviously at the musculus vastas medialis.

2. Tender spot in knee joint space. This is important in diagnosing meniscus injury. Rotation and crushing test (McMurray sign) is positive: With the patient lying on his back, the inspector, putting one hand on the affected knee and holding the ankle with the other, flexes the knee to the utmost, then makes abduction and outward rotation of the leg, and gradually stretches the knee joint to the full; in the same way, he makes abduction and inward rotation, adduction and inward rotation as well as adduction and outward rotation of the leg, then stretches the knee joint to the full. A pain felt or a snap heard would tell the location of the meniscus injury.

3. Friction test is positive: With the patient taking a prone position and flexing the knee joint, the inspector holds the foot, push-presses downward and twists to produce mutual friction between the tibia and the femur. A pain suggests the possibility of injury of the posterior apex of the meniscus.

4. Gravity test is positive: With the patient lying sideways with the affected leg suspended, flexing and extending the knee joint actively. Pain or a snap may be caused by crushing produced by the gravity effect of the leg on the injured meniscus. This is more common in the injury of discoid meniscus.

5. Locked joint: The knee joint may suddenly feel difficult to flex or extend at a certain position. It can only flex or extend freely when a sound is heard after massage treatment or passive movement. Locked joint is seen in about one-third of the patients suffering from meniscus injury.

Treatment

1. Acute injury: After a definite diagnosis is made, wrap the knee joint with a thick layer of cotton by applying pressure dressing to reduce swelling haemarthrosis, but the dressing should not be too tight lest the popliteal artery be compressed.

2. Manual reduction for acute locked joint:

a) Digitally press the acupoints Taichong (LR 3), Weizhong (BL 40) and Jiexi (ST 41) to relax the muscles and stop pain. (See Fig. 94)

b) Make the patient take a prone position, pull at the foot, flex the knee and rotate the leg with one hand and push-press along the articular spaces while extending the knee with the other. This treatment can also be performed with an assistant pulling at the foot and rotating the leg while the physician performs push-pressing manipulation along the articular spaces with both hands to restore the protruded meniscus. In case this manipulation is not successful, apply local anaesthesia with 2 percent procaine and perform manual reduction when the muscles get relaxed. The reduction may succeed in most cases and the knee joint will be able to flex and extend freely immediately after the treatment.

3. Manual treatment for old meniscus injury: Press, kneading and pull-grasp to relax the quadriceps muscle of the thigh and the anterior tibial muscle group. Perform push-pressing and plucking on the articular spaces deeply yet gently while

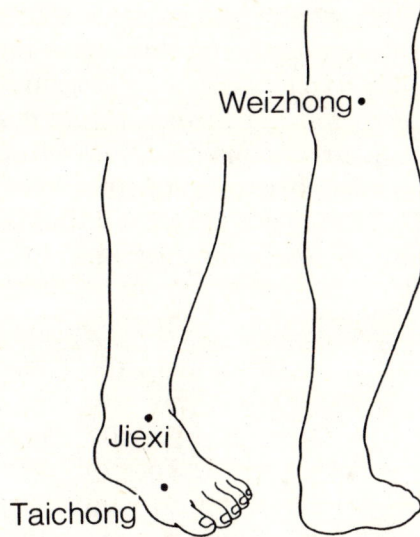

Weizhong•

Jiexi

Taichong

Fig. 94

flexing and rotating the knee joint. Pinch and nip the tissues around the patella to stimulate the diseased area and promote blood circulation and the restoration of the tissues. This treatment can yield satisfactory curative effect to crush injury of the meniscus. After the treatment, exercises should be performed on the quadriceps muscle of thigh to increase stability of the joint. For cases with distinct symptoms and repeated locked joint, it is advised to remove the ruptured meniscus by surgery.

5. Traumatic Synovitis of Knee Joint

Synovium of knee joint is the largest in area of all articular synoviums in the body. Being the lower end of the femur, the plateau of the tibia and the medial aspect of the patella are all covered by synovium, the traumatic synovitis of knee joint is most distinct.

Injury Mechanism

1. Acute injury: Impact by direct external force on the knee, falling, strain of the knee and trauma caused by other incidents may all crush, crunch and cause contuse to the synovium to cause hyperaemia, oedema and exudation in the synovial tissues, and hydrarthrosis may appear 6-7 hours after the trauma. Traumatic synovitis always exists together with other knee injuries, such as meniscus injury, ligament injury and cartilage fracture. The symptom of hydrarthrosis that appear right after a trauma is called haemarthrosis. It is often caused by serious injury in the knee, such as fracture and rupture of cruciate ligament. Though both articular exudation and haemarthrosis show signs of hydrarthrosis, the methods of treatment and prevention are not quite the same.

2. Chronic synovial strain: Long-term and strenuous activity of knee joint, such as sliding stride exercises with the knee being semi-flexed in basketball game, may crush and crunch the synoviums; free bodies and fracture in the joint may cause direct friction to synoviums, thus causing chronic inflammation and hydrarthrosis. As time passes, accumulation of dropsy may lead to sediment of cellulose, which, if not removed in time, may cause organization of fibre and articular adhesion. Due to long-term stimulation, the synoviums would turn thick gradually, thus impeding the normal motion of the joint, leading to disuse atrophy of the quadriceps muscle of the thigh and weakening the stability of the joint.

Symptoms and Diagnosis

1. After a trauma or when too tired, pain in the knee may appear. The pain become more serious when actively stretching the knee joint, especially when making resistive flexion of the knee. It may also appear when the knee is over-flexed to the extreme passively; and the knee often feels weak.

2. Swelling in the knee joint is an important manifestation of this illness. Apart from hydrarthrosis, thickening of synovium is one of the causes of swelling. At the initial stage, depressions on both sides of patella disappear, and in a serious case the whole knee is found swollen, so flexion and extension of the joint is hindered. Swelling in the joint is closely related to physical training: The swelling becomes more evident after excessive amount of training and improves after rest.

3. Floating-patellar test is positive: The massagist push-presses the top of patella with the part between the thumb and index finger of one hand to make the dropsy in the infra-patellar bursa flow into the joint capsule, while presses the patella swiftly with the index finger of the other. Then, the massagist can feel that the patella impacts on the femur and floats up. The more distinct this sensation is, the more dropsy there is.

4. Crushing test is positive: Stretch the knee joint straight, the massagist push-presses at the medial aspect of the knee upward from bottom with the palm, then push-squeezes at the lateral aspect of the knee from top downward. Now a wavy expansion can be seen at the front medial aspect of the knee. This is because the fluid is squeezed from the lateral aspect to the medial aspect. This method can help find out the small amount of dropsy in the articulation.

Treatment

1. Digitally press acupoints Futu (ST 32), Dubi (ST 35), Zusanli (ST 36), Weizhong (BL 40) and Chengshan (BL 57). (See Fig. 95)

2. Acute injury: Immediately apply pressure dressing to the knee to prevent bleeding and oedema, start manual treatment 24 hours afterwards.

3. Manual treatment for chronic strain:

a) Making the patient take a supine position and put a thin pillow under the knee, the massagist press-kneads and pull-grasps the quadriceps muscle of thigh to relax the muscles and prevent amyotrophy and adhesion.

b) Manipulation to remove articular dropsy: Manual treatment is more prefer-

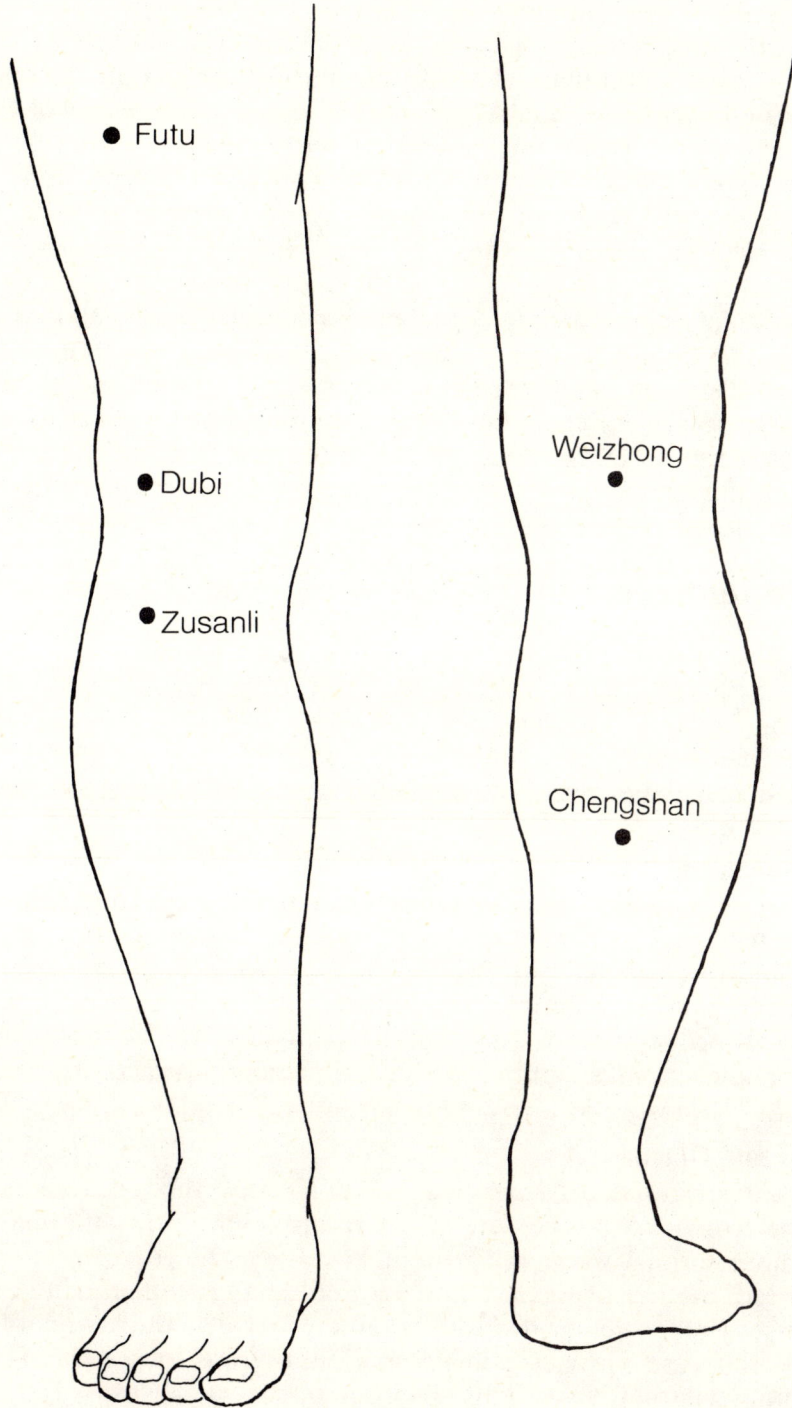

● Futu

● Dubi

● Zusanli

Weizhong
●

Chengshan
●

Fig. 95

able than repeated puncture in drawing out dropsy caused by chronic strain of knee joint, because dropsy may appear again after it is drawn out by puncture. The processes of manipulation are: The massagist push-presses the depressions on both sides of patella with the index finger for 1-2 minutes; for swollen soft tissues around the patella, perform the manipulation of scraping to stimulate the inflamed synoviums to promote the absorption of the dropsy by the synoviums. The scraping should be deep and forceful, but the force applied must not be abrupt lest it aggravates the swelling and results in more dropsy. Or, the massagist can repeatedly push-squeeze the dropsy from the distal end to the proximal end of the knee slowly yet deeply and strongly, supplemented with flexion and extension of the knee joint. The popliteal fossa should also be push-squeezed, but the force must be mild lest it causes subcutaneous extravasation of blood in the popliteal fossa. One round of treatment each day, better be given after physical training.

c) Adjustment of exercise amount: When there is swelling and too much dropsy, the amount of exercises have to be cut to promote absorption of dropsy. Keep the knee warm after recovery and prevent against exogenous cold and dampness.

6. Bursitis of Knee

The bursae of knee are distributed among skin, fasciae, tendons, ligaments and bony tissues. Their functions are to reduce mutual friction of the knee joint and increase the scope of motion of the soft tissues. In sports injuries, bursitis is more often seen than bursitis of other joints. Bursitis occurs most often at the propatellar bursa, suprapatellar bursa, infrapatellar bursa, bursa of semi-tendinous muscle and anserine bursa.

Injury Mechanism

This disease is divided into two types, i.e., chronic strain and acute injury. Their causes are mechanical friction due to repeated strenuous flexion and extension of the knee and direct impact on the bursae produced by external force. A case of acute injury may shows signs of haematocele in the bursae; while one of chronic strain reveals oedema and hyperaemia of synovium, thickening of the bursa wall and pale yellow glue-like fluid in the bursae, which may, after some time, result in sediment of cellulose, and a feeling of grain-like substance.

Symptoms and Diagnosis

1. Propatellar bursitis: Also called "miner's knee," there is a semi-global protrusion in the front part of the patella; there are slight pain and tenderness, which become more serious when the patient kneels down; there is a wavy sensation, when pressed, the size of the swelling does not change much. If it becomes smaller when pressed, it is articular dropsy. Palpation feels the thickening of the propatellar tissues. In a case with acute inflammation, there is local swelling and hot pain.

2. Suprapatellar bursitis: This disorder occurs at the superior aspect of the patellar and at the depth of the quadriceps muscle of thigh. The patient's chief

complaints are weakness, swelling and heaviness in the knee. There is a semi-circular tumefaction at the superior aspect of patella, more evident when the knee is flexed. When pushing with hand, the mass may become partially smaller but does not subside completely. The thickened bursa, and even the thickened border may be palpated. Slight amyotrophy may be found at the quadriceps muscle of thigh in a chronic case, more distinct at the musculus vastus medialis.

3. Infrapatellar bursitis: This bursa lies in the depth of the patellar ligament, linking the articular cavity. When the knee joint is semi-flexed, the pressure the bursa bears is the largest. Athletes who do more jumping movements from a semi-squatting position are more likely to contract this disease. The manifestations are: the knee feels weak at a semi-squatting position, the knee joint feels sore and aching, tumefaction appears on both sides of the patellar ligament, and there is pain felt on pressure at the depth of the ending point of the patellar ligament and at the upper border of the tuberosity of tibia when the knee is extended, as well as pain at the joint when the knee is flexed or extended passively.

4. Bursitis of pes anserinus: (See section on "Bursitis of Pes Anserinus")

Treatment

1. Digitally press acupoints Dubi (ST 35), Xiyan (Extra), Zusanli (ST 36) and Weizhong (BL 40).

2. Press-knead soft tissues around the knee joint to promote blood circulation and remove blood stasis as well as dredging the meridians and collaterals.

3. Manipulations at the bursitis area: First push-press the cyst with force. For suprapatellar bursitis, push-squeeze from the proximal end towards the inferior direction of the knee; for propatellar bursitis, push-press from the center of the patella toward all direction to reduce the fluid to the minimum. Then scrape on the wall of the bursa, exert stronger force on the hypertrophic border of the bursa wall to cause local hyperaemia to help in absorption of dropsy and repair of the tissues. Push-pressing and scraping are the main manipulations for treatment of this disease.

4. For acute trauma in the knee, pressure dressing should be applied immediately after the injury and removed after 24 hours. If there is too much dropsy in the bursa and tumefaction is distinct, puncture should be performed to draw out the fluid. For general tumefaction, however, manual treatment is recommended with push-pressing and scraping manipulations. For a case with marked symptoms in the knee, reduce or adjust strength exercises for the knee, avoid repeated doing of a single movement, and increase strength exercises for the quadriceps muscle of thigh to promote subsidence of tumefaction.

7. Popliteal Cyst

Popliteal cyst refers to swelling of bursa at the depth of popliteal fossa and the backward protrusion of the synovium of the knee joint. The content of the cyst is articular fluid or bursal fluid. Usually, the cyst locates at the medial aspect of the gastrocnemius and between the semi-tendinous muscle and the semi-membranous muscle. The cause of the disease is chronic inflammation resulted from repeated squeezing and pressing as well as friction of the synovial bursa or the synovium of the knee joint. In some cases, it represents a sort of symptom resulted from osteoarthritis of the knee or injury of the posterior apex of meniscus.

Symptoms and Diagnosis

1. At the initial stage, the posterior aspect of the knee joint feels uncomfortable and distending. When the cyst grows larger, squatting is limited and the patient cannot do full squatting movement.

2. Palpation may feel a smooth semi-circular cyst with fairly clear borders at the popliteal fossa. With the basal border being not so definite, its location is fixed.

3. When making overextension movement, the cyst grows larger and harder, but it still feels like a cyst. It can turn smaller when squeezed or pressed, and even disappears when the knee is flexed. Trans-illumination test is positive.

Treatment

1. Digitally press the acupoints Weizhong (BL 40), Chengshan (BL 57) and Dubi (ST 35).

2. Making the patient take a prone position, have the knee extended and put a thin pad in from of the knee, the massagist press-kneads the lower part of the posterior femoral muscle group and the upper part of the gastrocnemius; pluck the muscular tendons in the order of the semi-membranous muscle, the semi-tendinous muscle, and the biceps muscle of the thigh and the gastrocnemius.

3. Press the center of the cyst for 1-2 minutes to reduce the cyst and apply repeated push-pressing to promote the absorption of the fluid. As the skin at the popliteal fossa is thin without much subcutaneous fat, the force applied in the manipulation should not be too strong lest it may cause subcutaneous bleeding in the popliteal area. If the border of the cyst turns thick, apply gentle scraping with the thumb to stimulate the cyst for absorption of the fluid.

4. If there is too much fluid in the cyst, puncture it and draw out the fluid under the condition of strict sterilization. In doing this, be careful not to hurt the popliteal artery. To yield a still better curative effect, apply manual treatment the day after the puncture.

8. Bursitis of Pes Anserinus

Bursitis of pes anserinus is also called enthesiopathy of tendon of pes anserinus, pain of pes anserinus or inflammation of medial condyle malleolus of tibia.

Injury Mechanism

1. Anatomic characteristics: The sartorius muscle, the gracilis muscle and the semi-tendinous muscle run through the medial aspect of the knee joint and

terminates at the medial aspect of the tuberosity of tibia, assuming the shape of pes anserinus (anserine foot), hence the name of this area. The bursa between the deep part and the medial tibial ligament is called anserine bursa.

2. Overburden in medium- and long-distance running may cause muscular tension, spasm and even fatigue at the sartorius muscle, the gracilis muscle and the semi-tendinous muscle. Repeated pulling of these muscles can result in light injury at their attachment points. This is called in enthesiopathy. Stimulation on the anserine bursa can cause bursitis of pes anserinus, which is a sort of aseptic chronic injury.

Symptoms and Diagnosis

1. Pain at the medial aspect of the knee, force cannot be exerted when the foot holds the land; there might even be lameness in an acute attack.

2. There are tenderness and tumefaction at the medial condyle of femur and the tuberosity of tibia, as well as in the area of the three muscles, namely, the sartorius muscle, the gracilis muscle and the semi-tendinous muscle.

3. Pain felt when the knee joint is flexed or rotated outward, and when knee-flexion resistance is performed.

Treatment

1. Digitally press acupoints Xuehai (SP10), Weizhong (BL 40), Zusanli (ST 36) and Yanglingquan (GB 34). (See Fig. 96)

2. Making the patient lie on his side, the massagist press-kneads the muscles at the medial aspect of the knee with both palms, i.e., on the sartorius muscle, the gracilis muscle, the semi-membranous muscle and the semi-tendinous muscle, to relax them, increase their elasticity, improve their blood circulation and reduce

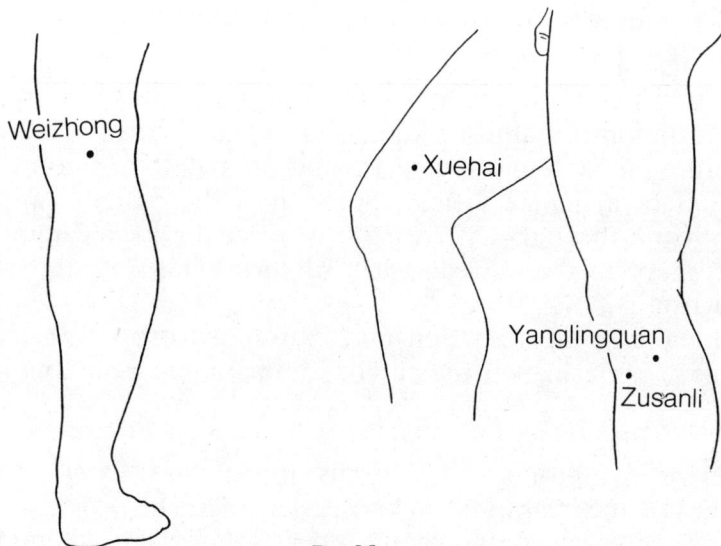

Fig. 96

pain at the soft tissues in the anserine area caused by muscular tension and long-time pulling; pluck to relax the tendons, increase muscle elasticity and reduce their pulling on the attachment points; then press along the trend of the tendons to restore the tissues.

3. Forcefully scrape or push-press the tuberosity of tibia with fingers to stimulate the affected areas and promote the cure of inflammation. This is a key step in treating this disease. The force applied at the acute stage should be comparatively light and that at the chronic stage should be relatively stronger.

9. Synovial Incarceration of Knee

Synovial incarceration of knee is a knee syndrome caused by compression of the synovial folds between the border of the patellar-femoral joint, the medial aspect of the medial condyle of femur the lateral aspect of the lateral condyle of femur.

Injury Mechanism

1. Direct trauma caused by impact on the anterior part of the knee and compression of synovium by the patella, which give rise to synovial hyperaemia and oedema.

2. Chronic strain due to repeated slight injuries in the knee, which lead to compression and friction on synovium. This in turn causes synovium hyperplasia. As a result, the synovium is apt to be incarcerated in the joint space when the joint moves.

3. Various kinds of pathological changes in the knee joint that can cause synovitis, such as osteoarthropathy, osteochondrosis, free bodies in the joint and atrophic arthritis, may lead to synovial hyperplasia, may render the synovium in valviform, nodular or cord form and make it apt for it to be incarcerated in the joint when the knee joint is excessively flexed, extended or rotated.

Symptoms and Diagnosis

1. Locked joint: This is the main symptom of synovial incarceration of knee. The major manifestations are limited knee flexion and extension, pain which often occurs at the border of the femoral condyle and the patellar-femoral joint, as well as a small amount of articular dropsy. Sometimes the patient can pull out the incarcerated synovium through self massage to relax the locked joint.

2. The knee feels painful and weak when squatting halfway, jumping, or going upstairs and downstairs.

3. Repeated long-term incarceration may cause amyotrophy in the quadriceps muscle of the thigh, tenderness at the patella and pain when making resistive knee extension.

4. Differentiating diagnosis: Synovial incarceration of knee has to be differentiated from locking symptoms in meniscus injury and from chondromalacia patellae. For synovial incarceration of knee, use 2 percent procaine for blockage at the painful area, the symptoms may disappear immediately. Digital-pressing at

the painful area for 30 seconds can also alleviate the pain.

Treatment

1. Digitally press acupoints Dubi (ST 35), Zusanli (ST 36) and Weizhong (BL 40).

2. Press-knead and pull-grasp the quadriceps muscle and the tibialis anterior of the leg to relax them.

3. Make the patient take a prone position, the massagist puts an elbow at the popliteal fossa of the affected limb and holds the ankle with the other hand, flexes the knee and pulls upward in conjunction with rotation of the leg so as to widen the joint space; and ask an assistant to scrape the soft tissues at the painful area from the center toward all directions to separate the synovium from the joint so as to relax the locked joint. The return of free movement for the joint indicates completion of the manual treatment. If one treatment fails to achieve this effect, change the pulling angle and turning direction until the effect is achieved. One other way is to perform blockage with 2 percent procaine in conjunction with pulling and scraping at the diseased area to re-locate the incarcerated synovium.

4. If the synovium is incarcerated in the patellar-femoral joint, the massagist can grasp the patellar with all five fingers of one hand and pull sideways to increase the patellar-femoral joint space and reduce compression on the synovium, then tract the soft tissues outward with force to pull out the synovium from the joint.

Repeated synovial incarceration may result in hyperplastic hypertrophy of the diseased synovium, thus causing dysfunction of the joint. Under such a condition, surgery is needed to remove the hyperplastic synovium which is liable to be incarcerated, or pull the incarcerated synovium out of the joint space and suture it onto the surrounding synovium.

10. Injury of Infrapatellar Fat Pad

Infrapatellar fat pad locates in the conoid space between the femur, tibia and the patella ligament, assuming a wedge-like shape and being covered by synoviums at the posterior aspect. Performing the cushioning and lubricating functions, it fills up at the anterior aspect of the femur and tibia, and prevent friction and stimulation. So, it plays a significant role to maintain the functions of the knee joint.

Injury Mechanism

1. Direct trauma: Normally caused by direct impact, such as kicking at the knee and compression of the fat pad by femur and tibia when the knee joint is over-extended.

2. Chronic strain: Compression and injury of the fat pad due to repeated over-extension of the knee joint with burden and repeated friction between the femur and tibia. The infrapatellar fat pad is more likely to be injured when the knee joint is flaccid and malformed due to over-extension. The injury of the fat

pad is an aseptic inflammation with such manifestations as hyperaemia, edema and thickening as well as stimulating the synovium to produce hydrarthrus.

Symptoms and Diagnosis

1. Pain: There is pain at the front part and in the depth of the knee joint. The pain becomes more severe after physical exercise and relieved after rest, and becomes more serious when the knee joint is extended and relieved when the knee joint is slightly flexed. For female patients, the pain becomes worse when wearing shoes with flat soles and is relieved when wearing a high-heeled shoes as they make the knees slightly bent. This is different from pain at the knee joint caused by other diseases.

2. Tumefaction: There is tumefaction on both sides of the patellar ligament; thickened fat pad, which feels rather soft, may be palpated; and protrusion of the fat pad becomes more distinct when the knee joint is fully extended. If tumefaction is observed at only one side, the possibility of other diseases should be considered. The symptoms become more evident when comparing the affected knee with the one that is not injured. Tumefaction of articular fat pad should be differentiated from hydrarthrosis. In the latter, floating patellar test is positive.

3. Tenderness: Tenderness is evident at the thickened fat pad; it also appears when the knee joint is extended passively.

4. Limited activity of the knee joint: The patient cannot do hyperextension movement of the knee joint. When the hypertrophic fat pad is compressed between the femur and tibia, there may occur locked joint with fierce pain. Active flexion and extension of the knee joint or rest may relax the pain, but manual treatment is necessary for locked joint caused by rupture of meniscus.

Treatment

1. Digitally press the acupoint Xiyan (Extra) on both sides of the knee joint.

2. The patient lies on the back, flexes both knees slightly with the affected knee being atop the healthy one, as in the posture to receive a knee reflex inspection, to widen the joint space with the weight of the leg, while the massagist press-kneads at both the depressions of the patellar ligament with both thumbs for 3-5 minutes to relax the fat pad tissues.

3. Press the surrounding regions of the patellar to relax the quadriceps muscle of thigh as well as the tissues besides the patella, then push the patella upward repeatedly to pull upward the infrapatellar fat pad.

4. The fat pad is protruded when the knee is extended, so the massagist may scrape and pluck it, with the force applied growing from light to strong. The treatment lasts two minutes each time, once a day. It is conducive to the absorption of inflammation and detumescence to promote blood circulation in the fat pad by forceful stimulation.

5. Treatment for incarceration of fat pad: Make the patient take a supine position with the hip and knee slightly bent, the massagist pulls at and makes outward and inward rotation of the leg while asking an assistant to push-press the

patella upward so the fat pad, incarcerated between the femur and tibia, may be pulled upward and out. The symptoms may disappear after repeating the manipulation 2-3 times while extending the knee gradually.

Patients suffering from injury of the fat pad should do more strength exercises of the quadriceps muscle of thigh, and avoid excessive extension of the knee joint. If the symptoms are serious, reduce the amount of knee exercises.

11. Epiphysitis of Tibial Tuberosity

Forceful contraction of the quadriceps muscle of thigh pulls at the tuberosity of tibia, causing degeneration, rupture and displacement of the epiphysis at the superior end of tibia. A disorder commonly seen in youngsters (between 11-18 years of age), it can recover by itself, yet may leave serious malformation.

Injury Mechanism

1. Epiphysis of the tibial tuberosity is also called lingulate epiphysis. Violent contraction of the quadriceps muscle of thigh may result in pulling at the epiphysis by the patellar tendon; repeated pulling at the epiphysis hinders its normal development, thus causing local injury, with such manifestations as local hyperaemia and edema, gradual hypertrophy, and enlargement and protrusion of the epiphysis, and even upward bending of the epiphysis in a serious case.

2. Direct trauma: Direct local crash at the epiphysis may cause injury to it. This cause is seldom, and sometimes serves only as a predisposing cause, as local protrusion is only found when the tuberosity of tibia feels painful after the injury. In fact, the cause of disease has been there for sometime. It has been overlooked and not arouse enough attention.

Symptoms and Diagnosis

1. Pain: The onset of the disease is slow and in most cases the pain is slight. It is felt only when the epiphysis is pressed by kneeling on the ground. Usually, pain is the earliest symptom. It is only felt when the knee is extended suddenly or resistively, or when kicking a ball hard. Normally, there is a sensation of distension and a uncomfortable feeling.

2. Swelling: Swelling is the major basis for diagnosis of this disease. The swelling develops slowly. Occasionally, swelling and protrusion are found at the tuberosity of tibia, as hard as the bone. Pain is felt when pressed, as in bone tumour. The protrusion develops slowly. In most cases there are symmetric swelling at the tibial area on both sides, and on one side in a small number of cases. A correct diagnosis can be made according to the position and characteristics of the protrusion.

3. The knee-extension strength reduces. As sudden contraction of the quadriceps muscle of thigh causes pain at the protrusion, in order not to cause pain the patient does not dare to extend the knee with force. This is a protective reaction, and as time elapses it may give rise to disuse atrophy of the quadriceps muscle of thigh.

Treatment

1. Digitally press acupoints Dubi (ST 35) and Zusanli (ST 36).

2. The massagist presses around the patella with the back part of the palm for five minutes to relax the quadriceps muscle of thigh and the tissues around the patella and raise the skin temperature; then press-kneads the anterior tibial muscle group and pluck at the patellar tendon 10 times to increase its elasticity and relax the pulling at the tuberosity of tibia. The force applied to pluck at the patellar tendon should not be too heavy.

3. Local manipulation: Press on the protrusion with finger for 3-5 minutes and the force applied should just be appropriate for the patient to stand; push-press towards all directions from the center of the swelling; scrape lightly or tap at the protrusion with finger tips for 2-3 minutes to promote local blood circulation, cure the inflammation and relieve pain. After the manipulation, the pain should markedly reduce when kneeling on the ground.

12. Painful Syndrome at the Lateral Side of Knee

Painful syndrome at the lateral side of the knee is also called friction syndrome of the iliotibial tract. It refers to pathological changes at the iliotibial tract of the lateral side of the knee, the upper and lower bursae and surrounding tissues of the collateral ligament of the lateral side of the knee joint as well as the hamstring.

Injury Mechanism

1. Friction of iliotibial tract: The iliotibial tract is at the lateral aspect of the knee joint. When the knee joint extends, it slips to the front of the external epicondyle of femur. There is a bursa between the external epicondyle of femur and the iliotibial tract. Excessively frequent movement of the iliotibial tract, i.e., too much extension and flexion of the knee joint with load, may give rise to hyperaemia, edema and exudate in the bursa, hence local pain. In a chronic case, degenerative contracture may occur at the iliotibial tract.

2. Trauma: Direct crush on the lateral aspect of the knee joint causes traumatic pain at the local soft tissues.

Symptoms and Diagnosis

1. At the early stage, most patients feel pain at the lateral aspect of the knee joint when flexing and extending the knee joint but feel no pain when walking with straight leg due to absence of friction between the iliotibial tract and the lateral condyle of femur. At the late stage, pain is felt in the knee when squatting or going upstairs and downstairs.

2. Snapping sound and frictional sensation: Denaturation, such as fibrosis or adhesion, is found at the iliotibial tract; a snap can be heard when the joint is flexed or extended; and palpation can detect a sensation of friction at the lateral aspect of the knee.

3. Tumefaction and pain when touched: Examination may verify tumefaction

and pain on pressure, and even painful masses.

4. Differentiation in diagnosis: This disease should be differentiated from the injury of the lateral knee meniscus and the injury of the lateral collateral ligament of the knee joint. For the injury of the lateral knee meniscus, there is an obvious history of trauma and evident locked joint and positive signs in McMurry test; and for the injury of the lateral collateral ligament of the knee joint, there is pain at the lateral aspect of the knee when the knee joint is stretched and the leg is pulled inward.

Treatment

1. Digitally press acupoints Fengshi (GB 31), Xiyangguan (GB 33) and Yang-lingquan (GB 34).

2. Make the patient lie on his side, the massagist presses the lateral aspect of the thigh to relax the tissues, plucks on the iliotibial tract from top downward several times to increase its elasticity, widen its range of movement, achieve spasmolysis and reduce adhesion; then press-pushes the thigh longitudinally to regulate and restore the iliotibial tract.

3. Push-pressing the painful area: Push-press or scrape the center of the painful area or the scleromata to remove them. Finally perform circular massage on the painful area with the thumb in conjunction with the flexion and extension of the knee joint. This can allay inflammation, alleviate pain and reduce tumefaction.

13. Osteochondritis Dissecans of Femoral Condyle

Osteochondritis dissecans of femoral condyle is often seen among people aged 13-25, most common among people between 13 and 15 years old. According to medical literature, the pathological change takes place more often at the medial condyle of femur than at the lateral condyle. Yet clinically, this author finds it takes place more often at the lateral condyle of femur than at the medial condyle, and more frequent at a single knee joint while changes at both knees being rare. Once, the author reported four cases and all of them occurred at the lateral condyle.

Injury Mechanism

1. The lateral condyle of femur is smaller than the medial condyle; the knee joint rotates with the lateral condyle of femur as the axis, and the medial condyle rotates around the lateral condyle. As the lateral condyle bears greater burden, repeated crushing, impact and friction may impede blood circulation at the still growing cartilage of condyle, thus causing ischemic necrosis.

2. The impact of aerial, side somersault, as well as circling and landing in gymnastics all act upon the lateral condyle of femur. The crushing and damage to the condyle will be more serious due to repeated failure of semi-squatting movements, particularly, squatting movements with the knee joint touching the ground.

3. At the initial stage of the pathological change, there is a bleeding zone at the ischemic area of bone; around this zone granulation develops. Later, the fibrosis of granulation causes stripping of bone and cartilage fragments resulting from ischemic necrosis. The injured area is often covered by fibrous tissues and cartilage tissues. The stripped cartilage fragments move into the joint and turn into free bodies.

Symptoms and Diagnosis

1. Medical history: Most patients are between 13 and 25 years old, that is, are at the stage for the development of epiphysis. There is no obvious history of trauma, but a history of long-term pain in the knee joint.

2. Pain: There is slight pain in the knee joint when going upstairs or downstairs or when at a semi-squat position. The pain is more serious when the amount of exercises is increased. The legs feel weak. There might be sudden lameness during physical training. The pain felt at the semi-squat position may disappear or be alleviated when the patient changes into a full squat position or after rest.

3. Tender spot: A limited tender spot can be found at the lateral condyle of femur. This point may be of significance for the diagnosis of the disease.

4. There might be slight atrophy of the quadriceps muscle of the thigh, about 1-1.5 cm. in size, with the complication of a small amount of hydrarthrosis that may repeatedly appear.

5. X-ray examination reveals an elliptical and uneven bone-density reduction at the articular surface of the condyle of femur, in which there may be small cystiform changes. At the initial stage, the articular surface is smooth, but unevenness may gradually develop at the articular surface. There might be a misdiagnosis as front and sideway X-ray photos do not show obvious change in the joint space. However, the pathological changes can be clearly revealed in X-ray photo taken with the knee joint being rotated inward at a 40-degree angle. Yet, the symptoms shown in X-ray photos should be differentiated from those for bone tuberculosis.

Treatment

1. Physical training must be suspended after an affirmative diagnosis is made. At the early stage, local immobilization by applying strapping with long-leg plaster support should be adopted as the main treatment. Physical training of other parts of the body may continue and static exercises of the quadriceps muscle of the thigh may be performed. Remove the plaster support at night and practise knee joint flexion and extension in bed to avoid joint adhesion. The strapping on the legs usually lasts three months without stop.

2. Manual treatment may be performed during the period of strapping by removing the plaster support temporarily. The key manipulations are press-kneading and pull-grasping the muscles of the thigh and leg as well as gentle pluck-poking at the belly of the muscles to maintain the elasticity of the muscles, prevent adhesion, relieve compression on the bone by muscular tone, promote

blood circulation in the tissues around the spot of pathological change for the healing of the bony tissues. In the local painful area, perform gentle scraping to stimulate and restore the local tissues. However, forceful scraping should be avoided lest the cartilage be further injured.

3. After the plaster support strapping is removed, it is necessary to strength exercises of the quadriceps muscle of the thigh in combination with static and other exercises, such as exercises at standing position, squatting and standing up exercises as well as jogging. For a short period immediately after the removal of the strapping, however, it is necessary to avoid activities that may cause impact on the knee joint.

Example: Miss Yu, 13, had been doing gymnastics training for five years. For no apparent reason, she felt pain at the lateral aspect of the right knee, which lasted for two years and became more serious, especially when the amount of exercises increased. The pain became more apparent at semi-squat position, and the leg felt weak when walking, going upstairs and downstairs. Sudden lameness may develop during training. Examination showed slight atrophy of the right quadriceps muscle of thigh; no tenderness at the joint space. Floating-patella test was negative; a limited tender spot was found at the lateral condyle of the right femur; there was pain when the knee was flexed at a 30-degree angle, but no pain was felt at a full squat position. Contrast examination of the knee joint revealed no meniscus injury. X-ray photo taken with the knee joint being rotated inward at a 40-degree angle showed an osteoporosis area 1.0 × 1.8 cm. in size at the lateral condyle of femur near the articular surface. Blood sedimentation is normal. Diagnosis: Osteochondritis dissecans of the right lateral femoral condyle. After strapping the knee with long-leg plaster support for one month, X-ray examination showed remarkable repair of the damage. During the period of strapping and after removal of the strapping, the patient was asked to make static exercises of the quadriceps muscle of the thigh every day while receiving manual treatment. Three months later, the disease went basically and the patient was able to participate in normal training and competition again.

14. Epiphysiolysis of Distal End of Femur

Epithysiolysis of the distal end of the femur is a serious but rare injury. Patients are usually teenagers 8-14 years old. Since it is often complicated with injury of the nerves and blood vessels in the popliteal area, so emergent manual treatment is necessary.

Injury Mechanism

1. The knee joint of teenagers is protected by strong ligaments, articular capsules and muscles, so it has a good stability. But the epiphysis of the distal end of femur is a comparatively weak part. Therefore, dislocation of knee joint is rarely seen but epiphysiolysis of femur is common in teenagers. Sudden turning of knee

joint caused by hyperextension due to brutal force may cause dislocation of the epiphysis at the distal end of femur. Due to the action of the posterior joint capsule, ligament and gastrocnemius muscle, the lower end of the epiphysis usually displaces forward while the comparatively separated distal part is squeezed between the patella and the femoral shaft. A serious epiphysiolysis may cause upward and eversion malformation.

2. In epiphysiolysis of the distal end of femur, the displaced end often compresses the nerves and blood vessels of the popliteal area, causing serious complications in the leg, which, if not given timely treatment, may result in serious blockage of blood circulation in the leg, which may even give rise to necrosis in the leg. Therefore, a case of this disease should be considered an emergency one calling for immediately treatment.

Symptoms and Diagnosis

1. Apparent traumatic history, severe pain in the knee, immediate loss of function, and inability to stand.

2. Deformity of knee joint, epiphysiolysis end is palpable, and abnormal movement in the knee.

3. In a case of serious deformity, the beating of pulse at the dorsal part of the foot disappears, the local sensation is impeded, the skin turns pale and the skin temperature drops — all indicate compression of the popliteal artery and nerve.

Treatment

1. As moving the patient and making preparations for anaesthesia might aggravate the injury and pain and lose time for treatment, it is recommended to start manual reduction without having a X-ray photo taken and applying anaesthesia so long a confirmed diagnosis can be made. Moreover, manual reduction will be made more difficult when swelling appears in the joint.

2. Traction: Making an assistant pull at the patient's thigh, the massagist holds the ankle with both hands and performs sustained traction along the trend of deformity in the leg and stretches the knee joint gradually when the fractured part is felt moving. Extend the leg by traction for another 3-5 minutes to fully separate the overlapping teratism.

3. Making an assistant still pulling at the thigh and another pulling the leg, the massagist push-squeezes on the fractured end back and forth at the lower end of the femur with both hands. If the displacement is lateral, push-squeeze from two sides towards the center. This method can effect a reduction for most cases. Then, the massagist assesses the result of the reduction with hand palpation. If the reduction is successful, ask the assistants to release their pulling. Afterwards, the massagist can feel the beating of the dorsal artery of foot. Normal beating of the artery indicates removal of compression on the popliteal artery. Finally, the massagist should inspect the skin temperature, and the sensation and movement of the foot. In a successful reduction, the skin turns red from a pale colour, the numb sensation is alleviated and the movement of the foot improved.

4. Reduce temperature of the knee joint with ice or chloroethane, and apply pressure dressing with a thick cotton pad and elastic bandage to prevent tumefaction, then send the patient to hospital immediately. In the hospital, take an X-ray photo to check the reduction, then apply strapping with long-leg plastic support for 4-6 weeks.

Example: Ouyang, female, 15, gymnast. On May 8, 1985, she got her left leg caught on the lower bar in landing during the pre-competition warm-up during the National Women's Gymnastics Championships in Hangzhou. As a result, her left knee joint was badly deformed, with the lower leg being bent upwards 180 degrees. The leg rested lateral to the thigh, the posterior aspect of the leg faces the front, and the foot rested at the lateral aspect of the buttock with the toes hitting the mat. The beating of the dorsal artery of foot was weak. In consideration of the situation, she was given emergency treatment without any anaesthesia. An assistant was asked to pull at her thigh, the massagist pulled the ankle with one hand and held the knee with the other to turn the leg downward by 180 degrees to make the toes point to the front. As there was lateral displacement at the fractured end, one assistant was asked to pull at the thigh and another pull the ankle gradually, the massagist pressed the fractured end with both hands to ensure a reduction. After the reduction, the beating of the dorsal artery of foot returned to normal. Pressure dressing was then applied and the patient was sent to hospital to take an X-ray photo, which showed that the fractured ends had been reduced precisely. She was able to take part in normal training and competition a year later.

15. Fracture of Patella

The patella is triangular in shape; it locates at the anterior aspect of the knee and forms the patellar-femoral joint with the femur. During the knee extension movements of the quadriceps muscle of thigh, the patellar serves as the main support. The tendon of the quadriceps muscle of thigh, the patella and the patellar ligament and aponeurosis constitute the knee-extension apparatus for enhancing the functions of walking, running and jumping.

Injury Mechanism

1. Direct hitting: Fracture may be caused by hitting the ground with the knee when falling down and by direct kicking or other direct impact; such fracture is often comminuted fracture (stellate fracture). Displacement is not obvious in such fracture. Yet, there can be serious injury at the articular surface and the femoral condyle, which may hinder the joint function later.

2. Indirect external force: Sudden and forceful contraction of the quadriceps muscle may pull the patella apart into two fragments. Sudden contraction of the quadriceps muscle of thigh by falling from a high-up place or violent kicking movement may cause fracture, which normally assumes transverse fracture accompanied by distinct displacement.

Symptoms and Diagnosis

1. Evident history of trauma, pain, swelling, ecchymoma and articular dyskinesia.

2. More serious pain when the quadriceps muscle of thigh contracts; palatable transverse depression in cases of transverse fracture, with the two fractured ends possibly displaced up and down; distinct pain on pressure.

3. X-ray examination may help confirm the diagnosis. An X-ray photo should be taken of the patellar at the tangential position if there is a fracture at the patellar border or not (the diagnosis of this kind of fracture can be easily missed).

4. The fracture of patellar must be differentiated from dichotomous patella in which the patella is divided into two or more parts due to congenital abnormal development, while its symptom of pain appears gradually, the border of the accessory bone is smooth and clear as may be shown in X-ray examination, and the bone trabecula is complete.

Treatment

1. Making the patient lie in supine posture and stretch the knee joint, the massagist applies anaesthesia with 2 percent procaine. If there is a large amount of haemarthrosis, draw it out under strict sterilization to make it easy for manual reduction and prevent articular adhesion which may happen after treatment.

2. Playing the thumb and index finger at the border of the patella, the massagist push-squeezes the fracture ends from the upper and lower border towards the center to unite the fracture. Feeling of the disappearance of the displacement indicates completion of the reduction. The usual practice is to fix the proximal part to the distal part, because the proximal part links with the quadriceps muscle of thigh and has good elasticity while the distal part links with the patella ligament and has poor elasticity.

For cases that receive treatment after a relatively longer period since the injury, there may be haemarthrosis and tumefaction. Therefore, it is necessary to apply anaesthesia, draw out the haemarthrosis and reduce the tumefaction by push-pressing the soft tissues around the patella from the distal part to the proximal part. If the tumefaction is serious, immediately apply strapping with the knee extending straight and raise the leg high for 1-2 days to perform manual treatment.

3. Knee-wrapping fixation: Make a knee-wrapping ring first—make a ring with thick lead wire according to the thickness of the knee, apply a thick layer of cotton around the ring and wind it with bandage. Put the ring around the reduced patella. Prepare a piece of long wooden board or a plaster support long enough to cover the length from the ankle at the bottom to the middle part of the thigh. And fix the knee-wrapping ring, with the knee joint being kept straight, onto the board or plaster support with a strip of cloth belt.

After the treatment, it is necessary to check the position of the patella now and then to see if there is relapse of displacement. Be sure to protect the skin around the patella from being ruptured by the board or the plaster support. Start to massage the quadriceps muscle of thigh a week later to avoid muscular atrophy and adhesion, improve blood circulation of the local tissues and promote union of the fracture. The patient must be warned not to do isometric contraction of the quadriceps muscle of thigh. He or she may be advised to do it and practise walking with crutches three weeks later. Remove the fixation 4-6 weeks later and take an X-ray photo to confirm complete union of the muscle. After this, exercises can be increased on the quadriceps muscle of thigh and knee joint gradually, along with continuous massage all over the leg to promote restoration of functions. However, such movements as semi-squatting and jumping must wait.

16. Traumatic Dislocation and Subluxation of Patella

Normally, neither inward or outward sliding displacement occurs at the patella when the knee is extended or flexed. It is the stability in structure which prevents such displacement. The stability of the structure is reinforced by the powerful pulling of the quadriceps muscle of thigh and the mutual engagement between the articular surfaces of the patella and femoral condyle. The pulling by the muscle vastas medialis and its sponeurosis at the superomedial aspect of the patella can also prevent the patella from dislocating outward.

The patellar dislocation is divided into three types, namely, congenital, traumatic and habitual. In sports, traumatic dislocation is the main form.

Injury Mechanism

1. Direct external force: The action of external force on the anteromedial, medial or lateral aspect of the patella can all cause patellar dislocation. This means that any violent foreign force can cause dislocation of the patella, with outward dislocation being the more often seen.

2. Indirect external force: In valgus and varus malformation of the knee joint, the turning of the knee changes the mechanical and linear relationship among the quadriceps muscle of thigh, patella and tuberosity of tibia. Under this condition, contraction of the quadriceps muscle of thigh would pull the patella to the lateral side, causing outward dislocation. Excessive twisting of the knee may also cause dislocation even if there is no valgus and varus malformation of the knee joint. For instance, failed landing in gymnastics and twisting of the body may lead to laceration of the musculus vastus medialis and the medial retinaculum, thus causing outward dislocation of patella. If not properly treated, it will develop into habitual dislocation of patella, which may seriously hamper the joint functions.

3. When the patella becomes dislocated, the patella and the femoral condyle may collide with each other, thus causing cartilage injury of the patella or the femoral condyle, and even fracture of the patella and femur, haemarthrosis and articular swelling. If not treated timely, it may lead to articular adhesion, uneven bony surface and, as times passes, osteoarthropathy.

Symptoms and Diagnosis

1. Obvious history of trauma; the dislocated limb assumes a flexed posture; and in a case of outward dislocation, there may be a projection at the lateral aspect of the knee and the patella may be felt to have moved outward. Yet, this typical symptom is rarely seen in clinical treatment, because the athlete or coach would immediately for a reduction. This is particularly true in subluxation when the patient would often push-press the patella for reduction himself.

2. Tumefaction at the knee: The tumefaction or haematoma caused by external force at the soft tissues of the knee are usually diffuse tumefaction and the skin appears cyanotic. Haemarthrosis may occur if there is rupture of the articular capsule or fracture of the patella or femoral condyle. Floating-patella test will achieve a positive reaction.

3. Articular dyskinesia of knee: Tumefaction in joint, injury of soft tissues and injury of the cartilage will hamper the movement of the knee joint and cause arthralgia. If not properly treated and the tissues not well repaired at the acute period, repeated dislocation will occur at the patella afterwards whenever there is slight injury. This is called habitual dislocation of patellar which may weaken the strength of the knee and seriously hinder all movements of the legs.

Treatment

1. For most cases of such dislocation, anaesthesia is not necessary and a reduction may be applied on the spot. Yet, if the reduction turns out to be difficult, local anaesthesia around the patella with 10 ml. of 2 percent procaine will be necessary. If there is haemarthrosis, tapping should be performed at the same time to lessen possible articular adhesion.

2. Manual reduction: With the patient taking a supine or sitting posture, the massagist holds and pulls at the ankle slowly with one hand to straighten the knee joint, and pinches the patella with the other hand to push-squeeze its outer border and pull the patella upward. By then the massagist should be able to feel the sliding of the patella. Check to see if the patella has been re-situated to the center of the knee. Flex the knee joint slightly, if the patella does not dislocate any more, it indicates the completion of the reduction.

3. Gently massage the thigh to relax the muscles and treat the tissues; gently thumb-push the lateral soft tissues of the knee to remove local spasm and reduce the outwardly pulling force on the patella.

4. Make the knee stretch straight to apply pressure dressing with elastic bandage or cotton mat to prevent tumefaction. Remove the dressing and start practising isometric contraction of the quadriceps muscle of thigh two days later. Keep the knee straight for three weeks until the tissues get completely repaired. Practise knee flexion and extension. However, the patient should remain patient lest the patella dislocates again. For habitual dislocation, surgery is necessary. But, knee joint dyskinesia may appear as a result, and it may seriously hinder the lower limbs in physical training.

17. Rigidity of Knee Joint

Joint movement plays an important role in the motor system. Hampered joint movement or joint rigidity may result in various degrees of harm to the functions of the limbs. Serious knee trauma may cause rigidity of knee joint to a certain extent due to denaturation of the peripheral soft tissues of the knee joint, joint adhesion and the loss of smoothness of the articular surface.

Injury Mechanism

1. Disuse joint rigidity: This is a common type of limitation of joint movement. Before the injury, the joint movement is normal, while unduly long-term immobilization of the knee joint after injury causes disuse atrophy, rigidity and adhesion, all of which in turn cause rigidity of joint. Long-term plaster immobilization is necessary after an surgical operation in the treatment of fracture of patella or knee joint. Yet, such immobilization would result in joint rigidity to some extent. Proper treatment can minimize the rigidity and help early restoration of functions of the knee joint.

2. Inflammation on and around the joint: Trauma or inflammation in the knee joint may cause tissue fluid exudate and haematocele. Usually, the exudate and haematocele may be absorbed and the joint function is not hindered along with the cure of the trauma or inflammation. Yet, if the primary disease is not cured timely or the articular surface is damaged, the exudate shall not be fully absorbed, and some fibrins may adhere to the joint and there will be lots of newly developed blood vessels between the fibrins, finally forming fibrous tissues and causing adhesion, which may cause limitations of joint movement and even lead to complete loss of joint function.

3. Synovitis and disease on muscular tendon: Attack of the knee by external pathogens of wind and coldness may cause gonitis and joint swelling and result in joint dysfunction. Besides, the lacerated muscular tendon may cause adhesion to peripheral tissues after healing. This may also result in limitation of joint movement.

Symptoms and Diagnosis

1. Different kinds of traumatic history in the knee joint, which include injury of meniscus, rupture of ligament, fracture of femur, patella and tibia, long-term immobilization of knee joint, surgical operation in the knee joint and delayed treatment of hydrarthrosis and haemarthrosis.

2. Impairment of extension and flexion of the knee joint is an important symptom of this disease. When normal, the knee joint may extend 180 degrees (functional position is zero degree) and flex more than 90 degrees. Failure to reach the normal range of flexion and extension is considered as a limitation in the joint movement. In a serious case, the patient will not be able to run or jump, and find it difficult to go upstairs and downstairs and squat.

3. Limitation in patellar movement. Normally, the patella is able to move

towards all directions. When there is adhesion between the articular surface of patella and femur, the leftward and rightward movement of the patella will be markedly limited and the range of movement, when pushed left and right, is small. Adhesion of the patella is often an important factor that hinders extension and flexion of the joint.

4. Tumefaction and pain in the knee joint: Tumefaction in the joint are manifested as hyperaemia and edema in the peripheral tissues and hydrarthrosis. If there is also atrophy of the quadriceps muscle of thigh, the tumefaction will be more distinct. In such a case, the patient often feels pain in the joint when walking and the pain turns more serious in night.

5. X-ray examination indicates that the joint surface is basically smooth, occasionally with spurs. If it shows the trabecula passes the articular surface, it is ankylosis of bone joint which cannot be treated manually.

Treatment

1. Treatment of disuse rigidity of joint: When the knee is injured, encourage the patient to do strength exercises on the quadriceps muscle of thigh as well as extension-flexion exercises of the knee joint. The duration for fixation of the joint (splintage, plaster immobilization and skeletal traction, etc.) for any knee injury should not be too long to avoid changes which make efforts to bring back the joint functions impossible. Repeated tumefaction may also affect normal function of the joint. So, in order to prevent tumefaction, lift up the affected leg at the initial stage, try ground exercises as early as possible to improve the elasticity of the blood vessels in the leg and reduce exudate and tumefaction; or apply elastic bandage dressing to prevent tumefaction. If there is haemarthrosis, perform tapping timely to avoid articular adhesion.

2. Manipulation to separate adhesion:

a) Make the patient lie on his back, the massagist press-kneads and pull-grasps on the anterior, posterior, medial and lateral aspects of the affected leg to relax different groups of thigh muscles. If there are cords and scleromata, perform forceful plucking or scrape-pushing to have them softened or removed. Perform the same manipulation on the anterior and posterior aspects of the leg.

b) Relax the soft tissues around the knee joint and move the patella. The massagist scrape-pushes on the soft tissues with the thumb to soften them, and push-presses the patella into all directions to expand the range of activity of the patella.

c) Holding the ankle with one hand and supporting the popliteal fossa of the affected leg with the other, the massagist presses down the ankle and at the same time lifts up the popliteal portion, i.e., makes the passive flexion of the knee joint. The force applied should first be light and turns heavy gradually and the angle of flexion should turn from small to large. Each round of this manipulation should last 3-5 minutes, with a total of 3-5 rounds, with a break of one minute between each two rounds. If the force applied by the hand is not strong enough to support the popliteal fossa, the massagist may put his elbow under it to lift up the knee joint. After the manipulation, perform press-kneading from the thigh, the knee to the leg to relax the soft tissues. (See Fig. 97)

d) The patient should practice active flexion and extension of the knee joint after treatment. He may also sit on the edge of a bed to flex the knee joint by hanging a heavy object on the ankle. (See Fig. 98)

e) Apply physiotherapy (keritherapy, hot bath and thermo-electromagnetic wave) to the knee and use fumigation or washing method with traditional Chinese medicinal herbs. The medicinal herbs used include: Frankincense, 20 grams; Myrrh, 20 grams; Peach kernel, 10 grams; Buck grass, 20 grams; Sperranskia Tuberculata (Bge.) Baill, 20 grams; and Safflower, 20 grams. Fumigate and wash twice a day, 20 minutes each time.

f) Manual separation: After the above treatment is performed, if the joint still remains rigid, it is necessary to force a separation with the leg being fully anaesthetized (local anaesthesia or dural anaesthesia). Indications: There is no inflammation around the joint; the state of the illness is stable; the joint surface is smooth as witnessed by X-ray photo; there is no damage to the bone and no synostosis. After the application of anaesthesia, an assistant holds the thigh and leg with both hands respectively to prevent fracture of the femur and tibia during the treatment, while the massagist flexes and extends the knee joint by force gradually to restore it. A sound of tearing may be heard at the adhesion area. The operation should never be brutal. If not correctly performed, it may result in fracture or injury of the soft tissues around the joint. Correct handling can widen the range of joint movement. The patient should make flexion and extension on his or her own the day after in conjunction with gentle massage. Otherwise, all previous efforts shall be wasted. This treatment should be repeated once or twice.

Example: Liu, female, hurdler. During a training session in 1986, she bumped her right leg on a hurdle and hit the ground with her left foot. As a result, she had

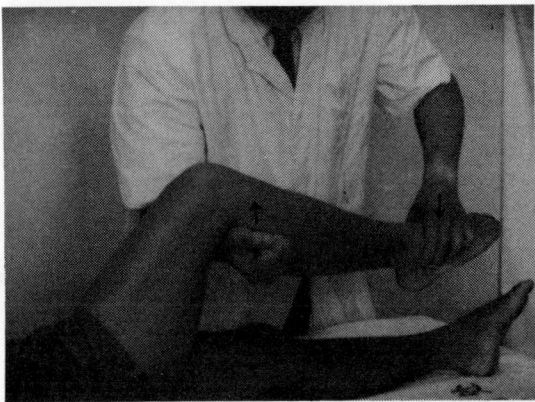

Fig. 97

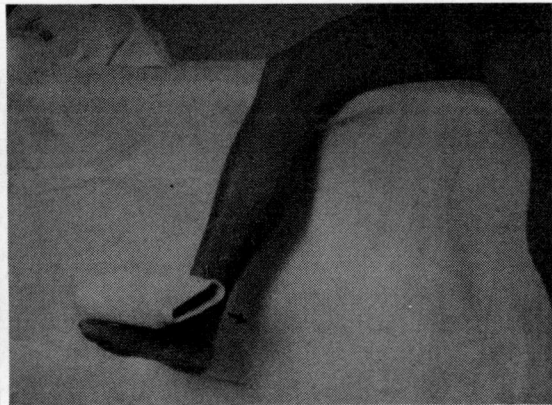

Fig. 98

her left knee joint sprained. The diagnosis confirmed an injury of the meniscus on the lateral aspect. She was given knee meniscectomy at the lateral side of the knee. After the surgical operation, the knee could extend by 170 degrees and flex by 90 degrees, which made it impossible for her to continue training. Later, a surgical operation was given to separate the adhesion. Yet, the result was not satisfactory. Then, she was given continues manual treatment and joint function returned to normal half a year later. Two years later, she broke the Asian record in women's 100-metre hurdling event and at the 1990 11th Asian Games she broke the record again.

18. Traumatic Gonitis

Traumatic gonitis is also called osteoarthritis, hyperplastic arthritis and hypertrophic arthritis. It is seen more often in athletes.

Injury Mechanism

1. Trauma is the direct cause of traumatic gonitis. For instance, in joint fracture although the fractured ends may unite, the relatively rough articular surface may injure the joint; and repeated grinding of the joint by ruptured meniscus and joint bodies may also injure the knee joint.

2. Chronic strain: Hyperosteogeny may rise due to overburden on the knee joint in running and jumping, impact on the knee, repeated injury of the joint and osteochondritis dissecans, etc.

3. Unstable joint may lead to further wear and tear to the bone surface, such as rupture of the cruciate ligament of the knee joint, flaccidity of the articular capsule and habitual dislocation of patella.

4. Heavy body weight also plays a part, because it increases the pressure on the articular cartilage during physical training.

Symptoms and Diagnosis

1. Pain in the knee joint is the most important symptom. At the early stage, there is aching or dull pain, and gradually the patient feels a grinding pain in the joint. In a serious case, the pain is lasting and disturbs sleep. For athletes, they only feel the pain when the amount of training is increased, and the pain will ease after some rest. The joint will also feel the pain if the patient stands or sits still for a long time. The pain is more serious in early morning due to lessened movement of the joint in sleep over the night, and it will be alleviated by walking. Pain in the joint is also referable to the change of weather. For instance, it may come in overcast and rainy days.

2. Dyskinesia of joint: As the initial stage, the joint feels stiff and cannot move limply, which will gradually develop into continuous dyskinesia. At this stage, a patient will find it difficult to go upstairs and downstairs. At an advanced stage, the patient may sometimes feel a sensation of friction or click in the joint. When a doctor presses the knee with one hand and flexes and extends the knee joint with

the other, he may also feel the sensation of friction and there is pressure pain.

3. The knee feels weak, particularly when going up stairs. Often there is lameness.

4. Tumefaction in the joint. Synovial hypertrophy or hydrarthrosis causes tumefaction and repeated dropsy in the joint. The tumefaction becomes more serious when the leg feels tired and it may subside after a long rest. In a chronic case, there may be slight atrophy of the quadriceps muscle of thigh.

Treatment

1. Digitally press acupoints Heding (Extra), Dubi (ST 35), Weizhong (BL 40) and Chengshan (BL 57). (See Fig. 99)

2. The massagist press-kneads the quadriceps muscle of thigh and the triceps muscle of leg with both hands to fully relax the muscles, remove spasms, and reduce pulling on the joint.

3. Pluck and push-press with both thumbs on the musculus vastus lateralis and the iliotibial tract to soften the stiffened muscles and fasciae. Spasm in the musculus vastus lateralis and the iliotibial tract may cause arthralgia. Essential to the treatment of this disease, this can yield satisfactory effect in the treatment of arthralgia. (See Fig. 100)

4. Scrape around the patella with a force that the patient can stand; stimulate the peripheral soft tissues with heavy manipulations to promote blood circulation.

5. Grasp the ankle with one hand and put the other in the popliteal fossa to flex the joint gradually. This is particularly important for those cases with joint dyskinesia. Note not to forcibly flex and extends the joint, and just do it gently.

6. Rehabilitation exercises: The major purpose is to increase the strength of the quadriceps muscle of thigh to enhance the stability of the joint, and reduce mutual friction between the bone joints.

a) Repeated squatting-down and standing-up: Patients advanced in age may place a hands on a chair or a wall for support. Three or four sets of this exercise should be done, with 20 squats per set. Young people may do this exercise with some sort of a burden on the back, such as sand bag or a barbell. For them, each set of the exercise may constitute 30-40 squats. After each set, there can be a break of 3 minutes.

b) Semi-squatting: Stand with the knee joint at an angle of 130-150 degrees, with the upper body being upright, neither facing upward nor bowing the head and bending the waist forward, till the thigh feels ache, then take a break of three minutes. This should be done once a day for 4-5 sets.

c) Sitting with legs crossed: For patients whose knee flexion and extension are limited, sit still in bed with their legs crossed till the knee joint feels ache. Then repeat this exercise 4-5 times, with a break of three minutes in between.

Example: Liu, female, 52, was formerly a track and field athlete. She suffered from pain in both knees for three months, which became more serious at night, swelling in the knee joints, and difficulty in going upstairs and downstairs and

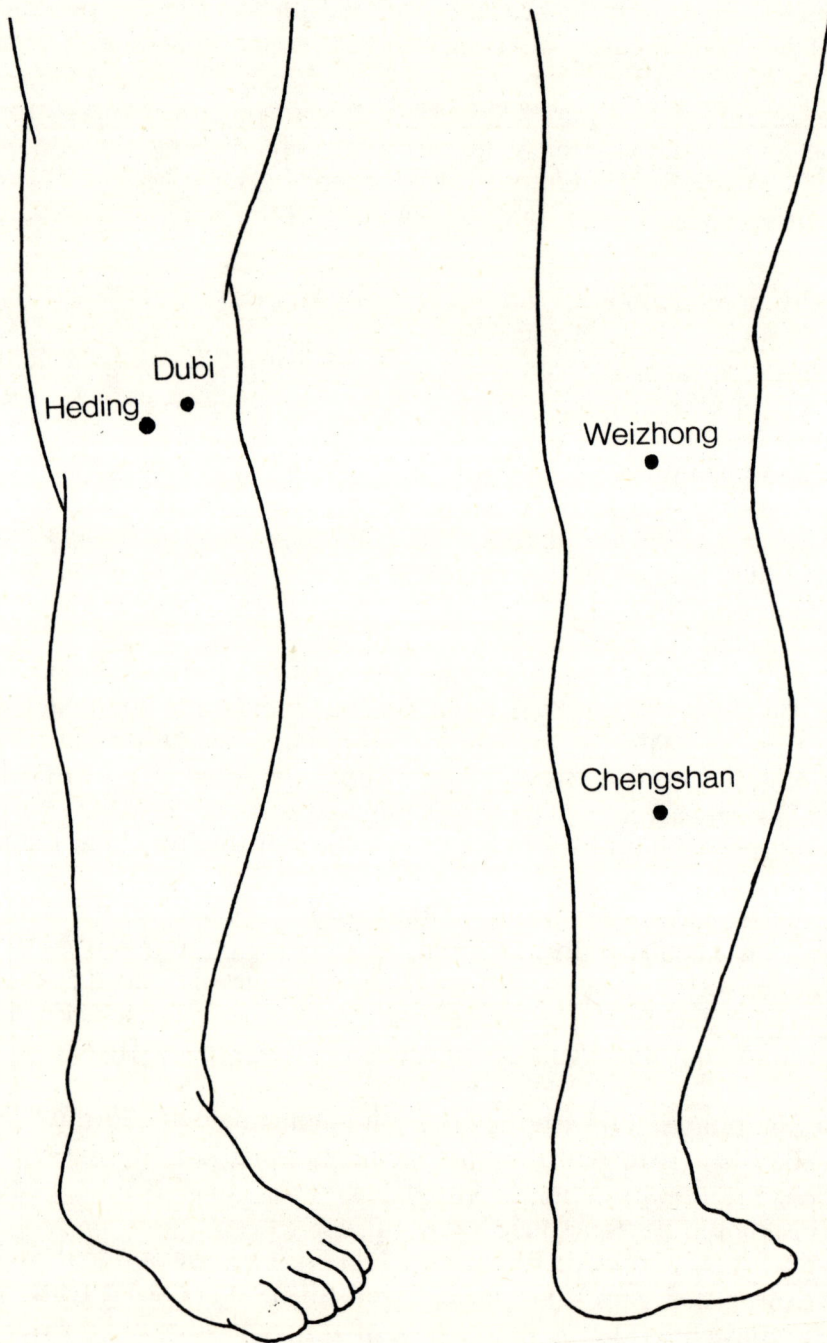

Fig. 99

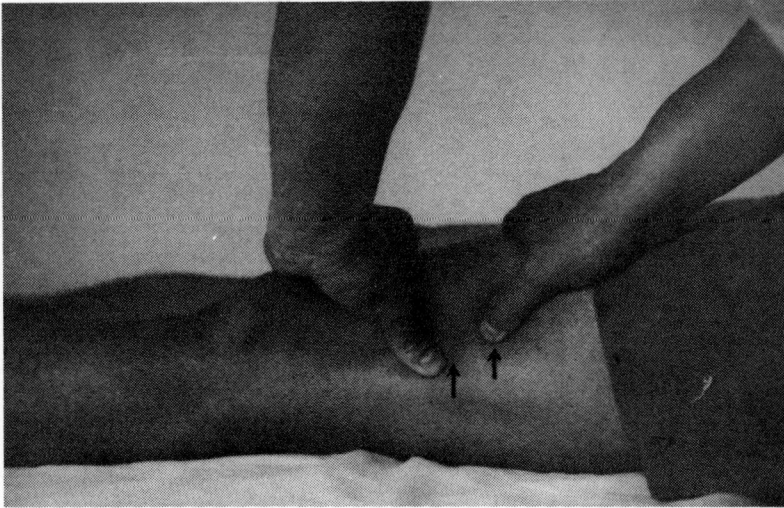

Fig. 100

bowel movement and urination. X-ray examination showed hyperosteogeny in both patellas. She had received physiotherapy and other treatment in the United States, which proved not effective. In the author's 1989 visit to San Francisco, she was given manual treatment in four sessions, After the treatment, the pain and tumefaction in the knees basically disappeared. She was then able to go upstairs and downstairs with ease, squat normally.

19. Fracture of Tibia and Fibula

Fracture of the tibia and fibula is a serious pathological condition in sports injuries.

Injury Mechanism

1. Injury due to direct external force: This disorder may result from direct kicking and crushing at or pressure by heavy objects on the leg. It may be divided into transverse fracture, short oblique fracture and comminuted fracture.

2. Injury due to indirect external force: Touching the ground with foot when falling down or from a high place may twist the leg violently. The tremendous torsional action may result in oblique fracture or spiral fracture of the tibia and fibula. When skating on natural ice, the skate may get stuck in a crack while the body is still rotating, thus causing fracture in the leg.

3. The tibia locates near the skin surface and it is protected by the skin only. So, the fracture of the tibia is often accompanied by an open injury and infection. The upper one-third of the shaft of the tibia is triangular in shape and the lower one-third is quadrilateral. And the middle one-third is the most vulnerable section where a fracture is most likely to happen.

4. Blood supply to the tibia mainly comes from three arteries, namely, the nutrient, metaphyseal and periosteal arteries. The nutrient artery enters the bone at the upper middle one-third, divides into numerous branches in the bone marrow and links up with metaphyseal artery at the metaphysis. The nutrient artery is often ruptured during the fracture of tibia and fibula, which makes the healing more difficult. Treating the fracture with both traditional Chinese medicine and Western medicine produces a very high cure rate, while open reduction and internal fixation with steel plate results in a rather high rate of non-union and delayed union of the fracture because it may rupture the periosteal artery. Therefore, non-surgical treatment is much more superior to surgical treatment.

Symptoms and Diagnosis

1. Apparent traumatic history. When there is the fracture, the affected leg suffers from severe pain; unable to stand up.

2. Malformation and abnormal movement of the leg: There is malformation when there is obvious fracture displacement, together with abnormal movement at the fractured part and bone crepitation and fraction when the affected leg is moved. The doctor should avoid making repeated checks of the abnormal movement as they may aggravate the pain and exacerbate the injury.

3. Swelling: Bleeding and edema appear soon after a fracture. Swelling soon appears in the leg, which, if serious, may increase the tension of the anterior tibial portion and the gastrocnemius, compress the nerves and blood vessels, as marked by the weakened beating of dorsal artery of foot and sensory disturbance. This is a kind of serious complication what calls for timely emergency treatment.

Treatment

1. Treatment of fracture of tibia and fibula without displacement: Gently knead the anterior and posterior aspects of the leg to clear the meridians and collaterals, remove blood stasis and promote blood circulation. Note not to press-push the leg and lift it too much so as to avoid fracture displacement. Apply splintage with four splints to the leg for 3-4 weeks, during which the patient may practise knee-extension and leg-lifting exercises in bed to promote the union of the fracture and relieve the tumefaction. The massagist may feel out the beating of artery at acupoint Chongmen (SP 12), press this point with appropriate force for one minute, then release it slowly; the patient may feel a sense of heat in the leg. The impact produced by the blood flow may promote blood circulation by removing blood stasis.

2. Treatment of fracture of tibia alone without displacement: Gently knead the leg; prepare 2-3 layers of hard paper board, soak them in water to soften them and apply them to the leg, and bind them up with bandage; dry them up with a source of heat to fix them into shape for 2-3 weeks. Or, apply a plaster support fixation.

3. When the fracture is of a transverse type or short oblique type, it is necessary to make manual reduction and apply splintage.

a) Local anaesthesia for manual reduction.

b) Manual reduction: Using traction method to correct angulation malformation and lateral displacement of fracture. The concrete procedures are as follows: making one assistant carry the ankle with both hands to pull towards the distal end with even and sustained force, and making another one carry the knee and pull towards the counter direction. Pressing manipulation: The massagist press-squeezes with both hands from the two sides towards the center to correct leftward or rightward displacement of fracture, and press-squeezes from the anterior and posterior aspects to correct forward and backward displacement of fracture. As the tibia is superficial, the hand may feel the contusions in the process of reduction. If it is fracture of both the tibia and fibula, the major purpose is to correct the fracture of the tibia while the slight fracture of the fibula may be neglected.

c) Small-splint immobilization: Altogether five splints will be used: two narrower ones are to be placed at the anteromedial and anterolateral aspects of the tibia; one is to be placed at the medial aspect of the leg with a length running from a point under the knee to the medial malleolus; one is to be placed at the lateral aspect of the leg with a length running from the small head of the fibula to the lower end of the lateral malleolus; and the last one is to be placed at the posterior aspect with a length running from the lower part of the popliteal fossa to the upper part of the calcaneus. Bone depressors are inserted along the original trend of displacement to prevent recurrence of displacement. Protect the small head of the fibula with small cotton mat to prevent compression on the common peroneal nerve and tie up with four cloth belts, with the tightness of binding being appropriate.

4. Functional exercises:

a) At the early stage, lift the affected leg to avoid excessive swelling. When covering the affected leg with a quilt in sleep, note not to cover the foot as the weight of the quilt may constrict the foot, inducing outward rotation and causing rotation deformity of the tibia.

b) At the early stage, the patient should be advised to make isometric contraction of the quadriceps muscle of thigh, i.e., repeatedly lift the patella and do flexion and extension movement of toes to improve blood circulation in the leg and promote the union of the fracture.

c) Do flexion and extension of the knee joint, and dorsiflexion and plantar flexion of the ankle joint with the help of the massagist one week after the injury. At beginning, the range of movement should be small. Note not to do any rotation movement of the ankle. The exercises should be done 2-3 times a day. Gradually, the patient should do the exercises on his or her own.

d) Practise walking with crutches three weeks later. At this stage, there should not be any burden on the affected leg. Try to walk with one crutch 4-6 weeks later. At this stage, the splintage can be removed everyday for gentle massage on the affected leg to promote blood circulation, increase the elasticity of the muscles, reduce muscle adhesion and prevent myotrophy.

Generally, splintage can be removed after 8-10 weeks. By then, the patient may begin walking, squatting and eventually jogging.

Example: Liu, male, a football player. One day when he kicked the ball hard with the body turning, he suddenly felt sharp pain at the lower left leg. Clinical examination revealed bone crepitation at the lower part of the fibula, and X-ray photo indicated an oblique fracture there with displacement. He was given manual treatment—traction, fracture reduction and restoration of soft tissues. After the treatment, plaster support fixation was used. Beginning from the third week, he was given massage treatment every day. Three weeks later the plaster support was removed and he could practise jogging. The condition returned normal after eight weeks.

20. Dislocation of Superior Tibiofibular Joint

The tibia and fibula form the superior and inferior tibiofibular joints. The superior tibiofibular joint is not a part of the knee joint. With a small range of movement, it is involved in the rotation movement of the leg, and around it are powerful fascia, articular capsule and interosseous membrane to maintain stability of the joint. Dislocation and subluxation of superior tibiofibular joint is a rare sports injury and has something in common with subluxation of the capitulum radii of arm.

Injury Mechanism

1. Indirect external force: In physical training, when the foot is suddenly set at plantar flexion and inverted position, the violent contraction of the long and short peroneal muscles and the extensor muscles of the great toe and other toes causes the upper end of the fibula being pulled forward, resulting in subluxation or dislocation of the joint. The dislocation often appears as an anterolateral one. For instance, kicking ball hard with the dorsum of foot and sudden turning of the body with the knee being semi-flexed may both result in dislocation of the superior tibiofibular joint.

2. Direct external force: Direct kick at the upper part of the fibula or direct bump on the lateral aspect of the fibula may all cause posteromedial displacement of the head of fibula.

3. Chronic strain: Repeated torsional movements of the leg as required in sport activities can result in flaccidity of the articular capsule of the superior tibiofibular joint. So, even a light traumatic injury may cause subluxation of the joint. This is seen more often in female gymnasts.

Symptoms and Diagnosis

1. Evident traumatic history, or a history of repeated torsional movements of the leg.

2. Pain, swelling and local tenderness at the small head of fibula. But the pain is not severe, and this is the difference from a fracture of the small head of tibia. There is apparent forward or backward displacement of the small head of fibula.

212

For ordinary patients, the small head of fibula may be felt sometimes moving back and forth, which is possibly due to the flaccidity of the articular capsule. A comparison with the other leg may make the diagnosis even more definite.

3. Dyskinesia of the knee joint: The knee joint cannot stretch straight and the pain turns worse when the leg is rotated.

Treatment

1. Digitally press acupoints Yanglingquan (GB 34) and Zusanli (ST 36). (See Fig. 101)

2. Ask an assistant to hold the ankle with both hands, pull downward slowly and make repeated inward and outward rotations of the leg, while the massagist presses the small head of the fibula with both thumbs. In the process, a click may be heard or the sliding of the fibula felt, showing the success of the treatment. Then, massage along the fibula longitudinally to treat the injured soft tissues.

3. Apply a circular plaster fixation at the small head of fibula, avoid violent rotating movement of the leg within one week of the injury and try to prevent recurrence.

21. Fatigue Periostitis and Fatigue Fracture of Tibia and Fibula

Fatigue periostitis and fatigue fracture of tibia and fibula are disorders frequently seen among athletes.

Injury Mechanism

1. Chronic strain: Excessive activity of the lower limbs with too much burden

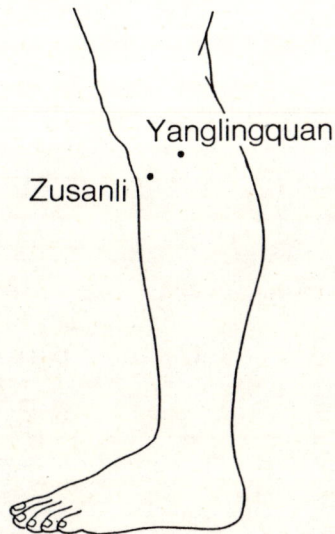

Fig. 101

213

causes repeated pulling on the tibia and fibula by leg muscles and interosseous membrane, thus stimulating the periost and inducing inflammation and thickening of the periost. This is commonly seen in teenagers.

2. Long-term tension of muscles: Leg exercises for a long time without enough rest causes lasting tension of the leg muscles, hence increasing the pressure in the fascial space of the leg and causing periosteal proliferation.

3. Repeated slight bending of the bone: Repeated impact from the ground, especially hard ground, or jumping down from a high place can cause very slight bending of the tibia and fibula and gradually result in periosteal proliferation. Since the anterior border of the tibia has no attached muscles, it is more likely to bend, and inflammation in the periost there can be more obvious. Such repeated bending may lead to fracture, and fatigue caused by them may be the major pathological cause for fatigue periostitis and fatigue fracture.

Symptoms and Diagnosis

1. Without an evident history of trauma, but with a history of fatigue in the leg.

2. Pain: Stimulation to the periost by inflammation causes pain; the pain at the medial aspect of the tibia and the lateral aspect of fibula is often manifested as sore pain, and in some cases, severe pain. The pain become more serious when the amount of physical training is increased and is alleviated after rest. Fracture of the tibia and fibula occurs gradually. So the pain of a fatigue fracture is milder than that of a traumatic fracture. A misdiagnosis is possible.

3. Swelling and tenderness: There are tenderness and diffuse swelling at the anterior aspect of the tibia, and a mass can be felt. When the inflammation is serious, there can be swelling at the soft tissues. At the advanced stage, callus and osseous tubercles can be felt, and sometimes a fracture space, i.e., a streaky depression may be palpated.

4. Tension of leg muscles: Between muscular tension and periostitis there is causality. Muscular tension may cause pathological changes in the periost and periostitis may bring spasm to the muscles.

5. Pain in leg driving: When the patient makes a power leg-driving on the ground with tiptoe, he feels pain in the leg, which in turn affects the running and jumping.

6. At the initial stage, X-ray examination does not show distinct pathological changes, while at the advanced stage it may reveal the shadow indicating the thickening of the periost. At the late stage of fatigue fracture, hyperplastic callus and a dim fracture line may be seen at the fractured part in X-ray photo. However, the displaced fracture end can rarely been seen.

Treatment

1. Digitally press acupoints Zusanli (ST 36), Sanyinjiao (SP 6), Chengshan (BL 57), Weizhong (BL 40) and Kunlun (BL 60). (See Fig. 102)

2. With the patient lying prone, the massagist first press-kneads the posterior aspect of the leg to relax the muscles; then pull-pinches the leg to stimulate the

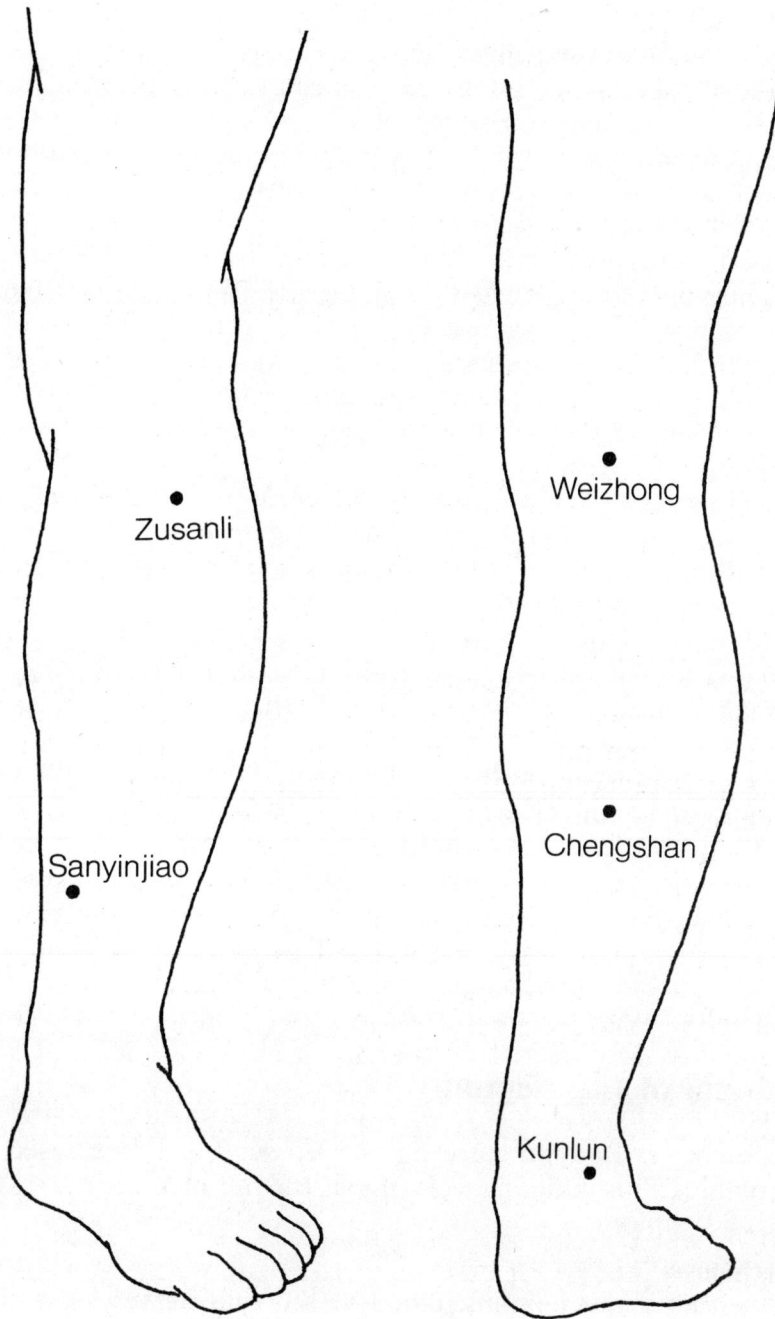

Zusanli

Weizhong

Sanyinjiao

Chengshan

Kunlun

Fig. 102

muscles and promote blood flow. These two steps are carried out alternatively for 5-6 rounds.

3. Use the thumb to press along between the tibia and fibula and at the anterior aspect of the leg to relax the interosseous membrane. Repeat this process from the distal end to the proximal end 5-6 times.

4. Scrape the anterior and medial aspects and the surface of tibia as well as the affected part in the fibula to stimulate the periost, improve local blood circulation and reduce exudation and inflammation.

To press the interosseous membrane and to stimulate the periost by scraping are two important steps in treating this disease. With one treatment each day, a course of treatment lasts two weeks. Usually, pain in the leg can be eased or removed after 2-3 courses. Patients with light symptoms can go on with physical training while receiving treatment, and those with serious symptoms of fatigue periostitis and fatigue fracture must reduce the amount of work or stop physical training until the full recovery.

5. Tin foil therapy: Apply 2 percent mercuric nitrate externally on the painful area, cover the area with foil (tin foil in cigarette box will do), and seal the periphery with wide adhesive plaster. Remove the foil the next day. This procedure should be repeated 10 times as one course of treatment.

Example: Zhang, female, 24, is a sprinter. After the 1988 Seoul Olympic Games, she suffered from pain at both legs and had to stop physical training. When the training was resumed in February 1989, she still felt painful at both tibiae. Then, she was given treatment while continuing training. During this period, she took part in the competitions at the 1989 Asian Track and Field Championships. Swelling appeared at both tibiae in January 1990 and the surface of tibia protruded forward. X-ray examination showed a fracture line at both tibiae, and bone trabecula was seen passing the fracture line. The case was diagnosed as fatigue fracture of tibia. With the confirmation of the diagnosis, the amount of training was reduced, a strapping with elastic bandage was applied, and fumigation and washing with Chinese herbal medicine was given. Massotherapy and physiotherapy were also applied. With the treatment, her condition has turned for the better.

22. Syndrome of Leg Septum

For different reasons, pressure on the leg septum is increased to block local blood circulation, thus inducing ischemia of the muscles and nerves and giving rise to a series of symptoms.

Injury Mechanism

1. Muscles, muscular tendons, blood vessels and nerves locate in different leg septa which are formed by bones, interosseous membrane, intermuscular septum and deep fascia of leg. In total, there are four septa and they are the anterior leg septum, the lateral let septum, the deep posterior leg septum and the superficial

posterior leg septum. The septum tissues have very poor elasticity.

2. Sharp increase in the volume of septum: Intense physical exertion, such as long-distance heel-and-toe walking and marathon running, can result in over-fatigue, which in turn can cause traumatic edema in muscles and a sharp increase in muscular volume. Yet, due to its poor elasticity, the septum restricts and compresses the muscles. This can induce ischemia and acute syndrome of septum.

3. Acute trauma: Heavy hit and crush in the leg or fracture of the tibia and fibula may cause acute tissue bleeding and edema, which in turn can compress the muscles, blood vessels and nerves in the septum, thus causing tissue ischemia.

4. Iatrogenic injury: This refers to injury caused by mishandling of the massagist in giving treatment. For instance, excessive tightness and too long a period in pressure dressing may compress the soft tissues. Too tight a splintage or improper location of the splintage, or too tight a plaster cast applied for leg fracture may all compress the swelling of the limb and obstruct the local blood circulation.

Symptoms and Diagnosis

1. Pain in the anterior or lateral aspect of the leg: Pain in the leg after intense physical training, which turns for the better when the leg is raised high and after rest; and swelling in the leg after physical training. In a small number of serious cases, severe pain, ischemia of tissues, and numbness in the leg.

2. Swelling in the leg, tenderness and stiffness in muscles, and exacerbating pain when making over-dorsiflexion or over-plantar flexion of the ankle.

3. Weakness and numbness in the leg: When there is weakness and numbness in the leg, the arteropalmus of dorsal artery of foot remains normal. Only when the blood vessels are seriously constricted, the arteropalmus of dorsal artery of foot or the posterior tibial artery vanishes and the skin turns livid and cold.

4. Sometimes, the chronic syndrome of leg septum must be differentiated from fatigue periostitis which may eventually give rise to the thickening of periost as may be observed in X-ray examination. Muscular fatigue in the leg can also show similar symptoms sometimes, yet with the soreness and weakness in the leg mainly at the posterior aspect.

Treatment

1. For patients with small splint immobilization and plaster cast fixation of leg fracture and with pressure dressing of traumatic injury in the leg, conduct frequent checks to make the tightness of the fixation and dressing is appropriate. If the symptoms appear, remove the fixation and dressing immediately.

This author once saw a patient who was given pressure dressing in the knee after an operation on the patellas to avoid haemarthrosis. But, as the dressing was too tight and the condition was not checked timely, he eventually contracted iatrogenic syndrome of leg septum, which then gave rise to long-term muscular ischemia in both legs and finally extensive necrosis of the muscles.

2. For patients with light symptoms, make the patient lie supine, have his affected leg raised and put something under it to facilitate the back flow of body

fluid. Digitally press acupoint Chongmen (SP 12). Press the femoral artery 30 seconds and release quickly, and repeat this process three times. This is to improve the blood supply of the ischemic tissues with the impact of blood flow. Massage the toughened leg muscles from the ankle to the knee. Repeatedly push-press along the lateral aspect of the tibia from the foot to the knee to promote detumescence and reduce the pressure in the septa. For patients with numbness in the foot, stimulate the acupoints Huantiao (GB 30), Weizhong (BL 40), Chengshan (BL 57), Taixi (KI 3) and Kunlun (BL 60) to relieve any congestion in the meridians and collaterals and restore the functions of the nerves. (See Fig. 103)

3. For patients with serious symptoms, raise the affected leg first and apply push-pressing for detumescence. If there are still not any signs of improvement in the symptoms and severe pain and dyskinesia are felt in the foot, timely fasciotomy in the leg is necessary to quickly reduce the pressure in the septa and improve blood circulation in the tissues.

Example: Zhao, female, 18, was a high jumper. Once, she felt pain in the antero-lateral aspect of the leg, which was so severe that she could not even continue the normal training. At first, the condition was diagnosed as fatigue periostitis of the tibia and fibula. Following observation failed to verify any pathological change in the periost. Further examination proved that her case was chronic syndrome of the anterior tibial septum of leg. Several rounds manual treatment removed the symptoms and she went back to her training and competition.

23. Systremma

A frequently occurring disorder in the leg, systremma is commonly known as

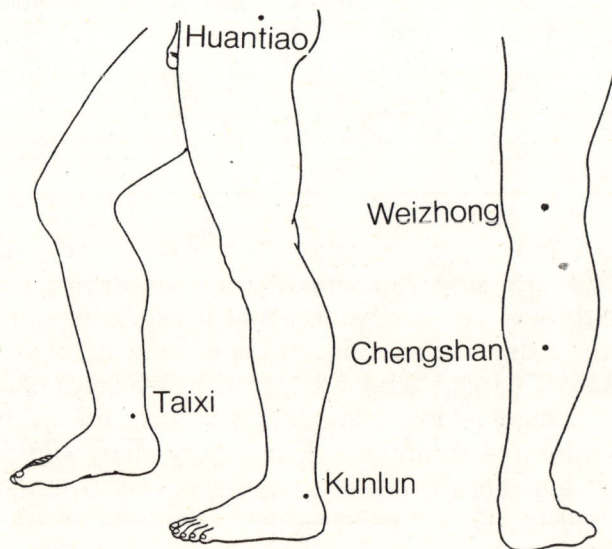

Fig. 103

"Spasm of the calf." It features a short course and can be relieved even without any treatment.

Injury Mechanism

1. Low temperature: This disease is related to temperature. It is likely to occur when taking part in physical training without adequate warming up in cold and damp weather. For instance, systremma occurs more frequently in winter when being in fast asleep.

2. Overfatigue: When the muscles are extremely tired after physical training, a sudden exertion of efforts may induce systremma. In fact, systremma can occur in any muscle. Once the author saw a 10-year-old girl gymnast who, due to excessive training, suffered from spasm in all four limbs as well as in the thoracoabdominal muscles. She was given manual treatment for half an hour before her muscles were relaxed, but it took much longer time to get the gastrocnemius of both legs relaxed.

3. General dehydration and salt loss: Too much sweating and emission reduce the content of sodium chloride in blood, thus causing systremma. For instance, in order to reduce body weight, weightlifters are often given long-term steam-bath, which leads to too much loss of water and salt, thus giving rise to myospasm. And marathon runners competing in hot weather may have too much sweat. If there is not enough salt-containing beverage to replenish water and salt, they are also likely to suffer from systremma.

4. Mental stress: Myospasm is also likely to occur when athletes worry too much that their muscles may be pulled in competition because they did not do enough warm-ups.

5. Calcipriva: For old people who suffer from osteoporosis and children who suffer from rickets, their blood calcium is usually below the normal value. Low blood calcium can increase the irritability of the nerves and muscles, and lead to myospasm.

Symptoms and Diagnosis

1. Pain: Sudden severe pain in the posterior aspect of leg, inability to walk; sudden awakening from sleep at night by myospasm.

2. Muscular tone, toughness and tenderness at the triceps muscle of calf, usually accompanied by spasm of muscles at the sole.

3. Spontaneous remission: Set the leg still without moving, the pain may abate without any treatment. Yet, there may be lingering pain when the spasm is relieved.

Treatment

1. Press acupoint Weizhong (BL 40) with finger.

2. Swiftly scrape the leg with both hands to generate heat.

3. Pull-grasp and press-knead the leg from the proximal end to the distal end to relax the spasmodic muscles. Note the strength applied must be appropriate lest it causes injury to the muscles.

4. Traction of muscles: With the patient have the leg stretched, the massagist

dorsiflexs the ankle with force to tract the gastrocnemius to passively relax the spasmodic muscles. (See Fig. 104)

5. Gently strike the muscles: When the spasm is relaxed, gently strike the posterior aspect of the leg with the palm or hollow fist to remove muscular fatigue and alleviate the aching pain in the muscles from the spasm.

After treatment, keep the leg warm and rest for several hours and cut the amount of exercises in the immediate following period. For patients with repeated recurrence of myospasm, it is necessary to find whether there are any other causes.

24. Injury of Triceps Muscle of Thigh

The triceps muscle of calf consists of the gastrocnemius and the soleus. The gastrocnemius is a powerful muscle among the leg muscles, with its medial and lateral head initiating from the posterior part of the medial and lateral condyles of femur. The soleus initiates from the posterior part of the proximal end of the tibia and fibula. The two muscles constitute the Achilles tendon at the lower end and terminates at the calcaneus. The triceps muscle of calf functions to flex the leg, lift the heel, stabilize the ankle joint and prevent the body from leaning forward. Injury of the triceps muscle of calf is a frequently occurring sport injury.

Injury Mechanism

1. When jumping off with the knee joint being stretched straight, the triceps muscle of calf may be pulled by a sudden and strong force. The muscle may also contract suddenly in the take-off of high-jump and long-jump events as well as when lobbing in badminton competition. In a majority of cases, the injury is of a pulling type, while in a small number it is of partial muscular rupture. The injury

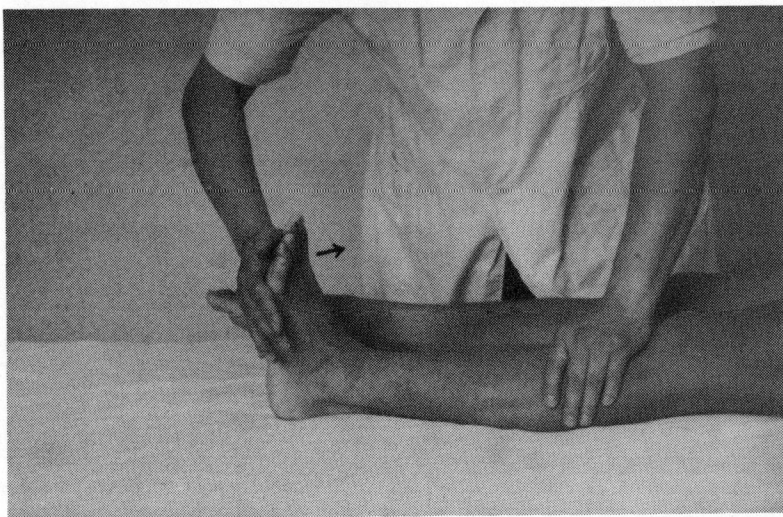

Fig. 104

can occur at the initiating points of the muscle, the attaching point of the Achilles tendon and the conjunction region between the muscles and tendons.

2. Passive pulling: The gastrocnemius may be pulled due to over-dorsiflexion from a fall.

3. Muscular fatigue: Long-time training and competition may cause fatigue to the leg muscles. The muscles are more likely to be pulled in cold weather when they are stiff and have poorer elasticity, if they are fully warmed up before training and if the amount of exercises increases suddenly.

4. Direct external impact: The impact of any external force, such as direct kicking on the leg, may cause injuries ranging from muscular contusion to rupture.

Symptoms and Diagnosis

1. Pain: The leg feels painful due to muscular injury, and the patient can only walk with the front part of the foot and does not dare to bear the body weight with the whole foot. There is also pain when lifting the heel.

2. Swelling: Direct trauma causes swelling at the posterior aspect of the leg. In a serious case, even ecchymoma can appear and the interspace of partial muscle rupture can be felt.

3. Tenderness and muscular tone: Tenderness is found at the injured area; scleromata or cords can be palpated; there is general muscular tone at the whole muscle group; and there is pain at the posterior aspect of the leg when making resistive dorsiflexion of the ankle joint.

Treatment

1 Digitally press acupoints Weizhong (BL 40), Chengshan (BL 57), Taixi (KI 3) and Jiexi (ST 41). The force applied in pressing the acupoint Chengshan should be gentle.

2. For a serious case, the massagist should apply cold compress and apply pressure dressing with elastic bandage on the spot immediately, with the ankle joint being flexed to relax the muscles. Manual treatment begins three days after the injury.

3. With the patient lying prone, the massagist puts a thin pillow under the anterior aspect of the leg and pull-grasps the triceps muscle of calf with both hands from the popliteal fossa downwards. The force applied depends on the depth of the pathological changes; it is sufficient so long as it can achieve the effect of relaxing the myospasm.

4. Pluck and digitally press the scleromata or cords to displace them, remove blood stasis and promote blood circulation; press knead and scrape the leg muscles till the skin turns hot. The force applied should grow from light to strong; it should not be brutal lest the injury be aggravated.

5. With the patient lying prone, the knee flexed and the leg muscles totally relaxed, the massagist gently and swiftly strikes at the muscles with the hypothenar, then rubs on the leg with palm five times. Generally, this treatment can relieve pain in the leg.

25. Peritenonitis of Achilles Tendon

The Achilles tendon is the largest tendon in the body. It has no tendon sheath but is surrounded by loosely connective membranous tissues, which are then called membrane around the Achilles tendon. These tissues function as tendon sheath and ensure the normal activities of the tendon. These tissues supply most nutrition to the Achilles tendon.

The Achilles tendon is repeatedly pulled when the ankle joint over-extends and over-flexes too much, and friction between the tendon and the peripheral tissues can cause peritenonitis of Achilles tendon. In a light case, there will be tension in the leg which feels painful and weak; while in a serious case, blood circulation of the Achilles tendon is impeded and there might be rupture in the Achilles tendon. Usually, peritenonitis of Achilles tendon occurs on both limbs.

Injury Mechanism

1. Acute injury: Violent contraction of or direct kicking at the leg may evoke, apart from injury to the triceps muscles of calf, injury to the peripheral tissues of the Achilles tendon. Some patients may have a medical history of acute injury in the leg.

2. Chronic strain: Most of the cases are of a type of chronic strain without a medical history of acute injury in the leg. When people run, jump or fall down from a high place, the Achilles tendon and its peripheral tissues as well, in order to keep balance of the body, are over-pulled and friction occurs between them. This may cause injury to the small blood vessels to the loose tissues and induce hyperaemia, edema, exudation in and denaturation of the tissues. Eventually, these tissues may turn thick or show adhesion. Denaturation of the tissues around the Achilles tendon may also impede blood supply to it, thus causing denaturation of the tendon itself and reducing its elasticity. Forceful pulling may even cause rupture of the tendon. In view of this last point, we may well say that peritenonitis of Achilles tendon serves as a sign of rupture of the Achilles tendon. So, it is of evident significance to prevent and cure the peritenonitis of Achilles tendon. According to my experience with the Chinese national gymnastics team, most gymnasts whose Achilles tendon has ruptured once suffered from peritenonitis of the Achilles tendon.

Symptoms and Diagnosis

1. Pain: Most of the patients develop tension and pain in the leg after physical training; sometimes they feel painful at the posterior aspect of the leg when jumping off or landing at the ground. In a serious case, pain can also be felt when walking.

2. Tension and tenderness in muscles: Tenderness can be found around the Achilles tendon, yet the tender spot does not focus at a certain point. Wherever there is evident tenderness, there are scleromata or cords. At the late stage, the Achilles tendon may be found to turn thicker due to hyperaemia and adhesion of

the peripheral tissues. The hand can feel the stiffness and tension in the triceps muscle of calf. This serves as a major point for diagnosis of this disease.

3. Sensation of friction: At the stage of acute inflammation, when the massagist holds the Achilles tendon on both sides and asks the patient to over-flex and over-extend the knee joint, he can feel a friction sensation around the Achilles tendon, a sensation like holding a handful of snow in hand. Thus, it is also called "snow-holding sensation." Usually, it is accompanied with pain.

4. Resistive test: There is pain at the Achilles tendon and its peripheral tissues when making resistive dorsiflexion or plantar flexion.

Treatment

1. Press acupoints Weizhong (BL 40), Chengshan (BL 57), Kunlun (BL 60) and Taixi (KI 3).

2. Relaxation of muscles and tendons at the triceps muscle of calf: Making the patient lie prone and putting a pillow under the ankle, the massagist overlaps both palms to press the leg hard downward a dozen times, then pull-grasps both sides of the triceps muscle of calf a dozen times. Making the patient flex the knee joint and relax the leg muscles, the massagist supports the foot with one hand and shakes the muscles left and right, or strikes the leg muscles gently and swiftly with the other hand to fully relax the muscles. Afterwards, the massagist holds the ankle with both hands to turn the ankle joint left and right quickly and at the same time shakes the leg muscles. Finally, the massagist holds the foot with both hands, flexes the knee and makes hard dorsiflexion of the ankle five times to tract the leg muscles, the Achilles tendon and its peripheral tissues.(See Figs. 105, 106)

3. Plucking the peripheral tissues around the Achilles tendon: The massagist

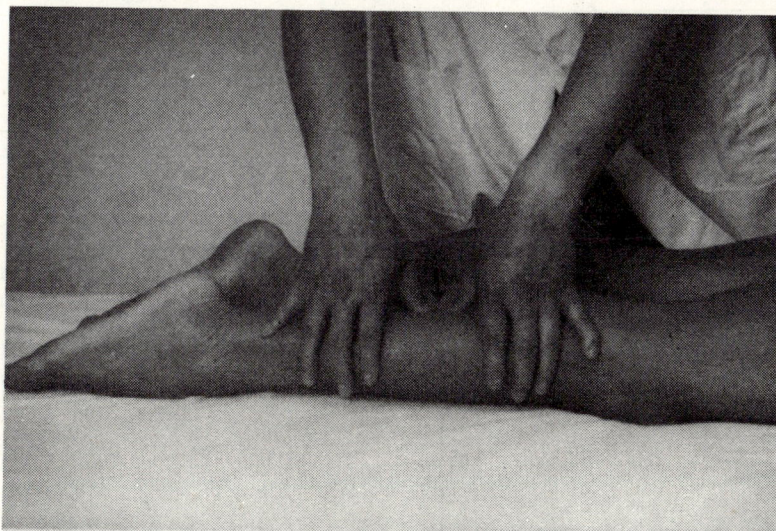

Fig. 105

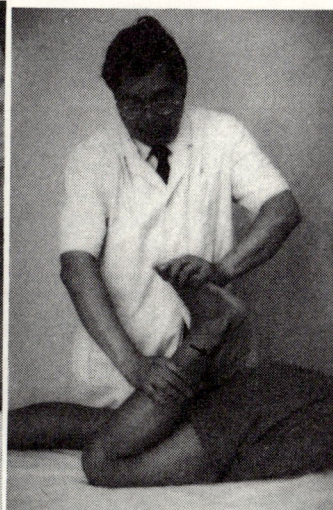

Fig. 106

223

push-presses the peripheral tissues with the thumb and index finger from the calcaneus along both sides of the Achilles tendon. This is supplemented with pinch to improve the blood circulation in the tissues and promote the absorption of inflammation. For scleromata, cords of tender spot, pluck, push-press or scrape hard with thumb to eliminate blood stasis and remove masses. To end the treatment, gently manipulate along both sides of the Achilles tendon to restore the tissues.

4. As a supplement to the above treatment, wash the leg with hot water or fumigate it with traditional Chinese medicines (20 grams of buck grass, 10 grams of safflower, 10 grams of earthworm, 10 grams of frankincense, 10 grams of myrrh and 20 grams of Speranskia tuberculata [Bge.] Baill), twice a day and 20 minutes each time.

5. Those patients who show evident symptoms around the Achilles tendon must reduce exercises in running and jumping. They must carefully protect the tendon — fold up several layers of adhesive plaster and apply it to the leg, ankle and foot to reduce pulling on the Achilles tendon and protect it from rupture. When the surface of the Achilles tendon is found unsmooth and there is scleromata and apparent tenderness, the patient must stop physical training immediately because this indicates the tendon might rupture.

Chapter 10
INJURY OF ANKLE AND FOOT

The feet and ankles are not protected by well-developed muscles. Yet, they are fixed by several small muscles, ligaments and tendons. They bear the full weight of the body, and in sports training such as running and jumping, the instantaneous impact they bear runs as high as several hundred kilograms. The rebound of the ground surface acts on the foot and ankle first. In the instant when the foot hits the ground, a quick take-off and turning of the body often follows immediately; and then falling from a high-up position, the foot and ankle are also responsible to keep balance of the body. All such violent movements may result in foot and ankle injuries, which rank the first in sports injuries. Among them, ankle sprain in particular is the most common.

1. Injury of Ankle Ligament

Also called ankle sprain, injury of the ankle ligament frequently occurs, ranking number one in terms of incidence of all ankle injuries. Abrupt turn of the ankle due to external impact, loss of the center of body gravity and hitting on hard ground may all cause injury to ankle ligaments.

In line with different location, the injury of ankle ligament can be divided into the following types: injury of lateral condylar ligament, which includes injury of the anterior calcanei ligament and posterior calcanei ligament as well as the calcaneofibular ligament; injury of the medial condylar ligament, i.e. injury of the triangle ligament; and injury of the inferior tibiofibular ligament.

In terms of severity of injury, it may be divided into light injury—partial laceration of ligament; which is also called stable injury because the stability of the joint is not affected; serious injury—the ligament ruptures completely; which is also called instable injury as the injury may be complicated by subluxation and even dislocation of the ankle joint.

Clinically, light injury of the lateral condylar ligament is more common. Manual treatment is mainly applied to this type of injury, i.e., partial injury of the condylar ligament.

Injury Mechanism

1. Sprain caused by eversion and inversion of ankle joint: In dorsiflexion of the ankle joint, excessive inversion pulls and injuries the anterior calcanei ligament first. Ankle joint sprain caused by walking downstairs is typical of this type. When the ankle joint is set at functional position, extreme inversion of the ankle joint

may injure the medial condylar ligament, i.e., the triangle ligament. Injury of the lateral condylar ligament is more than that of the medial ligament with the reasons being: first, the medial triangle ligament is pretty strong, but the lateral condylar ligament is comparatively weak; second, improper landing posture, often with the lateral side or instep of the foot hitting the ground, causes forced inversion, thus injuring the lateral condylar ligament.

2. Direct trauma: Ankle joint may be injured by direct kicking, stepping and pressing. For instance, football players may get direct kicks at the ankle when colliding with each other, and they also suffer from over-eversion of the joint caused by kicking the ball with the medial instep, thus harming the medial condylar ligament.

Symptoms and Diagnosis

1. An obvious history of sprain due to inversion or eversion.
2. Pain in the ankle, inability to walk and even to stand.
3. Swelling and blood stasis in ankle joint. Swelling appears soon after injury. When the anterior calcanei ligament and the lateral joint capsule are injured, the swelling appears mainly at the lateral and anteroinferior aspects of the ankle joint. If the injury occurs to more than one ligaments and is complicated by fracture, swelling around the ankle and local bleeding would appear, and cyanotic ecchymosis on the skin of the ankle can be seen the next day. Sometimes, the cyanosis may spread to the foot or the leg.
4. Tenderness: Tenderness is often found at the injured ligament, more evident in the joint space. Attention should also be paid to see if there is avulsion fracture at the medial and lateral aspects of the ankle. Other symptoms include obvious pain and bone crepitation which can be heard when pressing the bone surface; pain in the lateral side of the ankle when the middle and lower sections of the fibula are pressed.
5. Flaccidity of ankle joint: The ankle joint feels painful in passive inversion or eversion; the sensation of an "opening" at the lateral aspect of the ankle joint indicates a total rupture of the ligament. When the ankle joint is pulled, a moving sensation suggests a subluxation of the joint. A total dislocation of the joint gives rise to an obvious local malformation. However, a misdiagnosis is liable at the acute stage due to serious swelling and pain in the joint. If the subluxated joint is not strapped timely, it may result in the sequela of instable joint and frequent recurrences of ankle sprain and flaccidity of ankle joint during training, which may disrupt the athlete to complete some movements.
6. X-ray examination does not affect directly the diagnosis of ankle sprain, but can help rule out any fracture. When the physician suspects that the ligament is totally ruptured, he can make forced inversion of both feet to take a front-view X-ray photo of the ankle. Widening of the lateral joint space indicates a total rupture of the lateral ligament. If the front-view X-ray photo taken with both ankles being turned sideward shows a lateral displacement, it may be diagnosed as

a dislocation of the ankle joint.

Treatment

1. For an acute and serious case, make necessary local inspection only, avoid any over-traction of ankle and shaking of the joint so as to avoid further injury to the ligament. To present bleeding and swelling in the ankle, have the ankle soaked in cold water for 10-20 minutes or apply refrigerant spraying to evoke contraction of the small blood vessels. Apply traditional Chinese medicine and pressure bandage with thick cotton mat after treatment, lift the affected limb high and perform initiative limbering up of the toes.

2. For an emergent but light case, press the acupoints Jiexi (ST 41), Kunlun (BL 60) and Taixi (KI 3) to relax the muscles and tendons and promote the circulation of qi and blood in the collaterals and meridians; perform gentle kneading and scrubbing from the toes upwards to the leg for detumescence and stopping pain; gently pull at the ankle with both hands; put both palms at the medial and lateral aspects of the ankle to perform squeeze-pressing at the ankle toward the central region to restore the joint space; finally apply pressure dressing to the ankle, lift the affected limb high. (See Fig. 107)

Rehabilitation

1. For a light case in which the swelling does not get worse and the pain is somewhat relieved the day after the injury, the patient should be advised to do short-distance jogging or walking, and squatting with the heel not leaving the ground. To start with, do 10 squats the first time and increase gradually to prevent bleeding and joint adhesion.

2. For a serious case, apply flat-pushing 1-2 days after the injury. Push and pressing

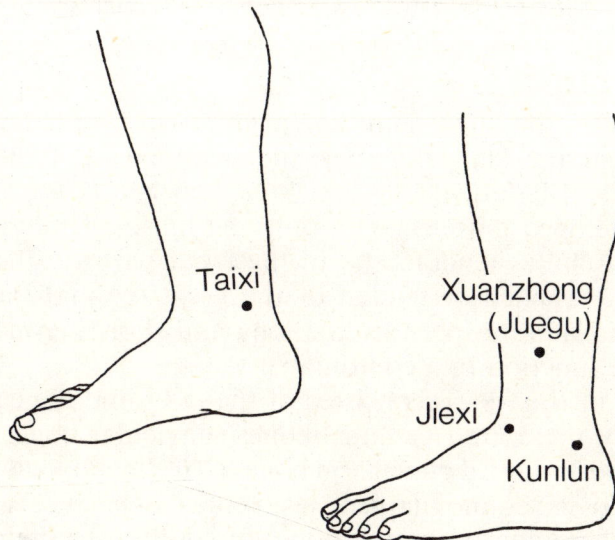

Fig. 107

with even force with both thumbs from the foot to the leg 10 times; perform petrisage on both sides of the Achilles tendon and the depressions of the medial and lateral sides of the ankle with the thumb and index finger to reduce detumescence and pain and relax the muscles and tendons to promote blood circulation.

3. For cases in which the stability of the ankle is not affected, perform traction and counter-traction and shaking. Make the patient take a supine position, the massagist carries the distal part of the foot and pulls upward with one hand, while pushing the ankle with the other. In the meantime, make inversion and eversion of the ankle, i.e., shake the foot left and right 10 times to widen the joint space to remove adhesion, with the force applied being appropriate for the patient to bear. Then, the massagist holds the foot and performs traction and counter-traction of the foot with both hands, makes plantar flexion and dorsiflexion of the ankle joint to widen the range of movement. (See Figs. 108, 109, 110 and 111)

A patient with serious symptoms may resume jogging and squatting one week after the injury. He should protect the ankle with ankle pad or adhesive plaster to avoid recurrence of the injury, do exercises to increase the strength of the leg muscles and ankle joint so as to enhance its stability.

2. Disturbance of Foot and Ankle Joints

The foot and ankle has many functions: The instantaneous force in running and jumping is mainly generated by the foot and ankle; and they also bear the brunt in rotating and kicking movements. So, the foot and ankle are liable to various dysfunction. Unlike sprain of ankle joint, the symptoms of foot and ankle joint can be immediately removed with manual treatment. Since this disease has been rarely recorded in medical literature, whether it is correct to use the name "disturbance of foot and ankle joint" remains to be discussed.

Injury Mechanism

1. In anatomic terms, the ankle joint comprises tibia, fibula and talus, and its main functions to bear the load, dorsiflex and plantar flex. It has three sets of ligaments (inferior tibiofibular, medial accessory and lateral accessory). It is not protected by well-developed muscles, with only the muscle tendons passing it. At the back part is the Achilles tendon, and in the front part are the anterior tibial muscle tendon, the long extensor tendon of the great toe and the long extensor tendons of toes. At its lateral aspect are the long and short peroneal tendons. All these muscle tendons function in a coordinated way.

The proximal part of the foot is consisted of the talus and the calcaneus. At the distal part of the foot, there are five tarsal bones (navicular bone, cuboid bone as well as the first, second and third cuneiform bones), five metatarsal bones, fourteen phalanges and a few ossa sesamoidia pedis as well as some accessory bones, such as the accessory scaphoid and triangular bone. In addition to the ossa sesamoidia pedis and accessory bones, there are 26 other small bones of different sizes and

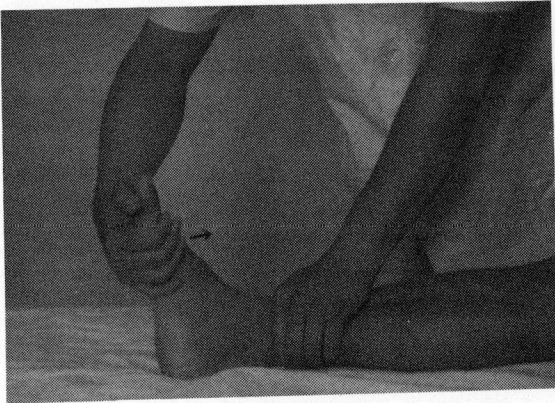

Fig. 108

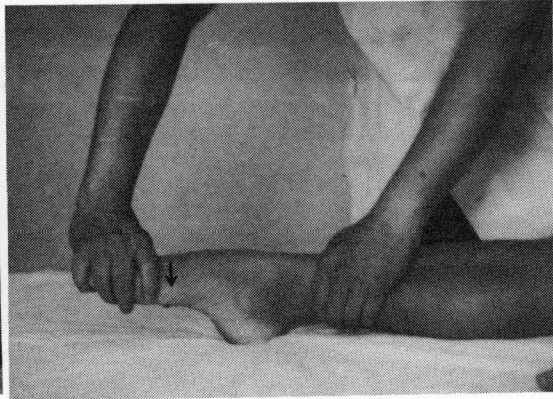

Fig. 109

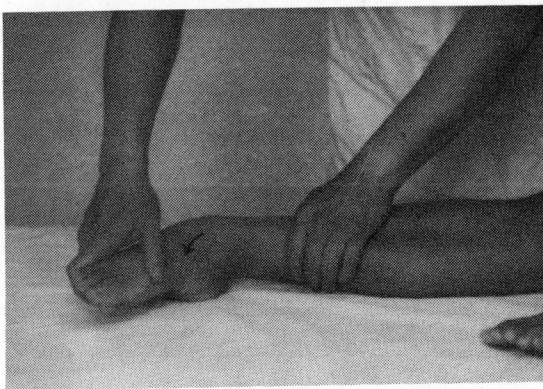

Fig. 110

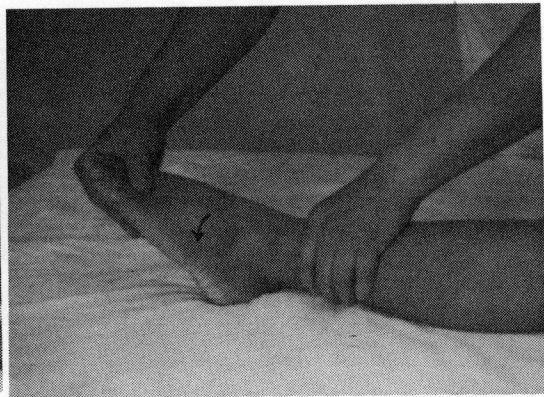

Fig. 111

shapes. They form 28 joints and are linked up as a whole by various ligaments, muscles, muscle tendons and aponeuroses. To meet the requirements of walking and bearing the load, there are three arches at the foot, namely, the medial, lateral and transverse arch of foot.

The structure of the foot and ankle is complicated. So, any improper exertion of force in landing, jumping or rotating may cause disturbance of the relations among the various parts, thus giving rise to symptoms at the foot and ankle.

2. Pathological dysfunction of the foot and ankle: Improper exertion of force or impact by external force may evoke locking (i.e., joint malposition) among the small joints of bones, pulling or squeezing of joint capsules and ligaments, as well as displacement of muscle tendons. All these can cause pain and impede the function of foot. Manual treatment may help reduce the joints and muscle tendons, thus remove the symptoms.

3. Flaccidity of foot joints and ligaments: When the foot and ankle are not

strong, the patient may feel flaccidity in them. This may lead to disturbance of small joints. Repeated malpositioning and displacement of the muscle and tendon may lead to chronic strain of the foot and ankle.

Symptoms and Diagnosis

1. Evident history of trauma: The manifestations include pain in foot and ankle, locked joint, dyskinesia. Clear tender spots and locking are absent, so repeated checking is necessary. There are no obvious swelling and blood stasis in the joint.

2. The symptoms improve soon after manual treatment. This is the main point for differentiation in the diagnosis of this disease.

3. Attention should be paid to differentiating this disease from sprain of ankle joint. The pain in this disease is mild, there is no clear tender spot and swelling, and no sensation of an "opening" at the joint. These symptoms are different from those for the sprain of the ankle joint.

Treatment

1. Digitally press acupoints Kunlun (BL 60), Taixi (KI 3) and Jiexi (ST 41).

2. Relax the lower leg muscles by kneading or grasping. This process can be omitted if time does not allow during a contest.

3. The massagist holds the distal part of the foot with one hand and the heel with the other to pull the foot downward and simultaneously rotate the foot and make dorsiflexion and plantar flexion of the joint. In this process, a click may be heard or a sensation of moving of the joint may be felt. This method, which can remove most of the symptoms, is essential in treating this disease. If the foot and ankle still feel unwell, pluck the painful tender spot to restore the tissues and squeeze the ankle from left and right and the foot back and forth to promote the restoration of the displaced tissues. For athletes who suffer frequently from disturbance of the ankle joint, it is essential that the massagist master different concrete reduction steps so that he or she can give timely treatment in sports training or competitions whenever a disturbance of the ankle joint occurs. (See Fig. 112)

Example: Zhuang, female swimmer. One day before the 11th Asian Games, she suddenly felt pain in the right ankle when going downstairs and turned lame. The author gave her an immediate treatment by the swimming pool. In the process, a click was heard in the ankle and the ankle joint was felt moving. Eventually, the pain disappeared and she was able to walk normally. She took part in the competition immediately afterwards and won a gold medal in the 100-metre free-style event.

3. Fracture of Ankle Joint

An injury that frequently occurs in sports, the fracture of the ankle is mainly caused by indirect external force, and only a small number are caused by direct external force.

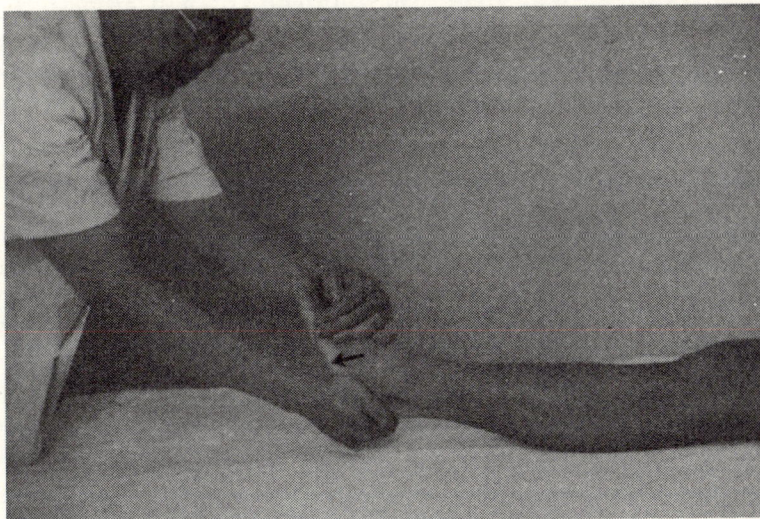

Fig. 112

Injury Mechanism

1. Incorrect landing when falling down from a high place can force outward rotation, eversion, inversion, dorsiflexion and plantar flexion of the foot, which in turn can result in different types of fracture of the ankle joint. According to the different areas where fracture occurs, the fracture of the ankle joint can be divided into the following types: single ankle fracture, fracture at the medial and lateral aspects of the ankle, fracture at the medial, lateral and posterior aspects of the ankle, T-shaped, Y-shaped and comminuted fracture of the lower part of the tibia, avulsion fracture and fracture of the ankle joint complicated by dislocation. Fracture due to outward rotation is more commonly seen.

2. Direct external force: Direct kicking or crushing at the foot and ankle or direct impact caused by body weight on the ankle when falling down from a high place may often result in T-shaped, Y-shaped and comminuted fracture or dislocation at the lower part of the tibia.

Symptoms and Diagnosis

1. Evident traumatic history, pain in the ankle, inability to walk and even to stand in a case.

2. Tenderness: Distinct tenderness at the injured spot, possibly accompanied by a grinding sensation. In fracture of the external malleolus, pushing and pressing at the fibula may induce pain at the lower part of fibula. Pain is also felt when gently striking the heel with fist. Tenderness and grinding sensation are the key points in the diagnosis of this disorder.

3. Swelling and deformity: Swelling and subcutaneous cyanosis are witnessed soon after injury. When the fracture is complicated by obvious displacement or

231

joint dislocation, deformity and abnormal movement will appear. This may serve to confirm the diagnosis.

4. X-ray photo of the foot and ankle can help reveal the exact location of the fracture, the trend of fracture displacement and the condition of the dislocation, and is therefore of some significance for manual treatment.

Treatment

1. Manual treatment: Any type of new fracture calls for manual reduction and external fixation. The fracture has to be reduced accurately. If not, there will be the sequela of osteoarthritis after the union of fracture, which in turn can impede the joint function. Manual treatment will be unnecessary if there is no displacement. In such a case, apply external fixation only.

a) Traction: This does not require anaesthesia. Make the patient lie on his back with the knee joint flexed, then ask an assistant to hold the knee joint and pull upward while the massagist holds the heel with one hand and the distal part of the foot with the other, and pull downward along the trend of the original deformity. In the process, a click may be heard or moving of the joint be felt, and this indicates completion of the reduction of the fracture and dislocation.

b) Rotation: While performing traction, the massagist makes gradual inward rotation or outward rotation of the foot and ankle in accordance with the specific type of fracture to correct the rotated deformity. This is followed by inversion and eversion movements of the ankle. For eversion fracture make passive inversion of the foot and for inversion fracture make eversion movement to correct the fracture.

c) Dorsiflexion: Dorsiflex the foot to correct displacement of the medial malleolus and the posterior malleolus.

d) Joining manipulation: The massagist holds the medial and lateral malleoli with both pals to perform squeezing on the malleoli towards the center to ensure better reduction. This method can help reduce the separated inferior tibiofibular joint, correct leftward or rightward displacement of the talus and restore the normal anatomic relations of the whole ankle joint. (See Fig. 113)

2. Fixation: Plaster support fixation is preferable. In addition to providing a fixation with the support going beyond the joint, it can make the ankle joint invert or evert slightly. It is conducive to the reduction and union of the fracture to set the ankle at a slightly everted position for an inversion fracture and set the ankle at a slightly inverted position for an eversion fracture. The length of the plaster support should run from the upper middle part of the lower leg to the metatarsophalangeal joint. This plaster support should be replaced by a central position one after three weeks. The total period of fixation is 6-8 weeks.

3. Rehabilitation treatment:

a) Start making active flexion and extension movements of the toe and knee joints the second day after the reduction fixation. Gently knead the legs and ankles to speed up blood circulation and promote the union. Practise walking with

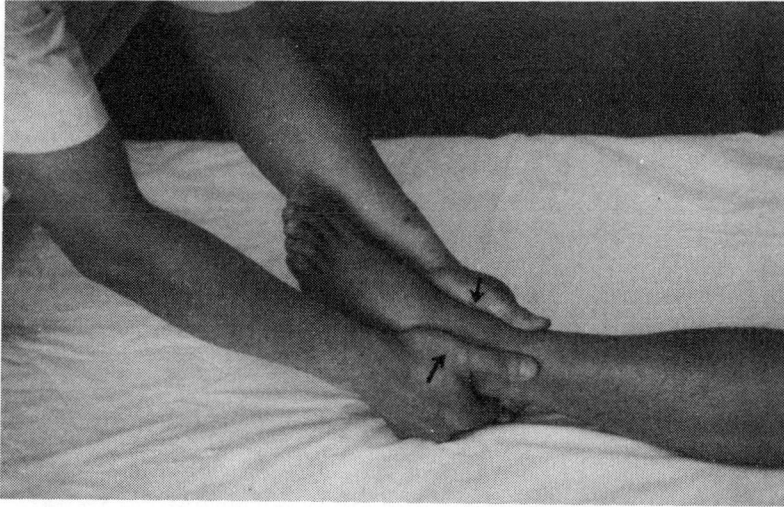

Fig. 113

crutches to reduce postural edema.

b) After the plaster support is removed three weeks later, the massagist does massage from the foot to the leg mainly by kneading and grasping to soften the stiffened muscles, and disperse scleromata by plucking. The patient can do ankle joint flexion and extension movements on his or her own, but not rotation or inversion and eversion movements of the ankle.

c) Soak the ankle in hot water every day, 20 minutes each time; or fumigate-wash the ankle joint with Chinese herbal medicine to remove the blood stasis, promote blood circulation and restore the joint function.

The plaster support is still needed when starting to walk. The external fixation can be completely removed six weeks later. Walking and squatting should be done on flat ground first, then running and jumping may gradually be practised. Protect the ankle with a supporting belt or an ankle pad in physical training.

4. Osteoarthropathy of Ankle

Osteoarthropathy of ankle is also called the "footballer's ankle." Its major manifestations are primary and secondary retrogressive pathological changes at the cartilage of the ankle joint, hyperplasia of new bone at the articular border, thickening of synovium and inflammation. The sports injury type of osteoarthropathy falls into the category of secondary pathological changes.

Injury Mechanism

1. Direct trauma: Rough articular surface left from union of fracture displacement or caused by callus developed at the fractured area. In addition, subluxation, dislocation and ligament rupture at the ankle joint may cause flaccidity of the

233

ankle and result in friction there, which in turn may injury the cartilage surface. All these may lead to osteoarthropathy as time passes.

2. Chronic strain: Overburden on the ankle may make it repeatedly dorsiflex, plantar dorsiflex and rotate to the extreme, causing mutual collision, friction and crushing among the tibia, fibula and talus, all of which result in minor injuries to the articular cartilage, synoviums and ligaments. In a long course, such minor injuries may cause denaturation and falling of articular cartilage and eventually hyperosteogeny. The ankle bears a tremendous impact when taking-off and landing in long jump; so the ankle joint is liable to injuries if it is not at a correction position. In football games, kicking the ball with different parts of the foot also likely causes injuries to the ankle, and this is why most footballers suffer from "footballer's ankle."

3. Repeated trauma in the joint can lead to flaccidity of the joint, which may lead to frequent joint malformation in physical training and the action of the shearing force may cause injury to the articular cartilage. Besides, rough and hard ground may also increase the chance of injury.

4. The pathological changes are mainly manifested as denaturation, chondromalacia and hyperosteogeny of the cartilage. Hyperosteogeny may give rise to spurs. Repeated crushing and stimulation on the anterior and posterior borders of the ankle joint can make the anterior border of tibia appear as osteophyte and the posterior protrusion of the talus become longer. Spurs can develop at the lower part of the medial and lateral malleoli and the bigger ones can get broken in a traumatic injury and turn into joint bodies. Friction between the exposed bony surface and the surrounding tissues can aggravate the pathological changes. In a chronic injury, the articular synovium thickens. When there are bony nodes, there may be hydrarthrosis and arthroncus. Repeated friction of the muscle tendons can also cause tenosynovitis, hence aggravating the condition at the ankle joint. The aim of the manual treatment is to avoid further injury of the ankle, relieve tumefaction, improve the function of the ankle joint and remove the symptom of locked joint.

5. Although teenager athletes may also contract osteoarthropathy, no symptoms will ever manifest in the ankle so long as they stop physical training, as their bony joint tissues have good plasticity and sound repairing ability. In some cases, however, no evident symptoms are found at the initial stage, and yet these symptoms and hyperosteogeny may develop when they reach middle age or old age.

Symptoms and Diagnosis

1. Pain: Pain is the most marked symptom of osteoarthropathy. At the initial stage, the ankle feels weak and more painful in the morning. The pain will abate and the ankle feel more relaxed after some time. But, exessive use of the ankle may cause pain that can become so serious that the patient will be unable to participate in physical training and competition. However, the severity of pain is not directly related to the size of spurs in the ankle, as revealed in X-ray examination.

2. Tenderness: Due to pathological changes in the bone and injury to the soft tissues of the ankle, there is tenderness around the ankle joint, with that in the joint space being more obvious. Moreover, to support the joint and ensure its movement, the leg muscles are in a state of tension. So stiffness and tenderness may be found together.

3. Swelling in the joint: Thickening of the synoviums, hydrarthrosis, tenosynovitis and spurs may all cause swelling in the ankle joint, mainly in the soft tissues. Manual treatment can reduce the swelling

4. Limitation of joint movement: At the early stage, the joint feels stiff, and at the late stage, the spurs grow larger and fibrosis of soft tissues may appear. Swelling in the joint may hinder joint movements, such as dorsiflexion, plantar flexion and rotation. Eventually, the patient cannot run and jump normally, the old-aged have to walk with crutches. When joint bodies are incarcerated in a certain part of the joint space, the ankle joint will feel painful and lose its normal functions temporarily. The patient will have to stop at once to move the ankle passively to alter the stance of the joint bodies in order to unlock the joint and restore its functions.

5. Sensation of friction in the joint: Due to the rough articular surface, displacement of the joint bodies in the joint and the wearing of muscles tendons and cartilages, a sensation of friction may be felt or a click heard in clinical examination of the ankle.

6. X-ray examination may not reveal any abnormal signs at the early stage while at the late stage it may witness hyperosteogeny at the articular border and narrowing of the joint space. This is an important basis for diagnosis of this disease.

Treatment

1. Digitally press Weizhong (BL 40), Chengshan (BL 57), Jiexi (ST 41), Taixi (KI 3) and Kunlun (BL 60).

2. When an athlete feels painful and weak in the ankle, he should, in addition to receiving timely treatment, readjust his training program to avoid doing such simple movements as dorsiflexion, plantar flexion, inversion and eversion, and cut those movements which need the ankle to bear a sudden force. After the treatment, he should be sure to have sufficient rest for the diseased part and soft tissues to heal.

3. Relaxation of leg muscles: The massagist performs kneading and grasping to relax the leg muscles and pull-grasp along both sides of the Achilles tendon with the thumb and index finger to loosen the pulling force at the ankle by the muscles and improve local blood circulation.

4. Holding the distal part of the foot with one hand and the heel with the other, the massagist pulls the ankle joint downward, makes forcible dorsiflexion, plantar flexion as well as inversion and eversion movement of the ankle to expand the joint space, separate adhesion and remove tendon contracture. For a case obviously with

spurs, the force applied should be appreciate lest it rupture the spurs.

5. The massagist push-presses along the joint space on both sides of the Achilles tendon, passing the lower part of the lateral malleolus to reach the dorsum of the foot; then nip and scrape hard at the painful area or anywhere pain occurs when moving the joint to relieve the pain by stimulating the diseased synoviums and ligaments; finally scrub the leg, ankle, and dorsum and sole of foot to generate heat, promote blood circulation, remove swelling and dispel dampness and cold. After the treatment, keep the ankle warm and away from cold and dampness. As a supplementary treatment, wash the ankle and foot with warm water or fumigate and wash them with Chinese herbal medicine, once a day and 20 minutes each time.

6. Treatment of locked joint: There will sudden dyskinesia of the ankle joint when joint bodies are incarcerated in the joint space. In most cases, the patient can remove the locking by turning the ankle joint slowly. Yet, there are some who cannot, and in these cases manual treatment are necessary. The concrete procedures are: The massagist hold the foot with both hands and turns the joint towards all directions to change the stance of the joint bodies to unlock the joint. In case that the treatment is not successful, make an assistant pull at the foot while the massagist push-presses the articular space or the tender spot with thumb to force the joint bodies to enter the articular cavity and unlock the joint. In a long-standing case, rest the ankle for 1-2 days.

5. Tenosynovitis of Ankle and Foot

At the ankle and foot region there are several muscle tendons and tendon sheaths. At the medial aspect of the ankle are the posterior tibial muscle tendon and the long flexor muscle tendon of toes; at the anterior aspect are the anterior tibial muscle tendon, the long extensor muscle tendon of the great toe and the long extensor muscle tendon of toes; and at the lateral aspect of the ankle are the long peroneal muscle tendon and the short peroneal muscle tendon. Each tendon is protected by a tendon sheath that performs the functions of lubrication and trochlea. Peritenonitis of the Achilles tendon at the posterior aspect of the ankle does not fall with the scope of this disease. Tenosynovitis of the ankle and foot occurs as often as that of the hand, and among them the most often seen ones are the tenosynovitis at the long flexor muscle tendon of the great toe, the posterior tibial muscle tendon and the long and short peroneal muscle tendons.

Injury Mechanism

1. Chronic strain: Running and jumping with great exertion, repeated movement with load and repeated external impact on the ankle can cause serious friction to the tendon in the tendon sheath, thus giving rise to inflammation and hyperaemia and exudation at the tendon and tendon sheath.

2. Repeated sprain of joint: Repeated sprain can cause flaccidity in the joint and give rise to constant joint malposition. To maintain the stability of the joint, the

muscles might contract protectively, thus increasing the burden on the tendon and causing tenosynovitis. When the ankle is kicked directly or pulled, the sheath on top of it can also be affected.

3. Tenosynovitis is characterized by tissue edema and thickening. When an injury causes the increase of exudate which cannot be absorbed, the exudate will accumulate at the affected area, forming thecal cyst and gradually causing stenotic tenosynovitis.

Symptoms and Diagnosis

1. Pain: Pain and weakness are often found at the medial and lateral aspects of the ankle and sole. These symptoms become more evident when the ankle exerts efforts. In a serious case, the patient are unable to run and jump even go lame, neither can he or she stand on one foot or on tiptoe. This is a unique feature of tenosynovitis of the long flexor muscle of the great toe. However, the pain can ease with rest and become serious when affected by cold.

2. Tenderness: Minimal swelling and tenderness at the affected area. Unique to stenotic tenosynovitis is the sensation of friction when moving the ankle tendon. Elliptical expansion at the instep indicates thecal cyst. Pain cannot be caused by backward driving of the foot. Local resistive pain appears in tenosynovitis of flexor hallucis longus and when the great toe is flexed.

Treatment

1. Digitally press acupoints Taixi (KI 3), Jiexi (ST 41), Kunlun (BL 60) and Zhaohai (KI 6, which is in the depression at the lower border of the medial malleolus). (See Fig. 114)

2. Push-kneading the posterior and lateral aspects of the leg 5-10 minutes to remove

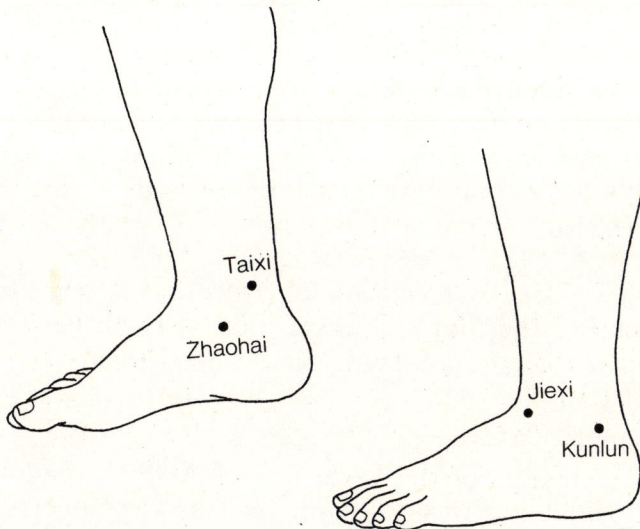

Fig. 114

obstruction in the meridians and collaterals and promote blood circulation; passively make dorsiflexion and plantar flexion of the ankle and tract the muscles and tendons to remove muscular tension and separate any adhesion in the tendon sheaths.

3. Perform hard plucking on the painful spot and in the area 5-10 minutes. This is the key to treat this disease. Scraping may also be performed, if necessary, to relieve inflammation. Then push-press along the trend of the tendons to relax them and the muscles and treat tumefaction. Finally, scrub the foot and ankle 5-10 minutes to make the skin red and hot. Keep the foot warm after treatment.

6. Injury of Posterior Talocalcaneal Articulation

At the posterior part of the talus is the posterior process of talus, the articular surface of which corresponds with the posterior lip of the tibia. At the posterior process of talus there is an accessory bone called triangular bone. The posterior talocalcaneal articulation is between the calcaneus and talus and its function is to ensure the completion of inversion and eversion movements of foot. In crush injury of posterior triangular bone of tibia, fracture of posterior process of talus and osteoarthropathy of posterior talocalcaneal articulation, the anatomic positions are similar and their injury mechanism, symptoms and manual treatment procedures are also the same. So, the three are grouped together as injury of posterior talocalcaneal articulation.

Injury Mechanism
1. Chronic strain of ankle: Collision and friction on the posterior talocalcaneal articulation in jumping, landing and falling from a high place may injure the articular surface, causing denaturation of the joint cartilages, hyperosteogeny, rough articular surface and synovitis, which is often complicated by tenosynovitis of the flexor hallucis longus.

2. Traumatic injury: Sudden plantar flexion of the foot caused by kicking ball with the dorsum of foot and incorrect stance of foot in landing when falling from a high place, for instance, may cause squeezing on the posterior process of talus by the posterior lip of tibia; and upward pushing of talus by the reacting force of ground may cause fracture of the posterior process of talus or squeezing on the triangular bone.

3. Repeated sprain of the foot and ankle, flaccidity of the joint and constant eversion and inversion of the foot and ankle joint at improper stance may cause malposition and moving of the joint and finally lead to injury of the posterior talocalcaneal articulation.

Symptoms and Diagnosis
1. Pain: Pain on both sides of the lower end of Achilles tendon; more serious pain when making overplantar flexion; pain when making inversion and eversion of the foot; and more serious pain when the triangular bone is injured by crush or fractured. In a case complicated by tenosynovitis of the flexor hallucis longus,

pain is also felt when touching the ground with tiptoe and jumping; and there will be resistive pain when flexing the great toe.

2. Tenderness and swelling: Limited tenderness is felt at both sides of the lower end of the Achilles tendon and at the upper part of the calcaneus, particularly at the joint space. Due to local exudation caused by synovitis, swelling may be found in the soft tissues at the tender spot and a sensation of friction may be felt or a click may be heard when moving the ankle.

3. X-ray examination helps confirm the diagnosis. Osteoarthropathy shows lip-like hyperplasia at the posterior border of the talus and calcaneus; a fracture line may be seen in a case of fracture of the posterior process; and in injury of the posterior triangular bone of the talus separated bone fragments with smooth borders may be seen.

Treatment

1. Digitally press acupoints Taixi (KI 3), Kunlun (BL 60) and Zhaohai (KI 6).

2. While making an assistant pull the foot with both hands to enlarge the joint space, the massagist press-kneads on both sides of the Achilles tendon with the thumb, nips or scrapes the tender spot or the upper part of the calcaneus along the joint space 5-10 times. As the tissues here are very thin, it is not difficult to locate the massage spots. The manipulations should not be too strong lest they cause pain and aggravate the local swelling at the rear part of the foot. For a case complicated by tenosynovitis of flexor hallucis longus, pluck and push the tendon to cure the inflammation.

3. For a chronic injury of the posterior talocalcaneal articulation, the patient may continue training while receiving treatment. However, a supporting belt must be used for protection when doing movements that require force from the foot so as to limit over-plantar flexion of the ankle and reduce compression on the posterior talocalcaneal articulation and the triangular bone. These methods may be supplemented by daily hot bath of the foot to relieve the local symptoms.

7. Injury of Scaphoid Bone of Foot

Injury of the scaphoid bone of foot refers to injury that happens at the middle part of the foot. It includes chondropathy of the scaphoid bone, fatigue fracture of the scaphoid bone and osteoarthropathy of the talovanicular joint. This disorder may hamper running and jumping.

Injury Mechanism

1. Injury to Epiphysis of the scaphoid bone of foot: This injury often occurs among young-age gymnasts when falling from a high place and jumping with great force. The pathological manifestations of this injury are similar to that of osteochondrosis, with the ossified center in the scaphoid bone turning rather flat. Continuous external impact may rupture the bone, forming ruptured bone chips and causing local swelling and pain. This disorder is more likely to occur among

children 4-6 years old, particularly boys. Sufficient rest and proper treatment may make the bone return to normal in two years.

2. Chronic strain: In running and jumping, the foot bears the major brunt, which may result in injury to the scaphoid bone. For instance, in long jump the impulsive force produced by the body weight and reacting force produced by the jumping board may both work on the scaphoid bone to cause fatigue fracture. When this happens, the scaphoid bone turns more flat, the articular surface becomes rough and new bone may grow. Repeated friction may wear out the talus, making the bone surface expose and turns hyperosteogenic, thus causing osteoarthropathy of the talonavicular joint, thickening of the articular synoviums and synovium incarceration in the joint space, hence pain.

3. Traumatic injury: Tremendous external impact on the scaphoid bone of foot may make the bone fracture. In this, the injury mechanism is similar to that of fracture of the scaphoid bone of wrist.

Symptoms and Diagnosis

1. Pain in the instep: Pain occurs in the instep when the foot exerts force to take off and forcibly stamps on the ground with the distal part; pain at the sole, which indicates injury in the palmar aspect of the talonavicular joint. In a case of fracture of the scaphoid bone, pain occurs in the foot when walking.

2. Tenderness: Solid protrusion and tenderness at the instep, and more evident tenderness at the talonavicular joint space. Pain will occur when the massagist holds the distal part of the foot and makes abduction of the foot with one hand to widen the joint space, and uses the thumb of the other hand to press the talonavicular joint space to push the synovium into the joint.

3. X-ray examination: Front-view X-ray photo of the ankle may reveal a fracture line of the fracture of the scaphoid bone of foot and show that the bone becomes flat, the joint surface has turned rough and there is lip-like hyperosteogeny at the border of the talus and scaphoid. It may help determine the type of the injury.

Treatment

1. Digitally press acupoints Taixi (KI 3), Jiexi (ST 41), Yongquan (KI 1) and Rangu (KI 2, at the depression of the lower anteroinferior border of the tuberosity of the scaphoid of foot). (See Fig. 115)

2. Traction is a suitable therapy for osteoarthropathy of talonavicular and fracture of scaphoid bone. The procedure is: The massagist holds the ankle with one hand and the distal part of the foot with the other to pull towards both sides to enlarge the talonavicular space and rotates the foot 10-20 times to remove articular adhesion and reduce pressure between the talus and the vavicular bones to relieve pain.

3. Push-press or scrape the protrusion of the instep to stimulate the thickened synovium and the diseased periosteum so as to promote blood circulation, remove swelling and relieve pain. The same can also be applied for pain in the sole. The force applied should not be too heavy lest it affects walking. Push-pressing and

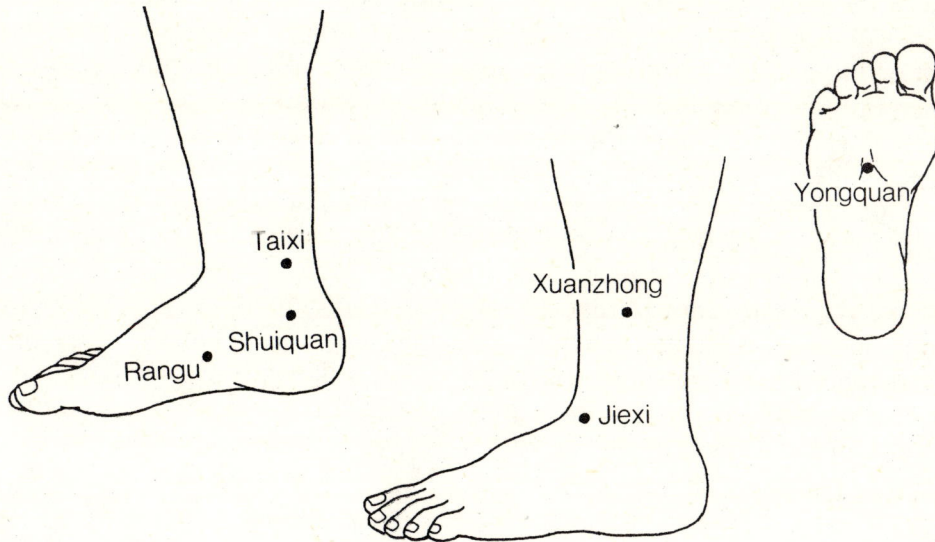

Fig. 115

scraping are the key manipulations to treat this disease.

Manual reduction will not be necessary if fracture displacement is not evident. Simply apply fixation by plaster support or paper board for 3-4 weeks. The patient should stop running and jumping for an appropriate period lest the fracture does not unite and develop into aseptic necrosis of the scaphoid bone or even osteoarthropathy.

Manual treatment should better be accompanied by daily hot bathing or fumigation and washing with Chinese herbal medicine. Patients suffering from serious pain in foot should stop physical training; those with light pain should apply adhesive plaster strapping during training. The strapping method is: wind 3-4 strips of cloth around the instep and sole transversely to limit the range of movement of the talonavicular joint and protect the foot.

8. Injury of Accessory Scaphoid Bone of Foot

The accessory scaphoid bone is linked with the scaphoid bone by soft tissues. Attached to the accessory scaphoid bone is the posterior tibial muscle tendon, which performs the function of plantar flexion and inversion of foot.

Injury Mechanism

1. Due to overinversion of the foot, the collision between the medial malleolus of foot and the accessory scaphoid bone may induce squeezing on the accessory scaphoid bone by the malleolus and the scaphoid bone, thus injuring the surface of the accessory scaphoid bone.

2. Passive pulling on the posterior tibial muscle due to sudden overeversion of

241

foot may cause avulsion of the tendon-attaching point of the accessory scaphoid bone. Forceful contraction of the posterior tibial muscle may also pull on the tendon-attaching point, thus inducing injury. For instance, touching ground with tiptoe when falling from a high place and hitting the jumping board with the distal part of foot can all generate violent contraction of the posterior tibial muscle, resulting in avulsion to the tendon-attaching point. Either caused by active contraction of or passive pulling on the posterior tibial muscle, the injury of the accessory scaphoid bone is an acute one. Direct kicking at the accessory scaphoid bone can also result in such injury, which is rarely seen however.

3. Chronic strain: In high jump and long jump, taking off with the front part of the foot or touching ground with tiptoe may cause excessive pulling on the accessory scaphoid bone by the posterior tibial muscle, thus giving rise to slight injury of the tendon-attaching point, edema of the soft tissues and inflammation at the periosteum and tendons, all of which are called enthesiopathy.

Symptoms and Diagnosis

1. There is pain at the tubercle of the medial scaphoid bone of foot, which becomes more evident when turned inward. The ankle feels weak when beating the jumping board and the tiptoe feels painful when touching ground.

2. Swelling: In an acute injury, there are edema, exudation, local swelling and tenderness around the accessory scaphoid bone. These manifestations are more evident when compared with the healthy foot.

3. There is resistive pain when making plantar flexion and inversion of the foot.

Treatment

1. Press acupoints Taixi (KI 3), Rangu (KI 2), Zhaohai (KI 6) and Shangqiu (SP 5, at the anteroinferior aspect of medial malleolus and mid-point of the line connecting the tubercle of the scaphoid bone and the medial malleolus). (See Fig.116)

2. Push-press from the medial aspect of the foot and the sole upwards to the superior aspect of the ankle with thumb 10-20 times to relax the pulling on the accessory scaphoid bone by the posterior tibial muscle to make the skin feel hot. This manipulation has the functions of relaxing the muscles and tendons, promoting blood circulation, and removing blood stasis and swelling. (See Fig. 117)

3. Scrape the painful area at the medial middle part of the foot 10 times. This is vital for treating this disease. After the treatment, wash the foot with hot water frequently or fumigate and wash it with Chinese herbal medicine. At the acute stage, cut jumping and running. During physical training, apply "8"-shaped adhesive plaster strapping to the ankle or adhesive plaster winding strapping to the middle part of the foot.

9. Enthesiopathy of Calcaneus

Enthesiopathy of calcaneus is also called osteochondrosis of the tuberosity of calcaneus. Continuous and repeated forceful contraction of the triceps muscle of

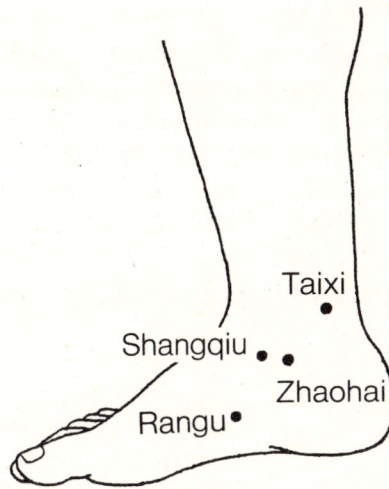

Fig. 116

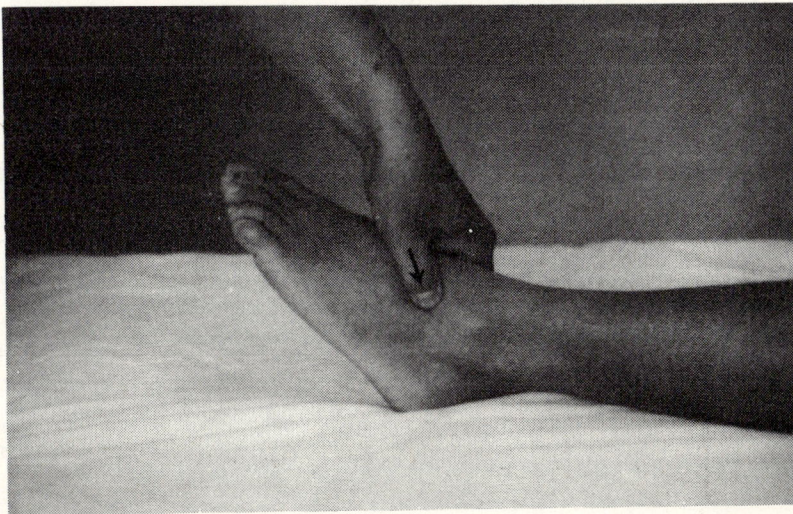

Fig. 117

calf pulls, through the Achilles tendon, the epiphysis of the tuberosity of calcaneus and leads to chronic injury and ischemic necrosis on it. A spontaneous cure may be achieved though physical training may be affected during the onset of the disease.

Injury Mechanism

1. Chronic strain: Continuous forceful contraction of the triceps muscle of calf

243

would naturally pull the tendon-attaching point, causing injury to the bone or the epiphysis of the tuberosity of calcaneus, and the terminating point of the Achilles tendon and its surrounding soft tissues. For adult athletes, although a union of the epiphysis of the tuberosity of the calcaneus has achieved, repeated over-load pulling on the Achilles tendon still can cause enthesiopathy at its attaching point. For instance, summersault in gymnastics and the take-off push in long jump may all pull the Achilles tendon hard, causing injury at the tuberosity of the calcaneus. With the passing of time, the above-described symptoms will appear.

2. Traumatic injury: Local symptoms may appear due to direct kicking at the heel, bumping against an apparatus by the heel as well powerful contraction of the Achilles tendon — all of which may pull at the tuberosity of calcaneus. Such cases are rare however.

3. The pathological manifestations of enthesiopathy of calcaneus include peri-tenonitis of Achilles tendon at its attaching point and chronic retrocalcaneal bursitis. Pull of the epiphysis usually result in an uneven appearance; in a serious case, however, the epiphysis may be ruptured into several pieces. Normally, union of the epithysis leaves no malformation. The enthesiopathy of calcaneus resulting from the union of the epithysis manifests as hyperosteogeny of calcaneus and backward protrusion of calcaneus.

Symptoms and Diagnosis

1. Pain at the heel: With a slow onset, pain at the heel may refer to the leg; jumping and running may induce pain; and in a serious case there may be lameness.

2. Swelling and tenderness: Deformation of bone and epithysis of tuberosity of the calcaneus as well as edema in the peripheral tissues of calcaneus, which appear as round swelling at the heel that feels hard and gives rise to evident tenderness and even pain when putting on shoes.

3. X-ray examination indicates that there is a swelling shadow of the soft tissues at the terminal of the Achilles tendon and the epiphysis appears uneven or is ruptured into several pieces. It is necessary to note the difference between these with a healthy epiphysis of calcaneus, both sides of which are similar and there is no tenderness. At the later stage, hyperosteogeny will appear at the calcaneus, with that at the back turning into spurs.

Treatment

1. Press acupoints Weizhong (BL 40), Chengshan (BL 57), Kunlun (BL 60) and Taixi (KI 3).

2. Press-knead or grasp the posterior aspect of the leg to relax the leg muscles and relieve pulling on the calcaneus by stiff muscles; and push-press both sides of the Achilles tendon with the thumb and index finger 5-10 times to increase its elasticity and relieve tumefaction caused by peritenonitis. This should be performed together with dorsiflexion and plantar flexion of the ankle joint.

3. Nip-pinch and scrape the tuberosity of calcaneus, or press it with finger-tip. The force applied should be strong to cause pain in the course of treatment. This, called "to cure pain by causing pain," is aimed at stimulating the local tissues to improve blood circulation, promote the healing of the affected tissues and disperse swelling. Usually, the patient will feel that the pain at the heel is greatly relieved and be able to walk normally after treatment. Use hot water to wash the foot after the treatment.

4. Acupuncture: Insert a needle at the diseased part and fumigate the tail of the needle with a moxa ball; keep the needle in place for 20 minutes each time, and apply the treatment once every other day.

Patients with obvious pain at the heel have to stop jumping and quick running exercises, and wear shoes with higher heels to reduce tension in the Achilles tendon.

10. Calcaneodynia

Calcaneus plays an important role in standing and walking. There is a synovial bursa between the Achilles tendon and the calcaneus, called the superior synovial bursa of calcaneus. Its function is to reduce their mutual friction. At the bottom of the tuberosity of the calcaneus is a fat pad which produces a cushioning effect. Between the fat pad and the calcaneus is the inferior synovial bursa of the calcaneus. Plantar fascia initiates from the tuberosity of calcaneus and runs forward, and its function is to support the longitudinal arch of foot. The pain occurring at the heel when standing and walking is called calcaneodynia, a common foot disease.

Injury Mechanism

1. Contusion of heel: Touching the ground with the heel in jumping generates a reacting force to the heel, while touching the ground with heel when falling down from a high place results in a sudden collision between ground and the calcaneus, hence causing injury to the fat pad of the calcaneus, the inferior synovial bursa and periost of the calcaneus, which will give rise to calcaneodynia. Calcaneodynia may also arise from fracture of calcaneus.

2. Epiphysitis of calcaneus among teenagers: Repeated injury of the calcaneus causes inflammation at the soft tissues of calcaneus, manifested as calcaneodynia in walking or standing.

3. Plantar fascia initiates from the tuberosity of calcaneus, the central part of which is hard and the medial and lateral aspects are thin and weak. Long-time walking with load or long-distance walking may cause strain in the plantar fascia. The lesion becomes more serious when the weather is cold and damp, as manifested in weakening elasticity of the plantar fascia and stronger pulling at the tuberosity of calcaneus while walking or standing. Local pain may arise from inflammation at the attaching point of the plantar fascia, followed by the formation of calcaneal

245

spur.

4. Long-time standing and walking and long-distance tip-and-toe walking as well as shoes with high and hard heels all can stimulate the inferior synovial bursa of calcaneus, causing bursal synovitis and calcaneodynia.

5. While reaching middle age, people will become physically weak and put on weight. People, who stay in bed for a prolonged course of illness and suffer from deficiency of the kidney qi, may find that their heel skin turns soft and their fat pad thinner. All these may result in calcaneodynia when standing and walking for a longer time. Such patients can also show such manifestations of kidney deficiency as weakness in the loin and legs, general lassitude, dizziness and poor eyesight.

6. For people advanced in age, calcaneodynia is often caused by calcaneal spur. When walking and standing with load, calcaneal spurs can stimulate the fat pad of the inferior synovial bursa of calcaneus to cause pain. The severity of pain is not directly related to the size of the spur but with its trend. In the case of a forward growing spur, the pain is not serious, while a downward growing spur can stimulate the soft tissues directly, thus causing serious pain.

7. For middle-aged and young people with rheumatoid calcaneities, there will be swelling and pain at the heel. The pathological symptoms are usually confined to the two sides of the calcaneus, at its tuberosity and the terminating point of the Achilles tendon.

Symptoms and Diagnosis

1. Pain in the heel: The onset of the pain is gradual. At the initial stage, the heel feels painful when landing and taking off in jumping movements; at the late stage, pain appears when standing or walking, even to the extent that the heel cannot bear any load. Standing up suddenly from sitting and lying may greatly aggravates the pain, which can, however, be relaxed somewhat after limbering up the foot for a while.

2. Swelling: In an acute heel injury, inflammation and edema in the soft tissues of the heel induce swelling around the heel.

3. Tenderness: Tender spots may be found at the calcaneus and on both sides of the Achilles tendon in a case of superior bursal synovitis of calcaneus, while in a case of inferior bursal synovitis of calcaneus, tenderness appears at the superficial part of the sole. Tenderness caused by spur goes deep; that caused by strain of the plantar fascia is found at the bottom of the heel and the underside of the arch.

Treatment

1. Press acupoints Zusanli (ST 36), Sanyinjiao (SP 6), Kunlun (BL 60), Taixi (KI 3) and Yongquan (KI 1).

2. Make the patient lie prone, the massagist puts a thin pillow under the dorsum of foot, press-kneads the leg muscles 5-10 times to relax them and the plantar fascia and warm up the tissues. For a case of serious pain in the foot due to cold, the

massagist scrapes the sole 3-5 minutes to promote blood circulation and relieve pain. (See Fig. 118)

3. Nip-pinch the painful areas in the heel with force to stimulate the calcaneus and its surrounding tissues. To increase the force, press the heel with the dorsal aspect of the phalangeal joint of hand within limits as can bear by the patient. This method of so-called "relieving pain by causing pain" is important in curing this disease.

4. Stepping-on-bottle method: Prepare a beer bottle, let the patient stand on it and roll it hard with the foot, particularly with the heel. This is an easy and simple method, which should be given once a day, 20 minutes each time.

5. Wash the foot with hot water or fumigate and wash it with Chinese herbal medicine in conjunction with daily physiotherapy—iontherapy. For patients with kidney deficiency, prescribe Chinese medicine to strengthen the loin and invigorate the kidney so as to relax pain in the heel. When early symptoms appear, cut the amount of training and avoid too much jumping and running on hard ground.

Middle-aged and old people should put on shoes with soft sole or soft insole or put a plastic "calcaneus support" at the heel area. For soft thick insole, cut a hole at the heel area to reduce pressure on the calcaneus.

11. Metatarsalgia

Metatarsalgia refers to pain occurring at the sole, and the trunk and head of the metatarsal bone. The disease is due to various causes, but is related to chronic injuries, such as chronic strain of the head of the metatarsal bone, strain of the

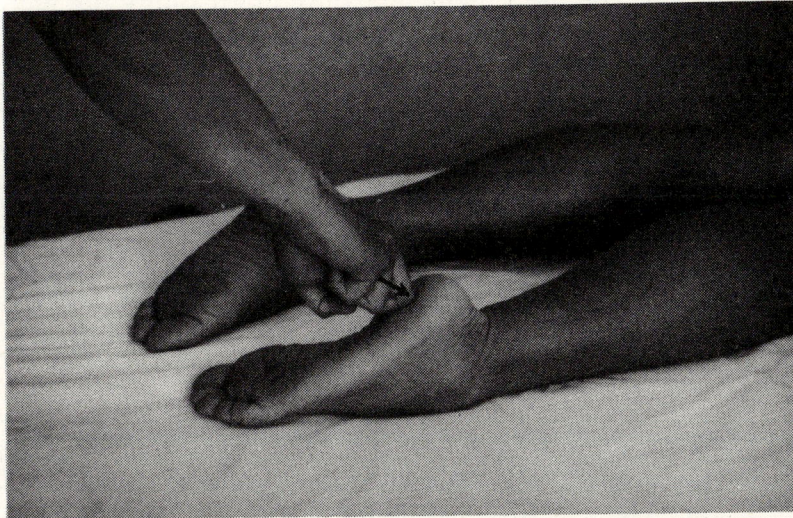

Fig. 118

plantar fascia, eversion or the metatarsus and aseptic necrosis of the head of the metatarsal bone.

The foot has a longitudinal arch and a transverse arch. The longitudinal arch consists of the calcaneus, talus, navicular bone, the first cuneiform bone and the first metatarsal bone, while the transverse arch consists of the five heads of the metatarsal bones. Both the arches are reinforced by muscles, ligaments and fasciae. While standing, the body weight mainly falls on the heads of the first and fifth metatarsal bones and the calcaneus, and while walking, the gravity moves from the calcaneus to the heads of the first and fifth metatarsal bones.

Injury Mechanism

1. Flaccid metatarsalgia: Malformation of the first metatarsal bone makes it lean towards the medial aspect of foot, so the ligament maintaining the transverse arch reduces in elasticity and turns flaccid, causing atrophy of the interosseous muscles, sinking of the transverse arch and dropping of the second, third and fourth metatarsal bones, so the major part of body weight falls on the heads of the second and third metatarsal bones, where pain consequently occurs when standing and walking. Pain can also be caused by jumping, pulling at the transverse ligaments of the head of the metatarsal bone and squeezing on the toe nerves by the head of the metatarsal bone, etc.

2. Injury of plantar fascia: This is injury commonly seen among running and jumping athletes. When taking off in jumping, the plantar fascia may be pulled and part of the fibres ruptured. As there may be cicatricial contracture after the union of the fascia, pain may occur in the soles of the feet while running or jumping. As this disorder is often complicated by calcaneal spur, there may also be pain in the heel.

3. Osteochondrosis of the head of metatarsal bone: Commonly seen in female athletes 14-21 years old, it is caused by long-time exertion of force with the distal part of foot, manifested as chronic injury of the head of the second metatarsal bone, falling of the cartilages, and even necrosis of the head of metatarsal bone. As osteochondrosis occurs at the metatarsophalangeal joint, pain is usually felt at the second metatarsal bone when standing, running or walking.

4. Eversion of the great toe: A kind of malformation in the foot, it is mainly manifested as eversion of the great toe, pain at the medial aspect of the front part of the foot when walking. The pain becomes more serious when landing with the front part of the foot in gymnastics and long jump. Any type of malformation in the foot may cause callus, corn and bursitis at the related part, which in turn aggravate the pain in the foot.

5. Flatfoot: The foot arch appears flat, the sole ligament is flaccid with reduced elasticity; the whole sole touches ground; the foot easily feels tired and painful when walking; even eversion of foot may be seen in a serious case.

6. Gout: It is mainly caused by obstruction in purine metabolism and increase of uric acid in the blood. Gout is often seen in the middle-aged and old people,

particularly males. It is manifested as swelling and pain in the first metatarsophalangeal joint, and lameness. The symptoms become more serious during night.

Symptoms and Diagnosis

1. Pain: At the initial stage, there is pain at the front part of the foot when running and jumping. At the advanced stage, pain appears at the metatarsus when walking and standing. A serious case produces stabbing pain, as that often accompanying a gout at night. Sometimes, it is necessary to pay attention to differentiating gout from angiitis of foot.

2. Tenderness: In most cases, there is tenderness at the head of metatarsal bone and the metatarsophalangeal joint. The tenderness become more serious when practising over-dorsiflexion and plantar flexion of the metatarsophalangeal joint. There is tenderness at the sole in an injury of planter fascia, and hard cords and scleromata may be felt at the healing area of a scar. Transverse squeezing at the front part of foot may also cause pain at the foot. Over-dorsiflexion of foot and pulling of the plantar fascia may cause pain in the sole. Swelling and thickening of tissues my be found at the metatarsophalangeal joint.

3. Change in outer appearance of foot: The transverse art in the front part of foot becomes flat; flatfoot, slight eversion of foot, eversion of the great toe, and thickening of skin and synovial bursa at the protruding part of the metatarsophalangeal joint. Complications by callus and corn may be seen at the sole.

4. At the early stage, X-ray examination reveals no evident changes, while at the late stage eversion of the great toe, inward displacement of the first metatarsal bone, rough bony substance at the head of the metatarsal bone and hyperosteogeny may be found. In case of gout of the great toe, injury of the bone and bony defects may be seen.

Treatment

1. Press acupoints Sanyinjiao (SP 6), Shangqiu (SP 5), Gongsun (SP 4, at the depression on the anteroinferior border of the bottom part of the first metatarsal bone), Taibai (SP 3, at the posteroinferior aspect of the small head of the first metatarsal bone), Rangu (KI 2, at the depression on the anteroinferior border of the scaphoid tuberosity of foot), and Yongquan (KI 1). (See Fig. 119)

2. Push-press the sole 10 times to relax the tissues at the sole; and pluck the tension area of the plantar fascia.

3. Tract the toe with one hand while pinch, nip and scrape the head of metatarsal bone and the metatarsophalangeal joint back and forth with the other hand to stimulate the surface of the bone and the articular capsule, promote blood circulation and relieve the inflammation. This method should not be used when the skin turns red, and the doctor should make sure whether the patient has contracted gout and infection of the toes. Finally, tract the toes, dorsiflex and flex the metatarsophalangeal joint to the most to relax articular adhesion and improve the elasticity of the sole. (See Fig. 120)

4. Perform push-kneading manipulation from the sole, via the metatarsophal-

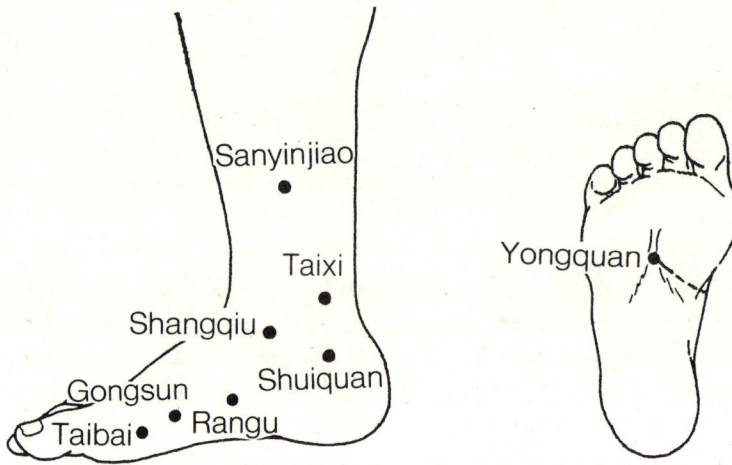

Fig. 119

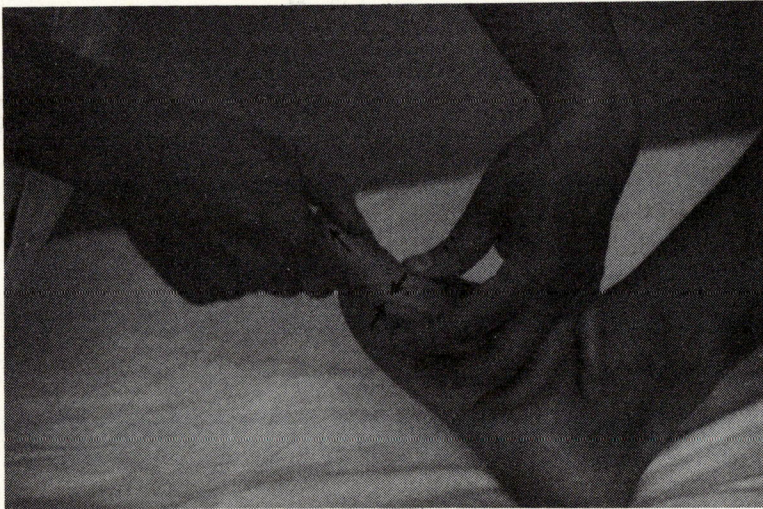

Fig. 120

angeal joint to the ankle 10 times, supplement this with scraping till the skin feels hot so as to relax the muscles and tendons and activate the flow of qi and blood in the meridians and collaterals.

After treatment, wear shoes with soft sole or loose shoes, do not walk too much. If there are obvious malformation of foot, surgery should be considered, such as surgery to correct the eversion of the great toe.

12. Fracture of Metatarsal Bone

Altogether, a foot has five metatarsal bones. Fracture of the metatarsal bone is mostly caused by direct external force. Of all fractures of the metatarsal bone, the fracture of the second, third and fourth ones are the most common. Fracture of the fifth metatarsal bone is often caused by contractive pulling of the tendon.

Injury Mechanism

1. Direct external force: When the foot is hit by a heavy object or run over by a car, the metatarsal bone may fracture. As the metatarsal bones are loosely structured, fracture may occur simultaneously at the second, third and fourth metatarsal bones.

2. Fracture of the metatarsal bones may also be caused by tremendous impact of the body weight when the front part of foot hits the ground or when ground surface is rough in a fall from a high place.

3. Basal fracture of the fifth metatarsal bone usually occurs alone, and it is normally caused by forceful pulling by the short peroneal muscle. The function of the short peroneal muscle is to ensure eversion and abduction of the front part of foot. Sudden inversion of foot may pull the muscle, resulting in avulsion fracture of the fifth metatarsal bone.

Symptoms and Diagnosis

1. Pain: An evident history of trauma; fierce pain at the foot, which makes the patient unable to stand or walk; if walking with effort, the patient can only touch the ground with the heel, but not the frontal part of the foot.

2. Swelling and malformation: There is local swelling after fracture, with that at the instep being more distinct. Ecchymoma may occur after a short time. When there is fracture displacement, obvious malformation is found at the instep.

3. Tenderness: There is evident tenderness, the sensation of friction or abnormal movement at the fractured part. If the fracture displacement is not very serious, pain is felt when pushing the toe longitudinally with a finger. In case the fifth metatarsal bone is broken, there will be pain, apart from tenderness, at the fractured area when the foot is inverted passively.

4. X-ray photo can help make a definite diagnosis and show the severity of the displacement. Attention should be made to differentiate the fracture of the fifth metatarsal bone from the epiphysis of the fifth metatarsal bone and from the sesamoidia in the long peroneal muscle tendon. When necessary, take an X-ray photo of the healthy foot for comparison. In epiphysis of the fifth metatarsal bone and sesamoidia in the long peroneal muscle tendon, the two feet look symmetrical.

Treatment

1. Digitally pressing acupoint Weizhong (BL 40) for two minutes for anaesthesia; then press acupoints Jiexi (ST 41), Kunlun (BL 60) and Taixi (KI 3).

2. Manual reduction: No manual reduction is needed for insignificant fracture displacement. For cases with serious displacement, make an assistant hold the ankle while the massagist holds and tracts the toe with one hand and squeezes the metatarsal bone from the instep and sole with the thumb and the index finger of the other hand to correct overlapping teratism and angulation deformity. Then squeeze-press the interosseous metatarsal spaces with the thumb and index finger to correct the lateral displacement. After treatment, examine the instep to see whether the fracture of the metatarsal bones has been reduced. (See Fig. 121)

3. Fixation: When the reduction is completed, apply a short plaster support for fixation, or put a soft board at the instep and the sole respectively and wind them with adhesive plaster transversely. For fracture of the fifth metatarsal bone, fix the foot with adhesive plaster at the aversion position to prevent inversion of the foot. Lift the affected leg, flex and extend the knee joint and ankle joint; practise walking with crutches one week later; and remove the fixation four weeks later.

13. Fatigue Periostitis and Fatigue Fracture of Metatarsal Bone

Caused by long-time and repeated slight injuries, fatigue periostitis and fatigue fracture of metatarsal bone is often seen among servicemen marching for long distances. So it is also called "marching foot." The injury often occurs at the second metatarsal bone, occasionally at the third and fourth metatarsal bones. Besides, it is also frequently seen in sporting events such as gymnastics, sprint, long-distance running and heel-and-toe walking.

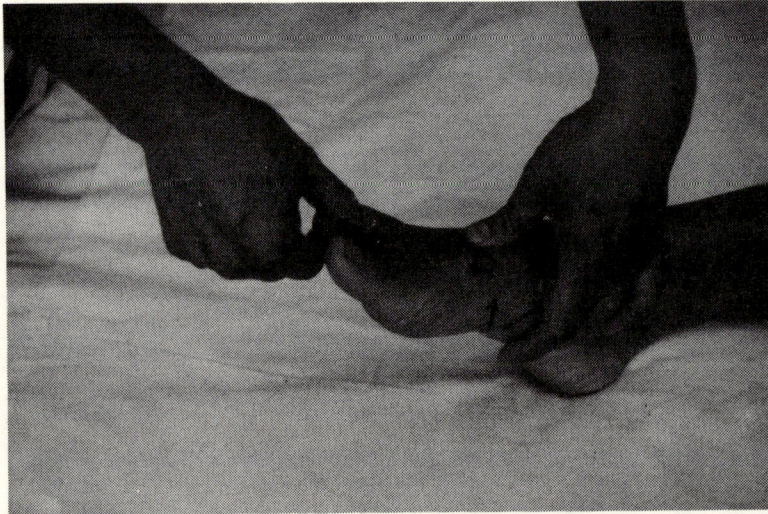

Fig. 121

Injury Mechanism

1. While walking, the body weight is mainly borne by the thick fist metatarsal bone. However, when the first metatarsal bone is short and small, the body weight will be shared by the thinner second metatarsal bone. The constant impact of the foot upon the ground when running or walking for long distance may act upon the head of the second metatarsal bone, causing injury to the distal part of its trunk and gradually inducing chronic fracture and callus. This is called fatigue fracture, which is common among athletes of adult age.

2. Over pulling by muscles and ligaments and repeated take-off drive may result in pulling at the periost of the metatarsal bone by the ligaments and interosseous muscle, causing slight stripping and gradually giving rise to such inflammatory symptoms as edema and bleeding at the periost. Inflammation at the periost may result in calcification, producing ridge-like hyperosteogeny. This is common among athletes of young age.

Symptoms and Diagnosis

1. At the initial stage, pain is only felt when walking and running for a long time. At the later stage, pain occurs in normal walking and is more evident when there is fatigue fracture.

2. Swelling and tenderness: Swelling or protrusion is found at the dorsum of foot; tenderness is felt in the metatarsal bones; and the bones give a thickened and rough feeling, which appears more distinct when compared with the healthy foot.

3. X-ray examination help confirm the diagnosis. For fatigue periostitis, X-ray photo may show that the periost of the diaphysis of the metatarsal bone turns thick, assuming ridge-like hyperplasia; for fatigue fracture, it may reveal the fracture space at the diaphysis, but no displacement. Labial hyperosteogeny may also be seen at the border of fracture.

Treatment

1. Foot and ankle relaxation: Push and scrape the instep and sole 10 times to make the foot hot and promote blood circulation; nip between each two metatarsal bones to relax the interosseous muscles; pull the toes and make plantar flexion and dorsiflexion of the metatarsophalangeal joint; and hold the front part of the foot to move the ankle joint in all directions.

2. Push and scrape areas in the instep and sole where there is hyperplasia at the periost or there is fracture 10 times to promote the healing of the bone and periost. This is a major method in treating this disease.

3. Apply 2 percent silver nitrate solution to the surface of the skin where there are pathological changes, cover it with tin foil, wrap the periphery with adhesive plaster, then bind up with bandage. Change the dressing every other day. One course lasts three weeks, and two courses of treatment are given all together.

When pain in the foot is serious, stop physical training. As a supplementary treatment, wash the foot with hot water, or fumigate and wash it with Chinese herbal medicine.

14. Contusion and Dislocation of Metatarsophalangeal Joint

Contusion of metatarsophalangeal joint is a common disorder, and more frequently it occurs at the first metatarsophalangeal joint. Although not a serious injury, it may result in long-time severe pain if not treated, and it may hinder physical training.

Injury Mechanism

Contusion of the metatarsophalangeal joint usually results from kicking an object with the tip of the great toe, such as kicking the ball. This injury is more frequently seen among secondary and primary school students,because they like to kick football with the tip of the great toe. In gymnastic event, hitting the ground with tiptoe can hurt the metatarsophalangeal joint, causing injury to the articular capsule and lateral ligament. A strong dorsiflexion force on the phalanx can also cause subluxation and dislocation of the metatarsophalangeal joint.

Symptoms and Diagnosis

1. Pain and tenderness: The first metatarsophalangeal joint feels painful and is unable to bear the body weight. Tenderness is found at the metatarsophalangeal joint, especially at the joint space and its two sides. If not treated timely, these symptoms may turn into old contusion. Pain can also be felt when touching the ground by toes.

2. Swelling: Swelling and ecchymoma appear soon after a serious injury. An old injury may be featured by ridge-like swelling, tenderness, dyskinesia of the joint and pain when bearing weight.

3. Dislocation of metatarsophalangeal joint is marked by displacement of the great toe towards the dorsal aspect, crispation of the great toe, hyperextension of metatarsophalangeal joint and flexion deformity of interphalangeal joint.

Treatment

1. Immediately after the contusion of the metatarsophalangeal joint, the massagist pulls the great toe with one hand and uses the other to push-press around the metatarsophalangeal joint gently 5-10 times to restore injured tissues, reduce compression on the joint capsule and promote subsidence of swelling. But, be sure not to make any rotation movement of the joint, let the diseased part rest for 2-3 days.

2. In a case of dislocation of metatarsophalangeal joint, the massagist pulls the great toe at the place where hyperextension deformity occurs with one hand and supports the head of the metatarsal bone with the other hand and presses the bone of the great toe. A snap or a sliding sensation suggests completion of the reduction. After this, the deformation should diminish, the pain relaxed, and the extension and flexion of the metatarsal bone resume. To ensure the healing of the joint capsule, be sure not to make the joint bear any weight for two weeks after injury.

图书在版编目(CIP)数据

中国传统手法治疗人体损伤:英文/许孟忠著 .—北京:外文出版社,1997
ISBN 7－119－01795－0

Ⅰ.中… Ⅱ.许… Ⅲ.软组织损伤－按摩疗法(中医)－英文 Ⅳ.R274.3

中国版本图书馆 CIP 数据核字 (95) 第 10116 号

责任编辑　刘文渊　余冰清
封面设计　李士仮
插图绘制　李士仮

外文出版社网址:
　http://www.flp.com.cn
外文出版社电子信箱:
　info@flp.com.cn
　sales@flp.com.cn

中国传统手法治疗人体损伤
许孟忠　著
崔树义　崔树芝　译
*
©外文出版社
外文出版社出版
(中国北京百万庄大街 24 号)
邮政编码 100037
北京外文印刷厂印刷
中国国际图书贸易总公司发行
(中国北京车公庄西路 35 号)
北京邮政信箱第 399 号　邮政编码 100044
1997 年(16 开)第 1 版
2000 年第 1 版第 2 次印刷
(英)
ISBN 7－119－01795－0/R·128(外)
08780(精)
14－E－3057S

3. Old metatarsophalangeal joint: The massagist pulls the great toe with one hand and push-presses from the joint to the metatarsal bone with the other hand 5-10 times, then pinches and nips on the metatarsophalangeal joint to stimulate the joint capsule and accessory ligament and rotates the great toe to prevent adhesion of the joint, promote subsidence of swelling and absorption of inflammation. After treatment, wash the foot with hot water and adjust the training program for the foot.